Atlas of Pediatric Cataract

Sudarshan Kumar Khokhar • Chirakshi Dhull
Editors

Atlas of Pediatric Cataract

Springer

Editors
Sudarshan Kumar Khokhar
Dr. R.P. Centre for Ophthalmic Sciences
All India Institute of Medical Sciences
New Delhi
India

Chirakshi Dhull
Dr. R.P. Centre for Ophthalmic Sciences
All India Institute of Medical Sciences
New Delhi
India

ISBN 978-981-13-6938-4 ISBN 978-981-13-6939-1 (eBook)
https://doi.org/10.1007/978-981-13-6939-1

This Springer imprint is published by the registered company Springer Nature Singapore Pte Ltd.
The registered company address is: 152 Beach Road, #21-01/04 Gateway East, Singapore 189721, Singapore

Foreword

It is often said that children are not just small adults. In no other area is that more true than in the care of patients with cataracts. For adults, everyone develops cataracts if they live long enough and having cataract surgery has become a normal part of aging. There is often no question about why the cataracts developed or what the cataracts are telling us about the genetic, developmental, or metabolic workings of the affected individual. The evaluation and treatment for those age-related cataracts vary little from individual to individual. In most of the world, emphasis is placed on efficiency and volume. Tremendous progress has been made and millions of aged adults have been restored to sighted, happy, and productive members of society. The surgeons who operate on cataract-blind adults can feel a tremendous amount of satisfaction for the positive impact they are having on the world.

For those who care for children, a special kind of dedication and compassion is required. While there are fewer children with cataracts compared to adults, each one represents 50 or more blind years that may be at stake. In addition, the cataract pattern may be a marker for alterations in metabolic, developmental, or genetic processes. Efficiency and volume may have to take a back seat to thoroughness and patience, exams that require anesthesia and treatment decisions that have to account for future growth, and the investigation of not only the whole eye but the entire child and family.

Professor Sudarshan K. Khokhar and his coauthors have produced an atlas and textbook that should be acquired by every ophthalmologist who sees and treats children. It is a work of art as well as a work of science. It is very visual and yet also contains concise and digestible advice from the literature and from the vast experience of the authors.

This book will teach the reader about the important implications of pattern recognition when examining a child with cataracts. We must describe the opacities we see in detail. The layer, location, density, and pattern must be appreciated. We must also answer many questions. Is it static or changing? It is co-natal or acquired? Is it unilateral or just asymmetrically bilateral? Is it familial or isolated? Is it genetic, metabolic, idiopathic, or related to infection, inflammation, or trauma? The questions go on and on, even before the surgical plan is developed. We learn to see that the cataract characteristics are a window into the past and future growth and development, as well as the systemic workings of the child and even the implications for the visual brain. We know that cataracts in young children often represent a pan-ophthalmic condition, not just a lens disorder. We prepare for the unusual surgical challenges that are before us and the long-term follow-up commitments we are embarking on.

I congratulate the authors for a book that I predict will be a must-have for every training program in ophthalmology and every practicing pediatric ophthalmologist who sees children with cataracts. It addresses an important and evolving area of pediatric ophthalmology and does so with startlingly clear photos and ultrasonic images made more amazing by the fact that children rarely hold still and must, at times, be subjected to general anesthesia multiple times.

An extra benefit of this book is that Professor Khokhar and the coauthors he has chosen have many years of experience and an enormous amount of credibility in the international community. When they speak, people listen. I also know that they have selected the images for this book from thousands they have taken over time so that the reader can see and learn from the best and most representative examples. I enjoyed studying this volume and the care of children worldwide will be positively impacted by its publication and dissemination.

M. Edward Wilson
Ophthalmology and Pediatrics, Storm Eye Institute,
Medical University of South Carolina,
Charleston, SC, USA

Contents

About the Editors

Sudarshan Kumar Khokhar is currently working as Professor at the Dr. Rajendra Prasad Centre for Ophthalmic Sciences, All India Institute of Medical Sciences (AIIMS), New Delhi, India. He has more than 20 years of clinical, teaching, and research experience at AIIMS, with particular expertise in pediatric cataracts and complicated adult cataracts. He is a well-published author with over 80 publications in peer-reviewed journals and numerous book chapters. Over the last decade, Professor Khokhar has offered instruction courses on pediatric cataracts at various national and international conferences, e.g., for the American Academy of Ophthalmology (AAO), European Society of Cataract and Refractive Surgeons (ESCRS), Asia-Pacific Academy of Ophthalmology (APAO), World Ophthalmology Congress (WOC), and American Association for Pediatric Ophthalmology and Strabismus (AAPOS). Professor Khokhar has designed a special cannula—Khokhar's capsular painting cannula—for phacoemulsification in white cataracts and was a pioneer in using the plasma blade in persistent fetal vasculature (PFV) eyes. He has received many achievement awards from international bodies, including the APAO and AAO.

Chirakshi Dhull is currently working as a Senior Resident in cataract and refractive surgery at the Dr. Rajendra Prasad Centre for Ophthalmic Sciences, All India Institute of Medical Sciences (AIIMS), New Delhi. A postgraduate from AIIMS, she has several publications in peer-reviewed journals and book chapters to her credit. She has presented papers at both national and international conferences, including the Asia-Pacific Academy of Ophthalmology (APAO) and Asia-Pacific Glaucoma Congress (APGC).

Morphology of Pediatric Cataract

1

Sudarshan Kumar Khokhar and Chirakshi Dhull

Pediatric cataract is a leading cause of childhood blindness. The incidence is in the range of 1.8 to 3.6/10,000 per year and the prevalence is about 1.03 per 10,000 children (0.32–22.9/10,000). There is no difference in the prevalence based on gender or laterality [1]. Untreated cataracts especially in children lead to tremendous social, economical, and emotional burden to the child, family, and society. Blindness related to pediatric cataract can be treated with early identification and appropriate management. Favorable outcomes depend not just on effective surgery but also on meticulous postoperative care and visual rehabilitation including glasses and amblyopia treatment.

1.1 Morphology of Pediatric Cataract

Examination of cataract morphology remains a challenge. The child is most comfortable in mother's lap and/or in the shoulder hold. The red reflex screening with direct ophthalmoscope kept at 30 cm and focused on each pupil separately (Bruckner's test) helps in identification of lenticular opacity in this position. For assessment of specific morphology, slit lamp examination, retroillumination examination, and ultrasound biomicroscopy (UBM) can be used [2–5]. Classification of cataracts on the basis of morphology is useful to ophthalmologists as it adds a clue to etiology and progression [2–3]. It also helps in better planning of surgery and avoiding certain complications associated with particular morphologies.

In this classification system, emphasis has been given on the location of opacity in relation to lens structures (Table 1.1). We have excluded traumatic cataract and persistent fetal vasculature from this classification and discussed them in detail as separate entities. Cataracts may be visually significant or visually insignificant. However identification of both remains of vital importance as visually insignificant cataracts may progress with age in certain cases. Certain miscellaneous morphology is described in this chapter which the author has encountered in last 20 years.

Table 1.1 Morphological classification of pediatric cataract based on location of opacity

Whole lens	Central	Anterior	Posterior	Miscellaneous
• Total • Congenital morgagnian • Membranous/partially absorbed	• Lamellar/zonular • Nuclear • Central pulverulent • Ant egg • Cerulean cataract • Cortical • Sutural	• Anterior polar (a) Dot like (b) Plaque like (c) Anterior pyramidal • Anterior subcapsular • Anterior lenticonus	• Posterior polar • Posterior subcapsular • Posterior lenticonus	• Oil droplet • Wedge shaped • Coralliform • Floriform • Dandelion like • Starry Sky cataract • Stud button • Reduplicated cataract • Linear opacities • Crystalline • Nodular • Stem of cactus • Barbed fence-like cataract

S. K. Khokhar · C. Dhull (✉)
Dr. Rajendra Prasad Centre for Ophthalmic Sciences, All India Institute of Medical Sciences, New Delhi, India

S. K. Khokhar, C. Dhull (eds.), *Atlas of Pediatric Cataract*, https://doi.org/10.1007/978-981-13-6939-1_1

1.2 Whole Lens Cataract

1.2.1 Total Cataract

Total cataract refers to opacity in whole of the lens where red glow is not visible from any part of the lens (Fig. 1.1a). Incidence varies from of all pediatric cataracts and it is more common in developing countries [6–8]. It is usually bilateral and sporadic in most cases although familial cases have also been reported [8–10]. It may be result of progression of cataract from zonular cataract, posterior lenticonus, or preexisting posterior capsular defect [11]. Since associated abnormalities may not be visible, UBM can help in identifying the same (Fig. 1.1b).

1.2.2 Congenital Morgagnian Cataract

Morgagnian cataract is a rare entity in pediatric population [2, 3]. It is characterized by liquified cortex with sunken nucleus (Fig. 1.2a, b) and can be confirmed by shifting head of the patient (Fig. 1.3) [12]. It may get absorbed with time and it has been reported in association with posterior capsular defect in children [13].

1.2.3 Membranous/Partially Absorbed Cataract

Membranous cataract occurs due to absorption of lens which may be secondary to infective or noninfective etiology

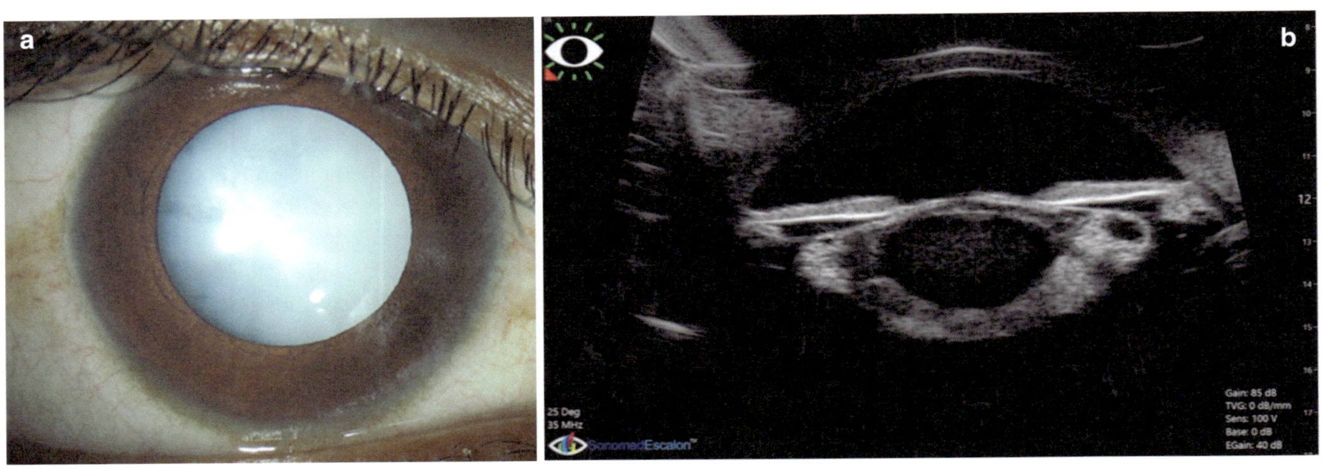

Fig. 1.1 Total cataract. (**a**) Clinical picture, (**b**) UBM of the same showing involvement of all layers with center relatively clear than periphery. Posterior lenticonus and posterior capsular defect have been ruled out

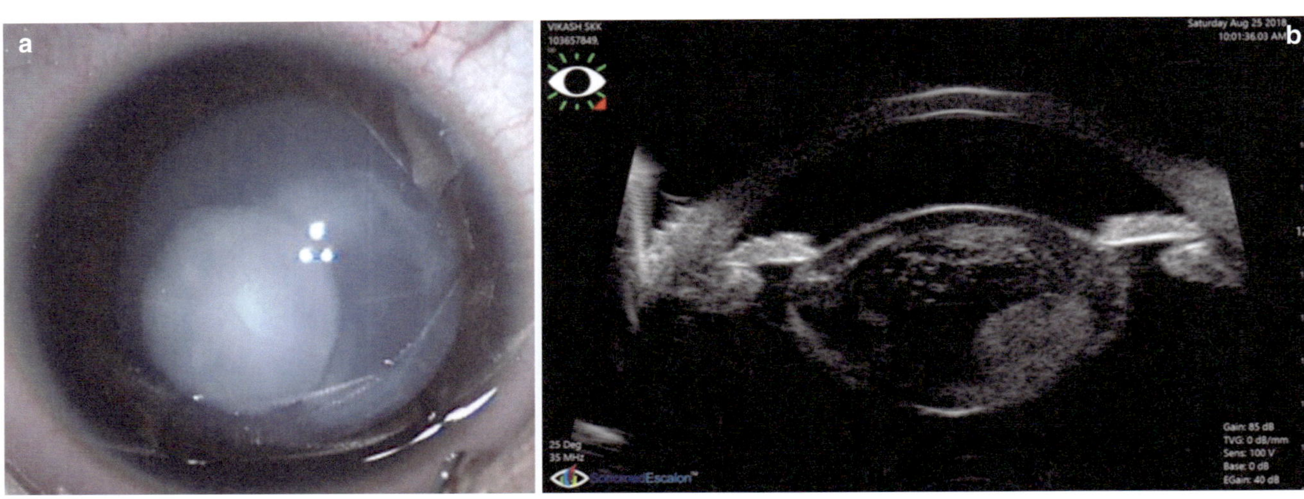

Fig. 1.2 Congenital morgagnian cataract. (**a**) Clinical picture showing liquefied cortex and sunken nucleus, (**b**) UBM of the same patient confirming the findings

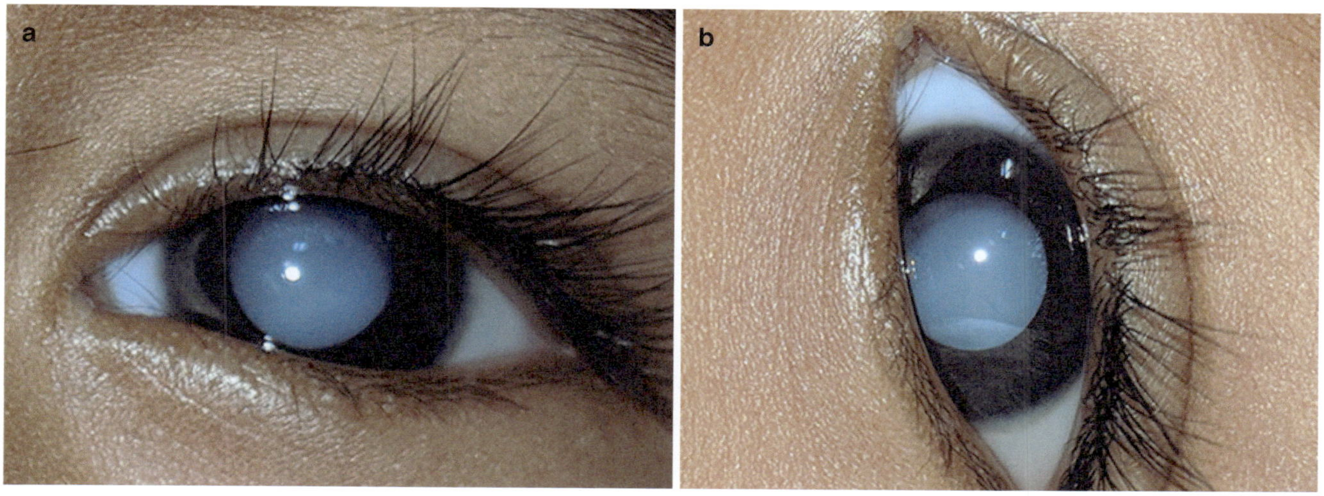

Fig. 1.3 Congenital morgagnian cataract. (**a**) Sitting position, (**b**) left lateral position. Note the change in position of nucleus as it moves along gravity due to liquefied cortex

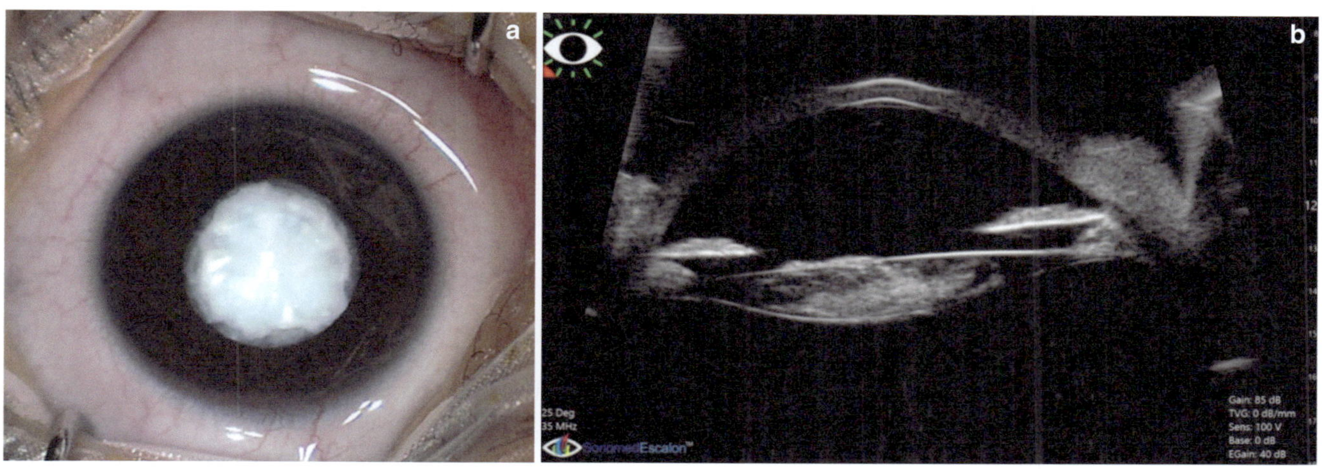

Fig. 1.4 Membranous cataract. (**a**) Clinical picture with partially absorbed cataract and anterior capsular plaque, (**b**) UBM of the same showing anterior capsular flattening and loss of lens volume

(Fig. 1.4). While congenital rubella syndrome and leptospirosis have been implicated as infective etiology; persistent fetal vasculature, posterior capsular defect or syndromes like Hallermann–Streiff syndrome and Lowe syndrome are implicated as non infective etiology [14–20].

1.3 Central Cataract

1.3.1 Lamellar/Zonular Cataract

Zonular cataract is commonly a type of development cataract involving one or more layers of lens fibers. It is secondary to insult to specific layers of lens fibers which were metabolically active at the time of insult [21]. The central nucleus generally remains clear [21]. Presentation may vary from minimal cataract to dense opacity, involvement of complete layer to incomplete involvement and isolated zonular cataract or associated with other morphology (Fig. 1.5a–k). Visually insignificant zonular cataracts may progress with time. Riders may be seen in association with zonular cataract. Pathogenesis of these riders is not clear. We have given terminology "reverse cuneiform cataract" for riders in zonular cataract as a hypothesis based on their presentation and evolution pattern [22]. Good visual prognosis is seen in most cases with this morphology.

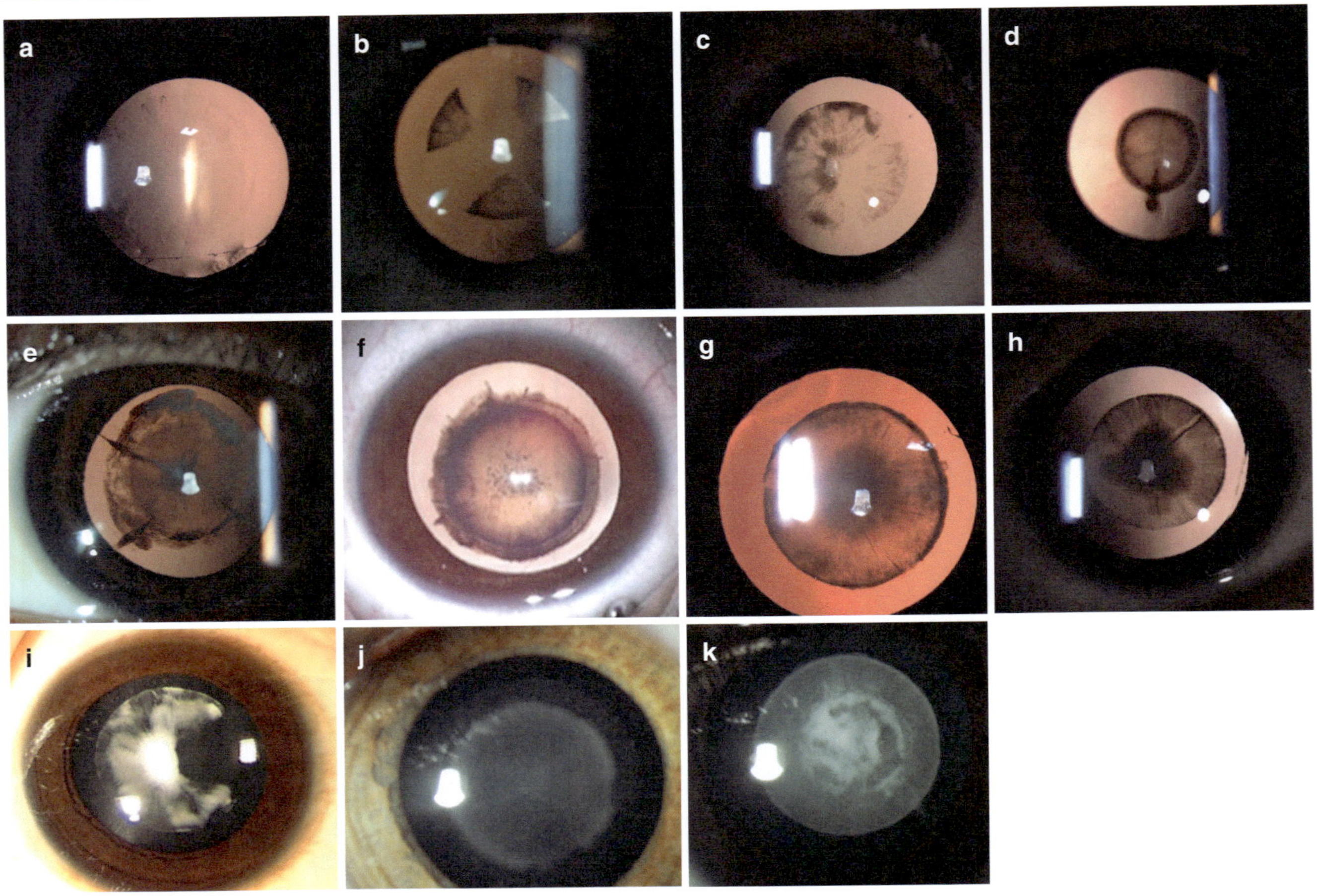

Fig. 1.5 Variable presentation of zonular cataract ranging from visually insignificant cataract to dense cataract. (**a**–**k**) Riders may or maynot be present

1.3.2 Nuclear Cataract

Opacity involving embryonal or fetal nucleus is referred to as nuclear cataract. It may be isolated or associated with zonular or cortical cataract (Fig. 1.6a–d). They are commonly bilateral and may have autosomal dominant inheritance [21, 23]. Congenital rubella syndrome is also known to be associated with nuclear cataracts [2]. They are common in developing countries and are generally visually significant [6].

1.3.3 Cataracta Pulverulenta

The term "pulverulent" means powdery or consisting of fine particles. This type of cataract is generally visually insignificant. It may be located in central nucleus which was initially described as Coppock cataract (Fig. 1.7), may involve a zone or it can be diffuse which may be visually significant [24, 25] (Fig. 1.8).

1.3.4 Ant Egg Cataract

This refers to a unique morphology of congenital cataract where larger grainy well-defined dots are seen in the lens. Location may vary. It could be central with associated nuclear or cortical cataract (Fig. 1.9). Cataract in the form of pure ant eggs is also observed (Fig. 1.10). It may be a result of secondary calcification in the lens [26]. Such cases have been reported to have unique composition of proteins including cytokeratin and Matrix-Gla [27].

1.3.5 Cerulean Cataract

Cerulean Cataract or blue dot cataract refers to congenital cataract which have greenish or blueish hue (Fig. 1.11). They are usually bilateral and nonprogressive [21, 28]. Vision is not affected in most cases.

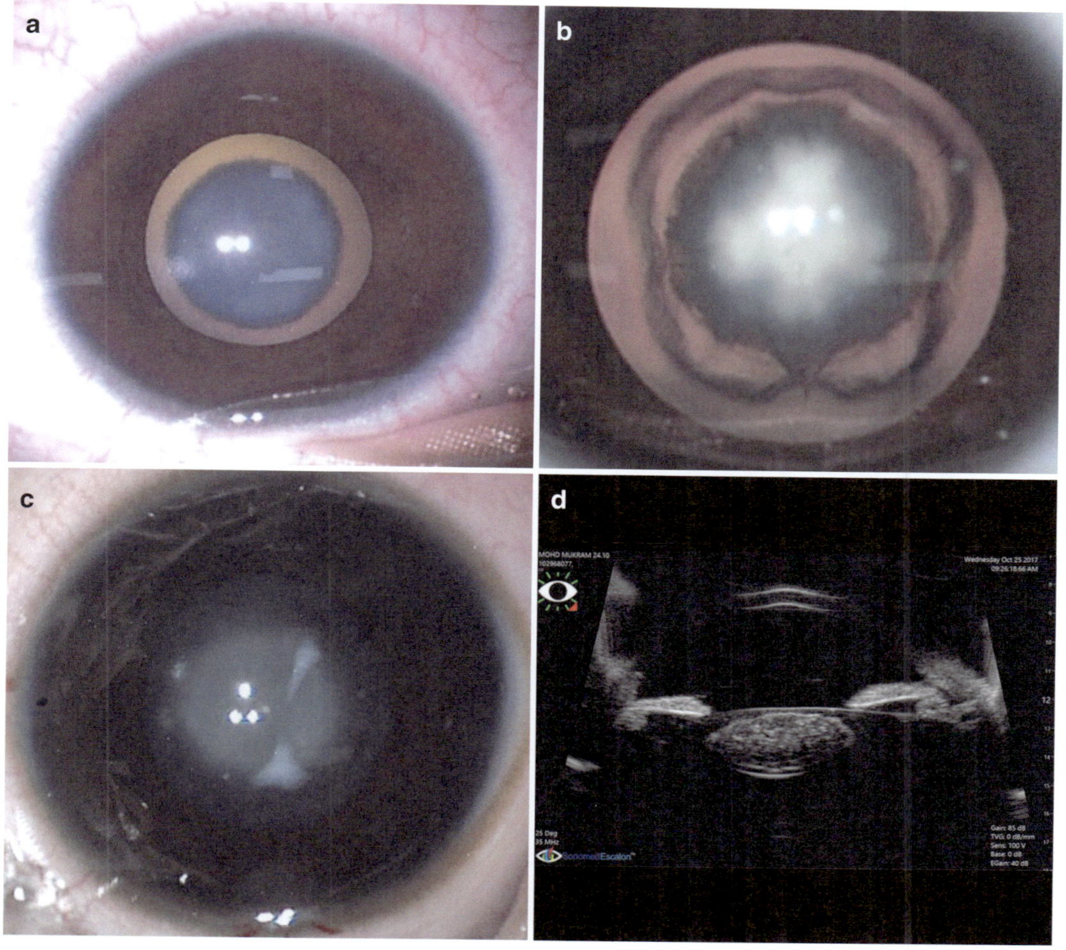

Fig. 1.6 Nuclear cataract. (**a**) Central dense nuclear cataract with periphery clear. (**b**) Nuclear cataract with associated zonular and cortical opacity (**c**) Nuclear cataract with anterior subcapsular cataract (**d**) UBM of (**c**) showing involvement of nucleus

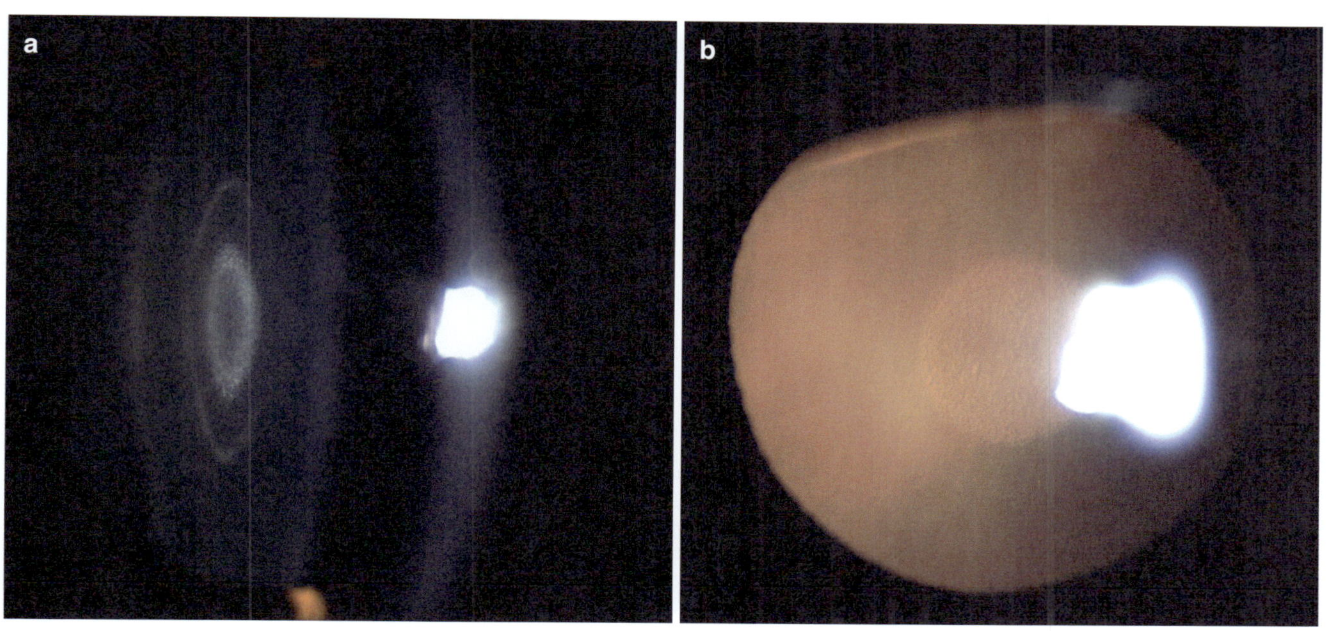

Fig. 1.7 Coppock cataract—central pulverulent cataract. (**a**) Slit picture showing involvement of embryonal nucleus, (**b**) retroillumination picture showing visually insignificant cataract

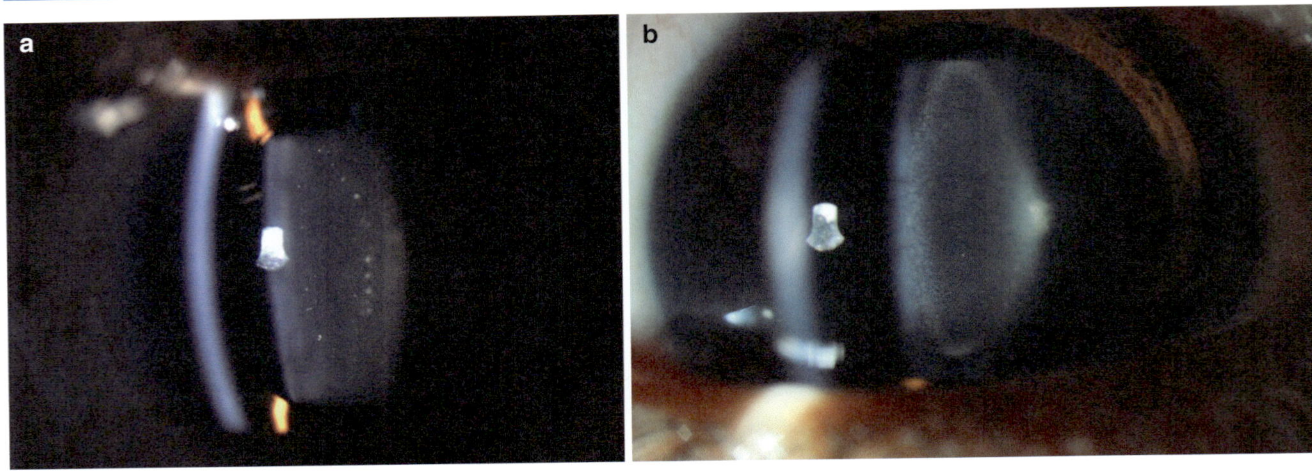

Fig. 1.8 Pulverulent cataract. (**a**) Minimal pulverulent cataract with involvement of specific zone, (**b**) diffuse pulverulent cataract

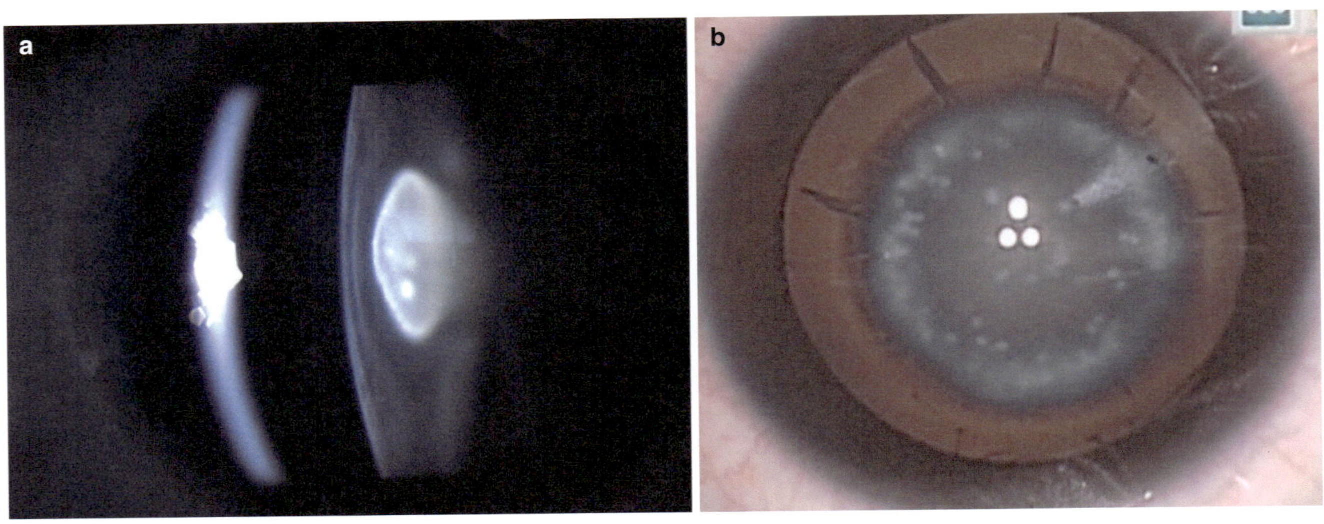

Fig. 1.9 Ant egg cataract. (**a**) Nuclear cataract with central ant eggs, (**b**) zonular cataract with riders with dispersed ant eggs

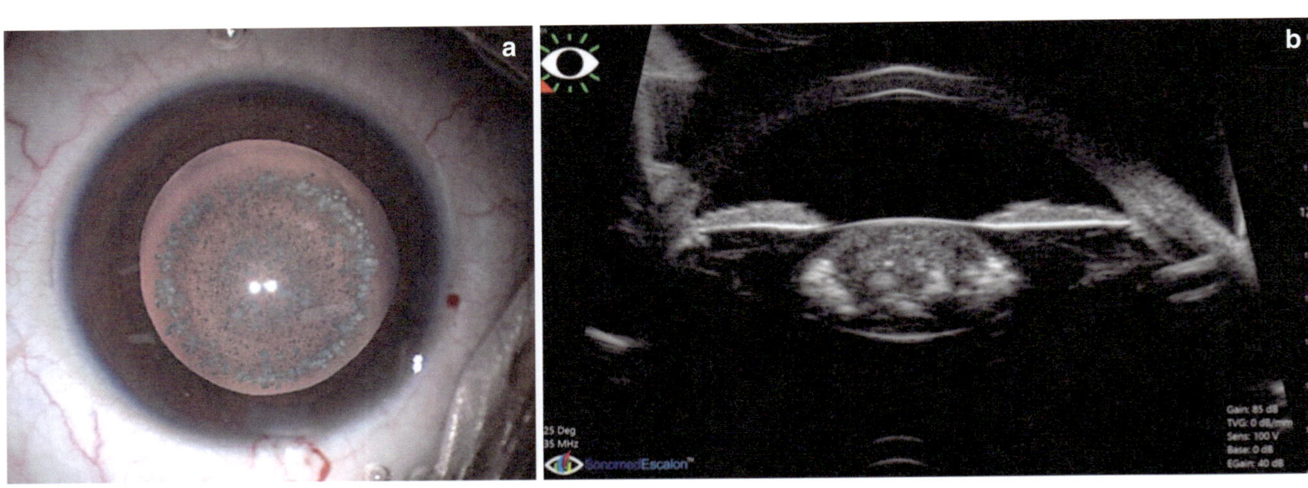

Fig. 1.10 (**a**) Clinical picture of ant egg cataract, here presence of these opacities is the principle cause of visual loss, (**b**) UBM of the same showing hyperechoic ant eggs

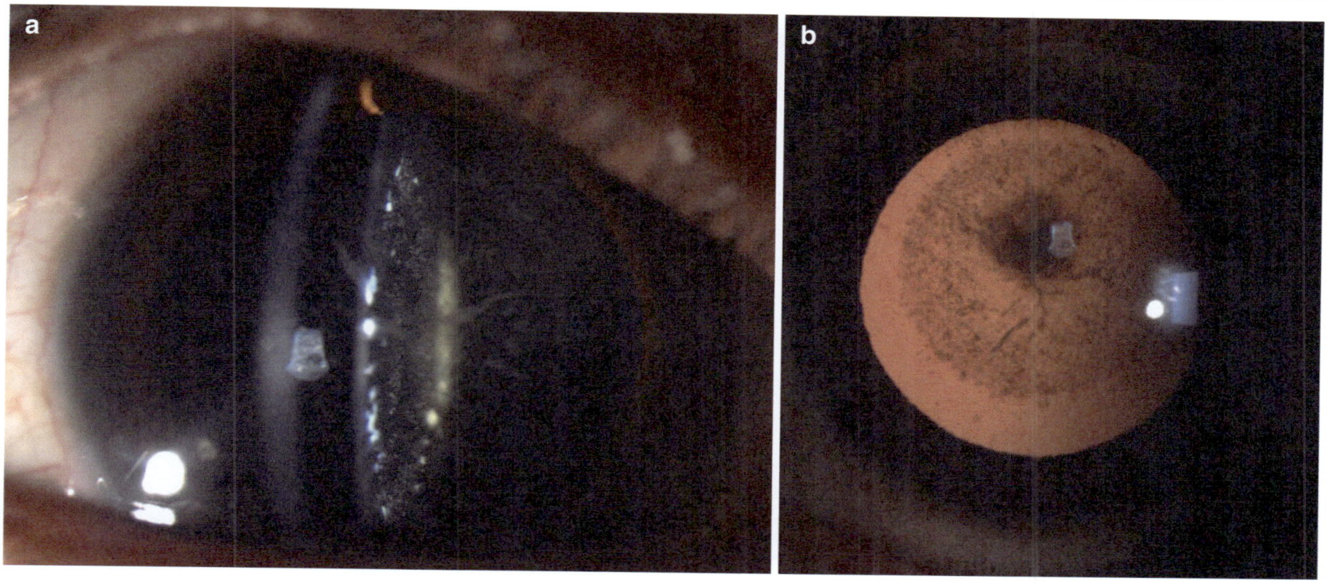

Fig. 1.11 Cerulean cataract. (**a**) Slit lamp picture showing multiple bluish opacities, (**b**) retroillumination picture of the same

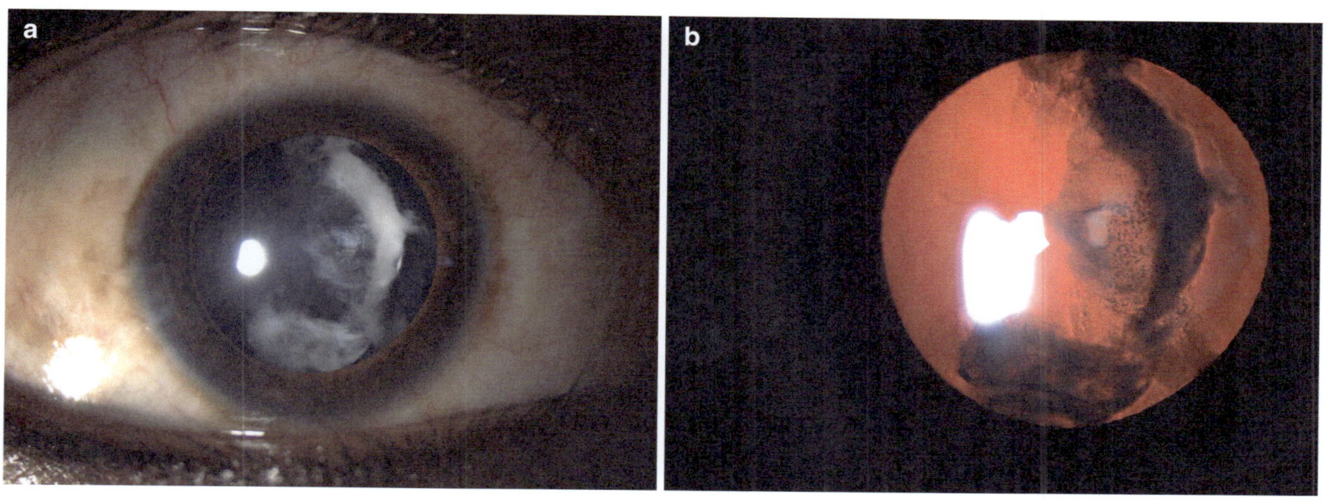

Fig. 1.12 Congenital cortical cataract in a 6-year-old child detected during routine examination. (**a**) Diffuse illumination picture showing nasal and inferior cortical cataract, (**b**) retroillumination picture of the same

1.3.6 Cortical Cataract

Although commonly seen in adult age related cataracts, it is a rare morphology in congenital cataracts. Center is clear in these cases and outer cortex is generally involved (Fig. 1.12).

1.3.7 Sutural Cataract

Sutural cataracts are congenital lens opacities that affect the Y sutures of the nucleus of the fetal lens. Generally, sutural cataracts are nonprogressive, bilateral and visually insignificant but severity may vary (Fig. 1.13a–d) [21, 23]. They may be associated with nuclear, lamellar, or pulverulent cataract which may require intervention.

1.4 Anterior Cataract

1.4.1 Anterior Polar Cataract

Anterior polar cataract involves the central pole of the lens anteriorly. They may range from small dot-like opacity to plaque type or less commonly more dense pyramidal type. Small opacities are generally visually insignificant but they may cause refractive error and amblyopia in untreated

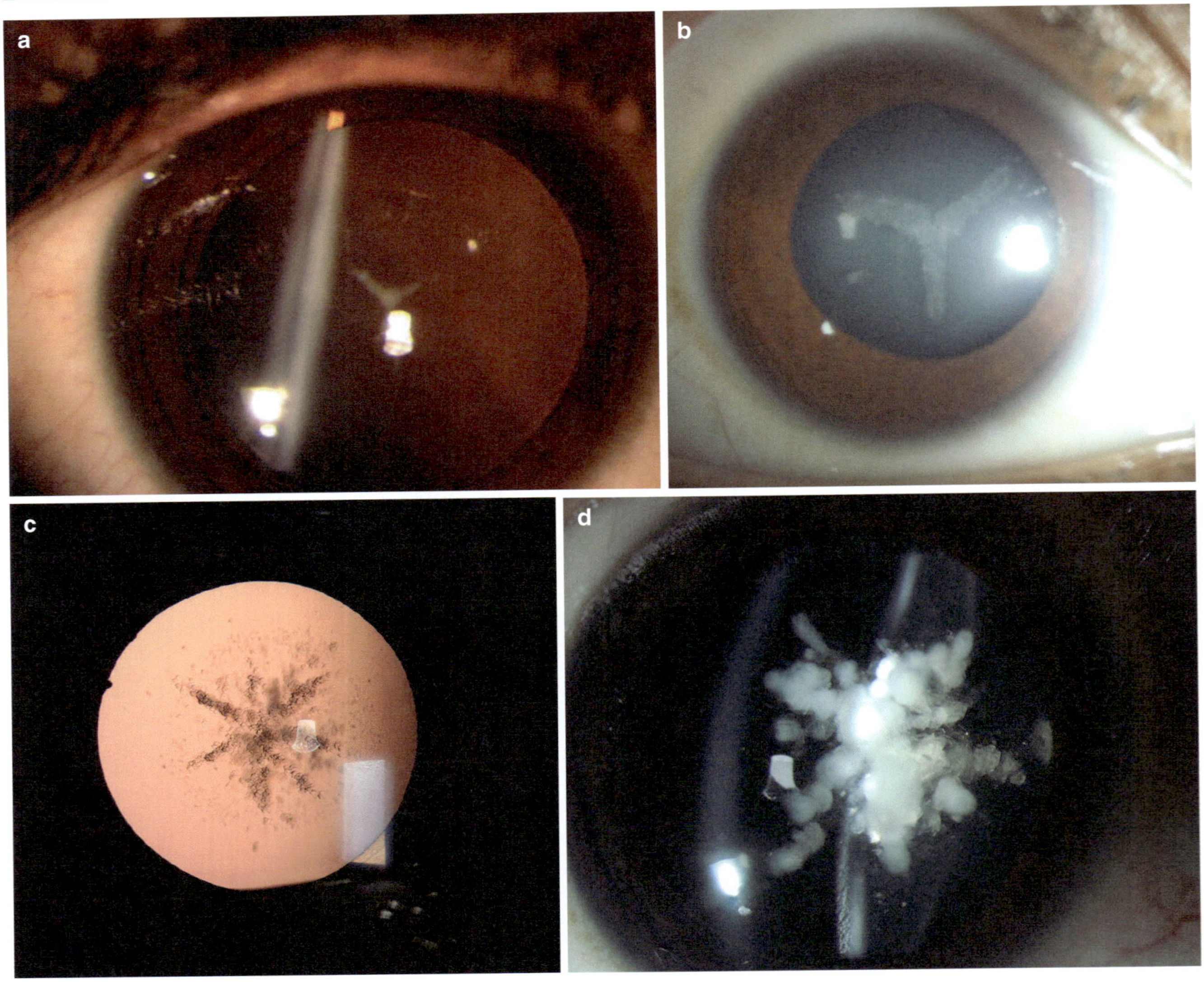

Fig. 1.13 Sutural cataract. (**a**) Minimal anterior sutural cataract, (**b**) broad Y-shaped anterior sutural cataract, (**c**) pearly droplet-like sutural cataract involving both anterior and posterior-stellate cataract, (**d**) fleshy visually significant sutural cataract with associated nuclear opacities

cases [29, 30]. Pathogenesis is not completely understood. They may be seen in association with persistent fetal vasculature which may have a role in pathogenesis [21, 31].

(a) *Dot-like cataract*: It refers to visually insignificant central opacity of lens capsule.
(b) Plaque-like cataract: It refers to opacity associated with central fibrosed and flat anterior capsule (Fig. 1.14). It may be isolated or associated with total or membranous cataract.
(c) Anterior pyramidal cataract: In this type of cataract, central opacity is noted in the anterior capsule with elevation resembling shape of pyramid (Figs. 1.15 and 1.16). These are generally visually significant and may be associated with anterior subcapsular or cortical cataract.

1.4.2 Anterior Subcapsular Cataract

Anterior subcapsular cataract may be seen in association with anterior polar cataract in congenital cases. Isolated congenital variety may have visually insignificant cataract and vacuoles may be seen in such cases (Fig. 1.17). More commonly acquired type of such cataract is seen in uveitis, trauma, drug induced cases, etc. which may be visually significant (Fig. 1.18).

1.4.3 Anterior Lenticonus

It is a form of disorder of lens and generally not associated with cataract (Fig. 1.19). Rarely seen in isolation, systemic association with Alport syndrome (most common), Lowe's

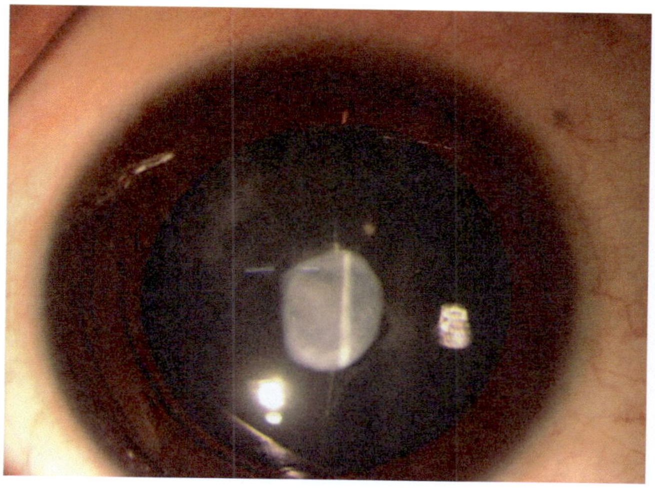

Fig. 1.14 Anterior polar cataract—plaque type with flat and fibrosed anterior capsule

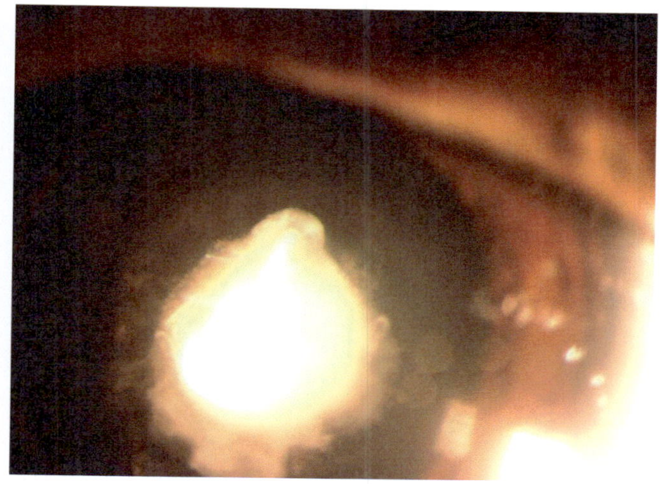

Fig. 1.15 Anterior polar cataract—pyramidal type with dense raised opacity

Fig. 1.16 UBM of an infant with anterior pyramidal cataract along with morgagnian cataract. Note the central elevation resembling shape of a pyramid

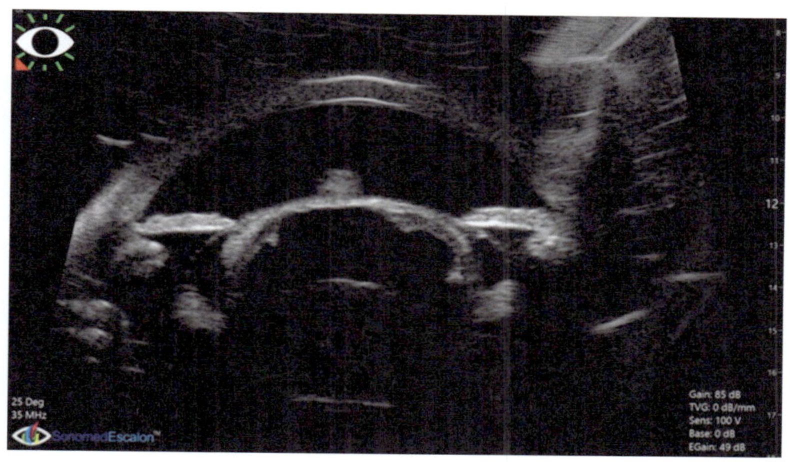

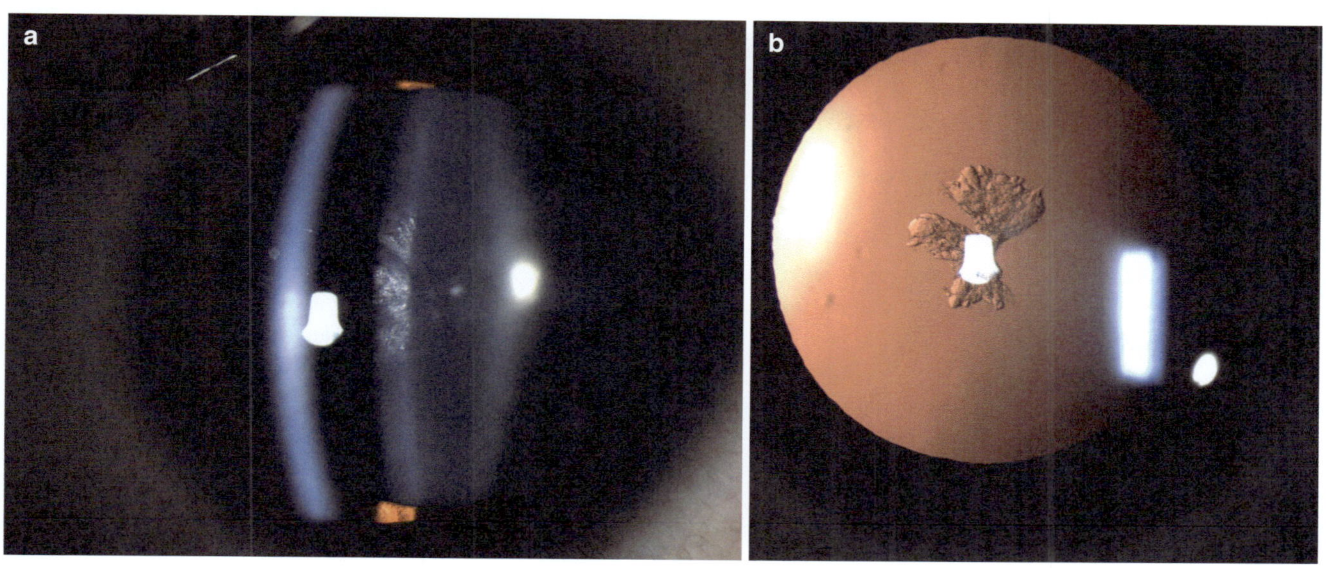

Fig. 1.17 Visually insignificant congenital anterior subscapular cataract. (**a**) Slit examination picture, (**b**) picture of the same in retroillumination. Notice presence of fluid pockets

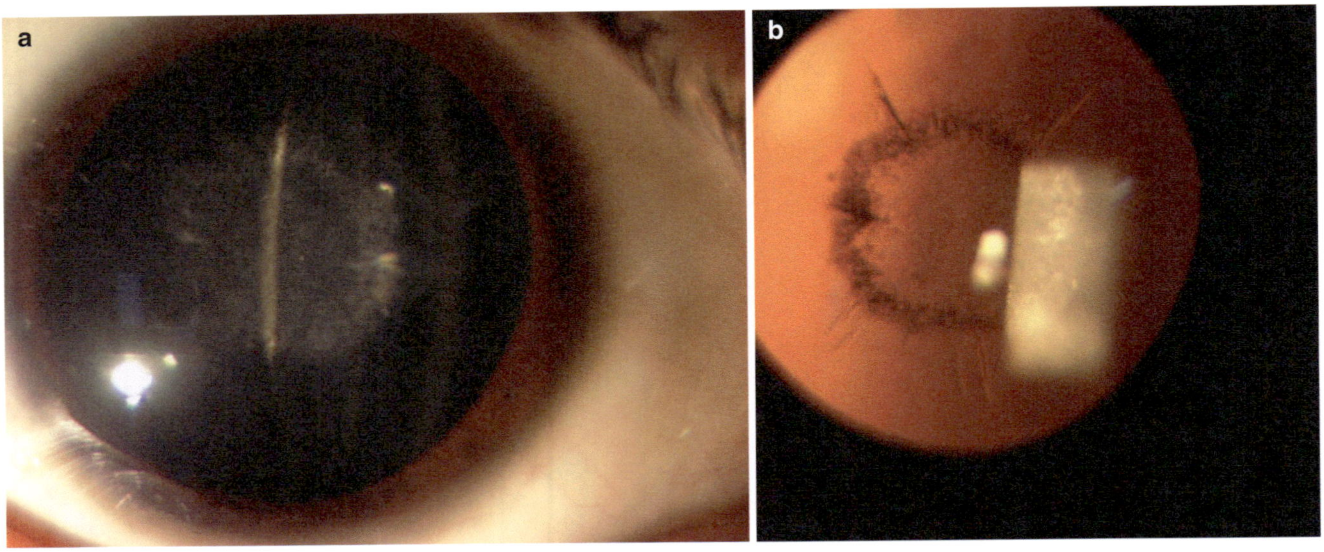

Fig. 1.18 Visually significant complicated anterior subscapular cataract. (**a**) Slit examination picture, (**b**) picture of the same in retroillumination. Also note the presence of polychromatic lusture and associated folds in the anterior capsule

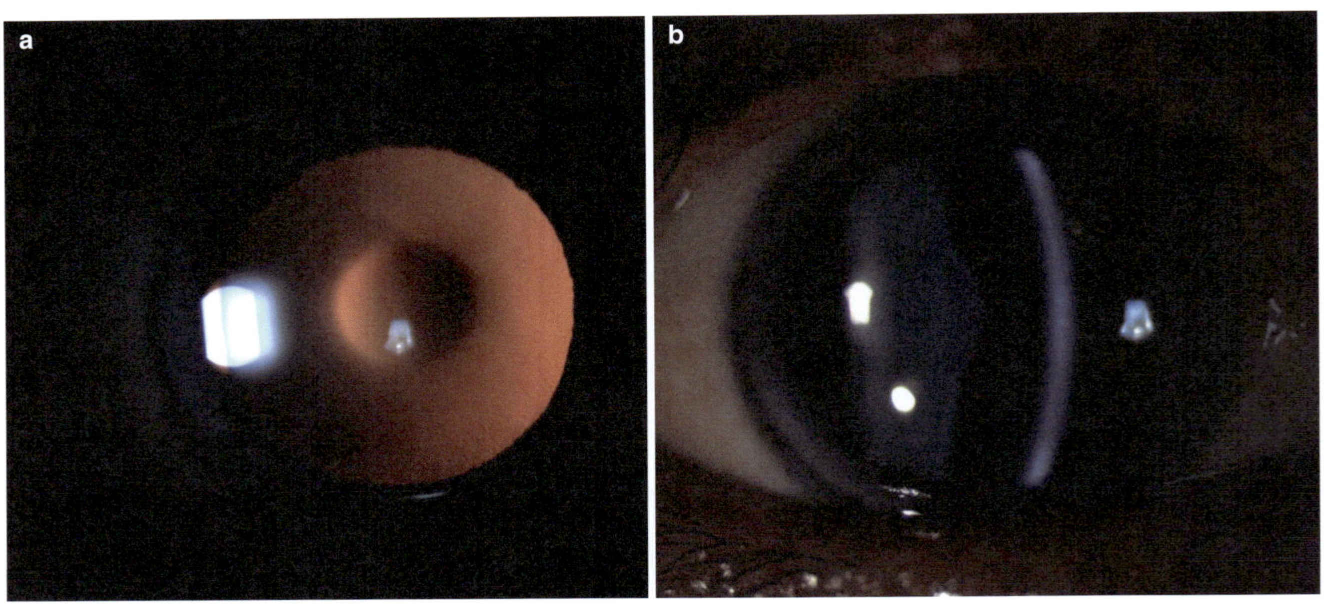

Fig. 1.19 Anterior lenticonus. (**a**) Slit illumination picture showing bulge in the anterior capsule, (**b**) retroillumination picture of the same showing oil droplet reflex

syndrome, and Waardenburg's syndrome is seen [32–34]. High lenticular myopia and astigmatism may warrant surgery in these cases.

1.5 Posterior Cataract

1.5.1 Posterior Polar Cataract

Just like anterior polar cataract, posterior polar cataracts include opacities involving posterior pole of the lens (Fig. 1.20). They are peculiar due to predisposition of posterior capsular defect during surgery [35]. Some cases may have prexisiting posterior capsular defect which is discussed in the respective chapter (Fig. 1.21). Trivial blunt trauma may also cause rupture in posterior capsule in such cases (Fig. 1.22).

1.5.2 Posterior Subcapsular Cataract

Posterior subcapsular cataract may be congenital or acquired in pediatric age group. Morphologically it may be vacuolar

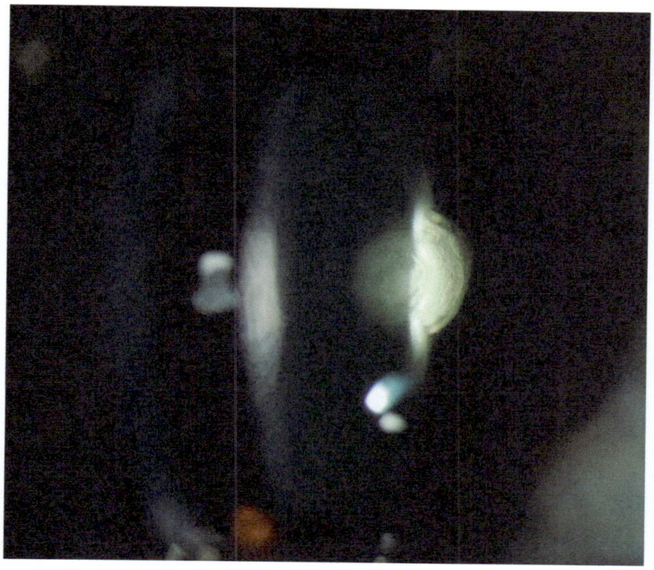

Fig. 1.20 Posterior polar cataract with typical onion ring appearance

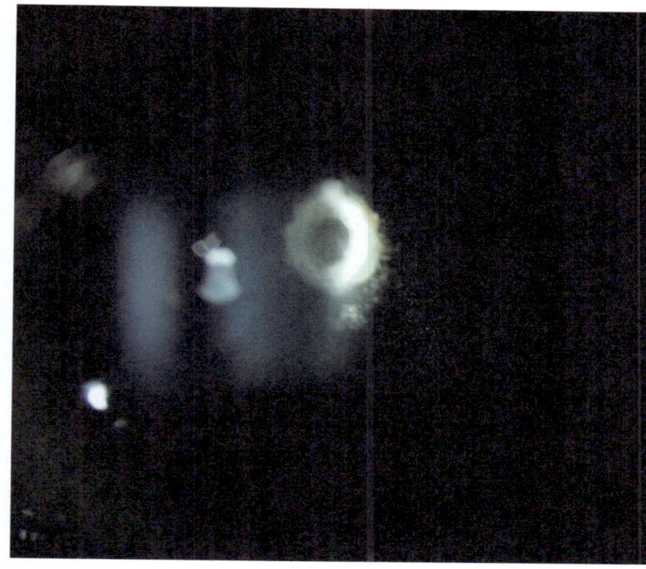

Fig. 1.21 Posterior polar cataract with typical onion ring appearance with preexisting posterior capsular defect with white dots seen in anterior vitreous

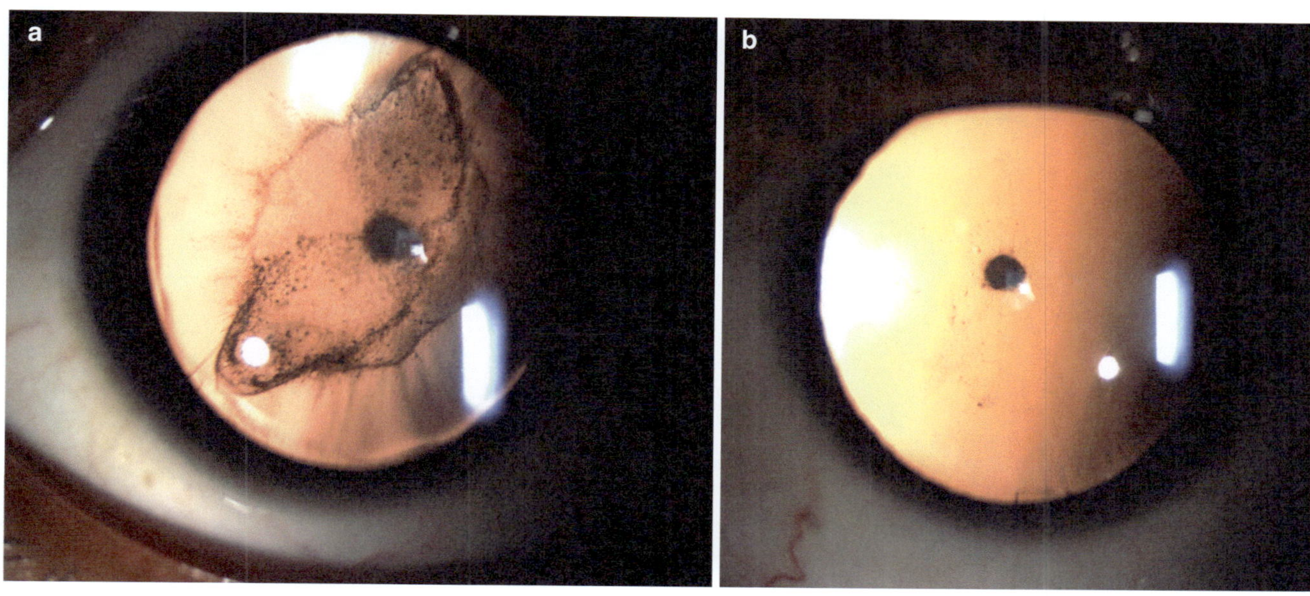

Fig. 1.22 Bilateral posterior polar cataract, retroillumination. (**a**) OD Post traumatic rupture in posterior capsule in posterior polar cataract, (**b**) OS Posterior polar cataract with no defect

or plaque like [36] (Figs. 1.23 and 1.24). It may be seen in traumatic, uveitic, or drug related cases and these causes have been described in respective chapters.

1.5.3 Posterior Lenticonus

Posterior lenticonus is associated with posterior bulging in the posterior capsule [37]. It is more common than anterior lenticonus and may be unilateral or bilateral. It is also a form disorder of the lens but it is more commonly associated with cataracts than anterior lenticonus [37, 38]. Lens may be clear initially and can progress to cataract later on [38] (Fig. 1.25). Subcapsular, cortical, or nuclear cataracts may be seen (Figs. 1.26 and 1.27). Persistent fetal vascular is hypothesized to have cause association with this type of disorder [39, 40] (Fig. 1.28a–c). It is also hypothesized to occur secondary to thinning in posterior capsule.

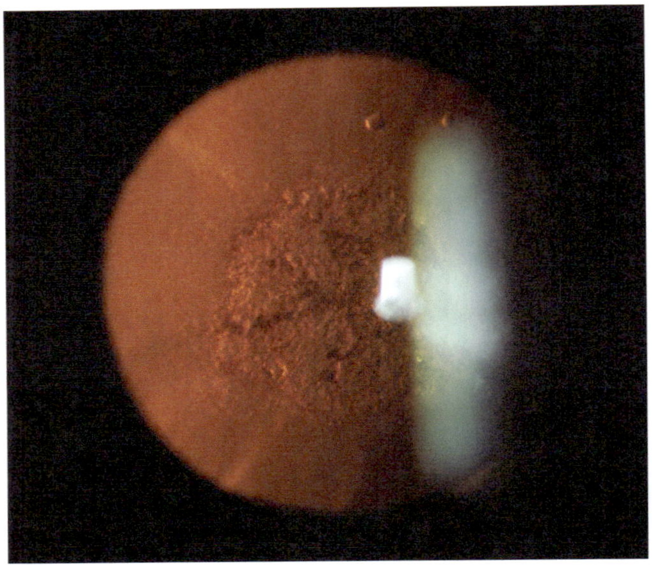

Fig. 1.23 Retroillumination picture of posterior subcapsular cataract—vacuolar type

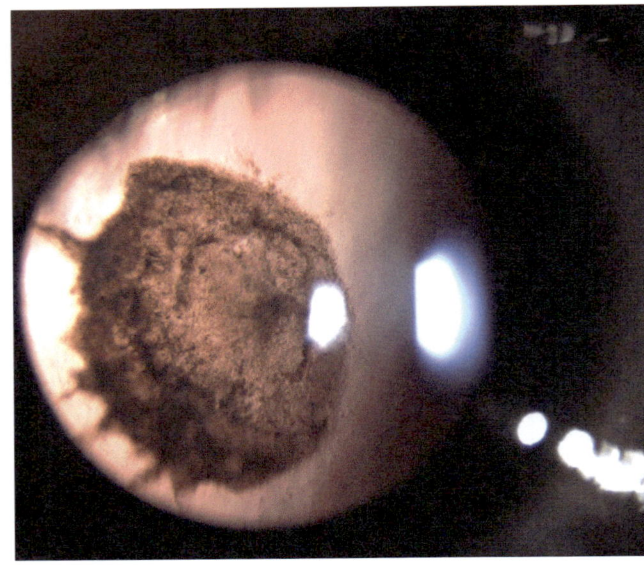

Fig. 1.24 Retroillumination picture of posterior subcapsular cataract—plaque type

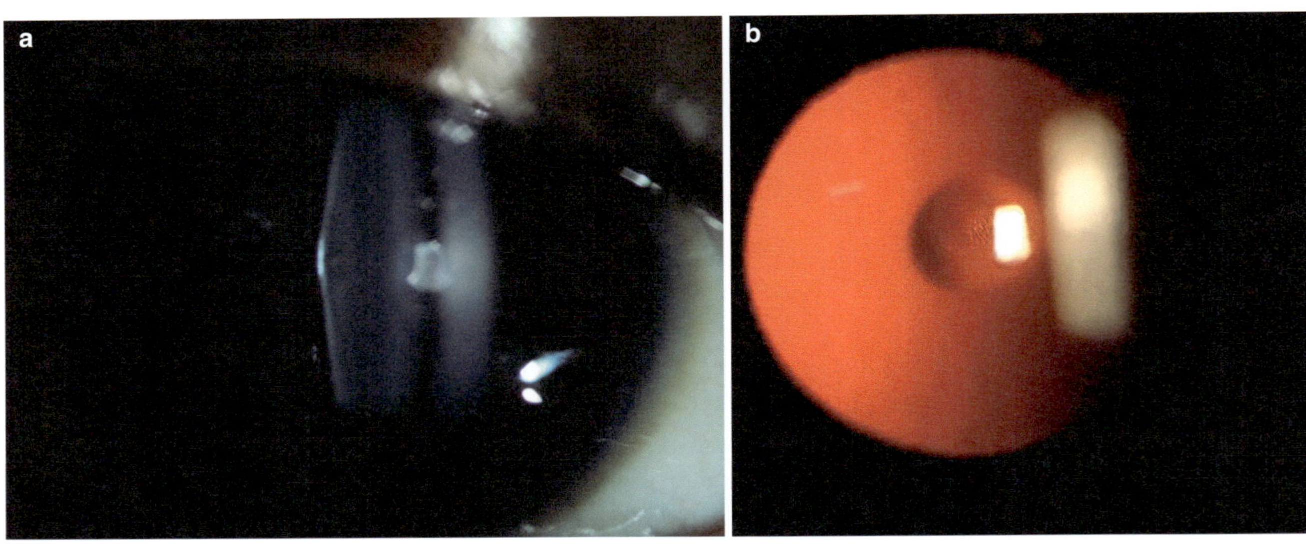

Fig. 1.25 Posterior lenticonus without cataract. (**a**) Slit illumination picture showing posterior bowing of the posterior capsule, (**b**) retroillumination picture of the same showing oil droplet sign, no cataract and few folds in the posterior capsule

1.6 Miscellaneous Cataract

The following include relatively rare morphology that we have encountered over the years. They are mentioned here in order to aid in diagnosis and better management of such pathologies.

1.6.1 Wedge-Shaped Cataract

These are generally visually insignificant cataracts. They are peripheral and may involve any quadrant (Fig. 1.29a, b). They are generally bilateral and may be specific to diseases like Stickler syndrome and Conradi Hunermann syndrome [41, 42].

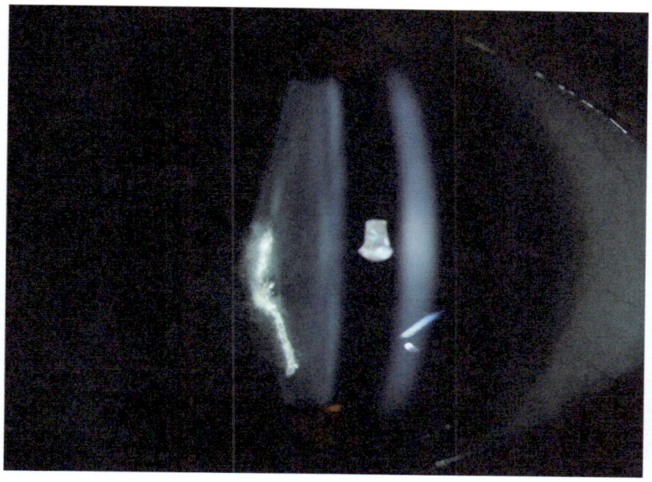

Fig. 1.26 Slit illumination picture of posterior lenticonus with associated localized posterior subcapsular cataract

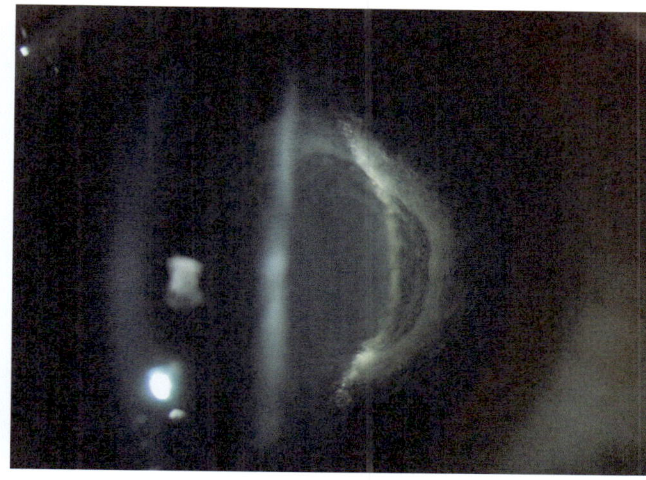

Fig. 1.27 Slit illumination picture of posterior lenticonus with associated posterior subcapsular cataract and cortical cataract

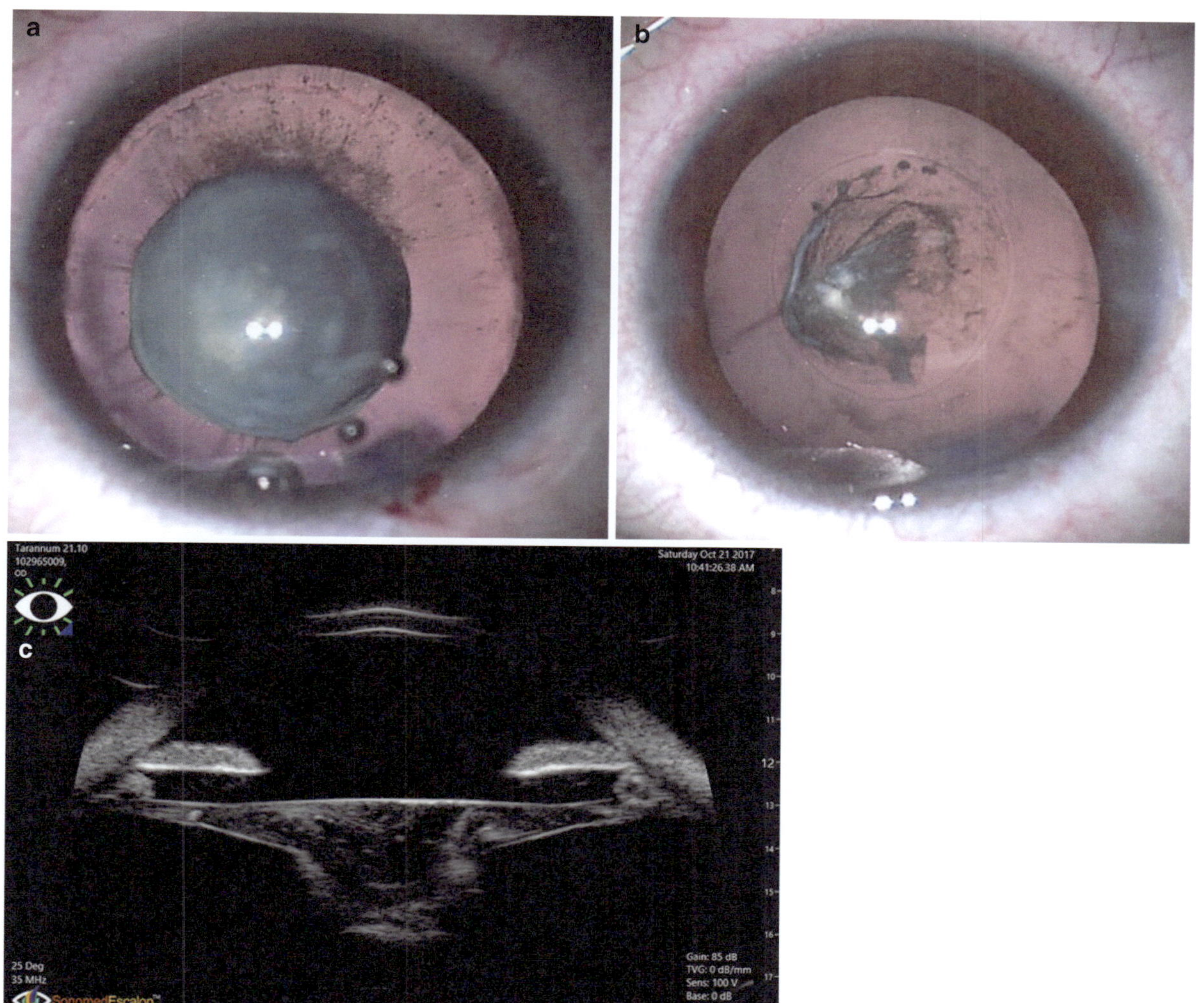

Fig. 1.28 Posterior lenticonus with persistent fetal vasculature (PFV). (**a**) Clinical picture of the patient showing posterior lenticonus with nuclear cataract, (**b**) intraoperative picture of the same showing attachment of stalk of PFV attached to posterior capsule after lens aspiration, (**c**) UBM of the same patient confirming posterior lenticonus

1.6.2 Oil Droplet Cataract

Although a rare morphology, it is typically seen in cataract related to galactosemia [43]. Central lens has change in refractive index which causes appearance of oil droplet on distant direct examination (Fig. 1.30). It is reversible in most cases. In long-standing cases, permanent opacification of lens may occur in galactosemia [43, 44].

1.6.3 Coralliform

Coralliform or coral-like cataract is seen as opacities of lens fibers radiating from the center in linear or fusiform pattern (Fig. 1.31) [45]. They are generally bilateral and may have autosomal dominant inheritance [2, 45].

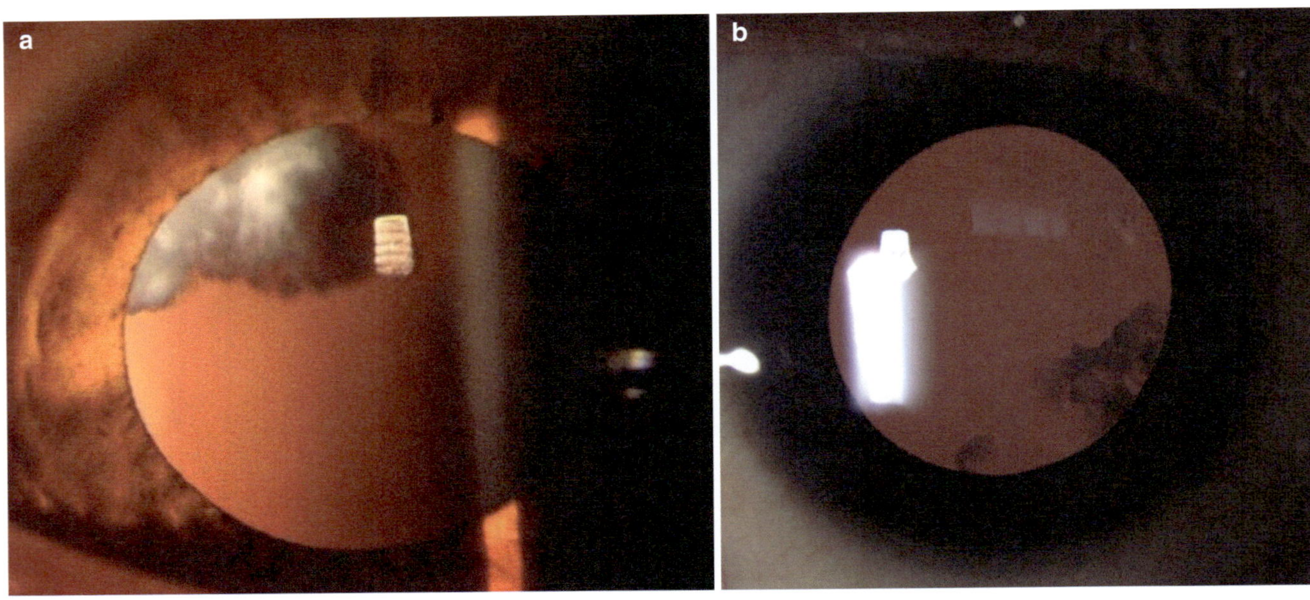

Fig. 1.29 Wedge-shaped cataract. (**a**) Superotemporal wedge-shaped cataract with predominantly cortical involvement. (**b**) Visually insignificant sectoral cataract seen inferonasal quadrant. Small speck seen in inferotemporal quadrant

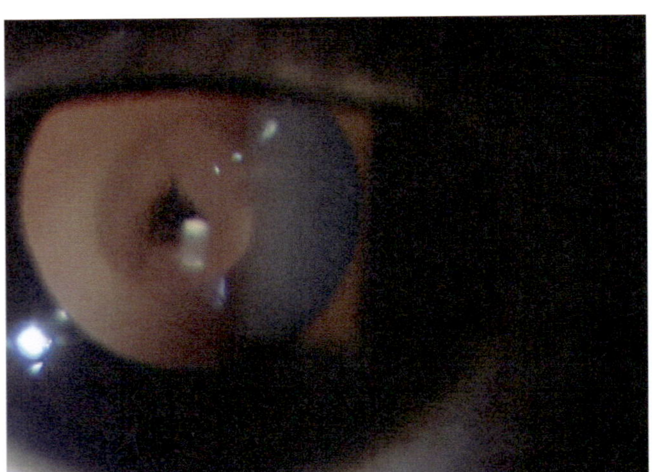

Fig. 1.30 Oil droplet cataract in an infant with galactosemia. Notice small central nuclear opacity along sutural lines

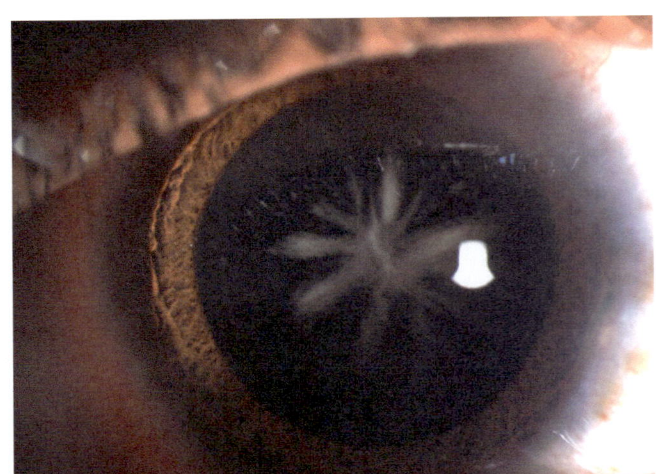

Fig. 1.31 Coralliform cataract with fusiform opacities radiating from center to periphery

1.6.4 Floriform Cataract

It resembles petals of a flower. There is a central opacity around the sutures with oval or circular shape [46] (Fig. 1.32). Similar opacities may be seen around nuclear or posterior subcapsular cataract which resembles floriform cataract.

1.6.5 Dandelion-Like Cataract

These are rare fluffy opacities seen in the lens nucleus. They may not be central in location or may be associated with polychromatic luster in some cases (Fig. 1.33).

1.6.6 Starry Sky Cataract

Multiple opacities are seen in subcapsular or cortical lens resembling shinning stars (Fig. 1.34). They are generally bilateral and visually insignificant.

1.6.7 Stud Button Cataract

It is like a reverse pyramidal cataract where circular opacity is seen attached to anterior capsule with pyramid pointing

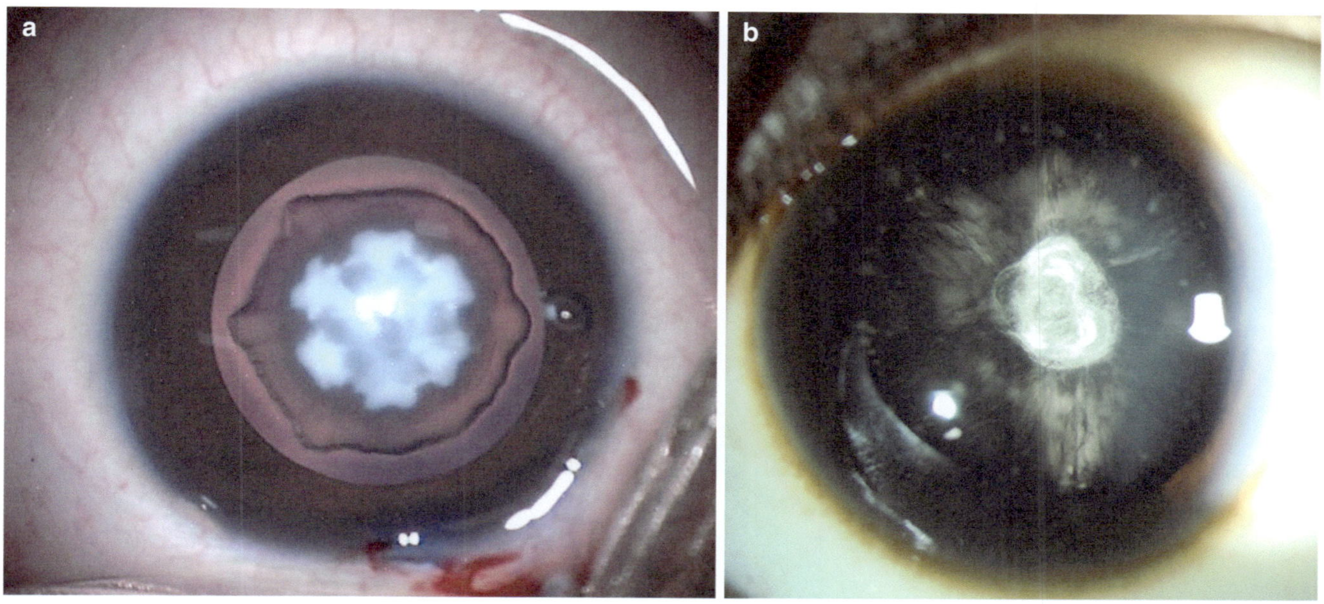

Fig. 1.32 Floriform cataract. (**a**) Koby's floriform cataract with petal-like opacities around sutures, (**b**) floriform cataract around posterior subcapsular cataract

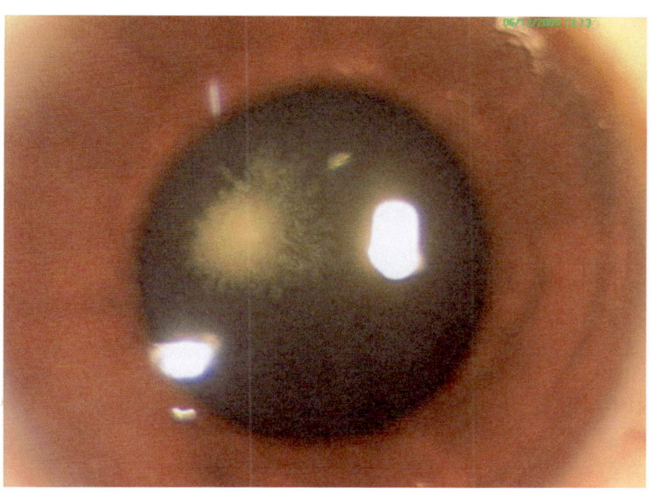

Fig. 1.33 Dandelion-like cataract

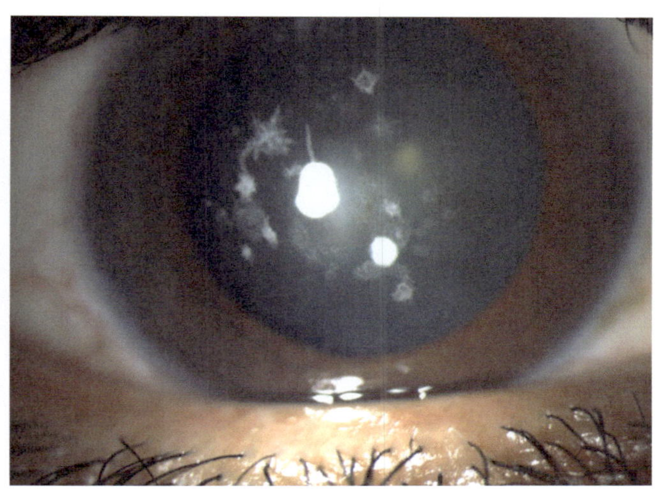

Fig. 1.34 Starry sky cataract

towards the center of lens (Fig. 1.35). It is also visually insignificant and nonprogressive but sometimes it may be associated with reduplicated cataract.

1.6.8 Reduplicated Cataract

In this type of cataract, two opacities are seen in the eye with clear zone in between (Fig. 1.36). First opacity is generally capsular and second one is behind this opacity and is called an imprint [47].

1.6.9 Linear Opacities

Linear opacities or slit-like opacities, although less common, are similar to punctate opacities and mostly nonprogressive and visually insignificant (Fig. 1.37).

1.6.10 Crystalline Cataract

Crystalline cataracts are associated with clumped, crystal-like appearance and haphazard arrangement [21, 23, 48]

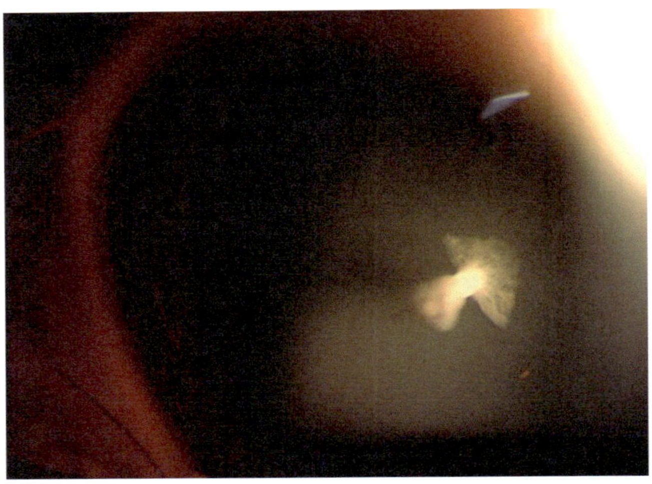

Fig. 1.35 Collar stud button cataract

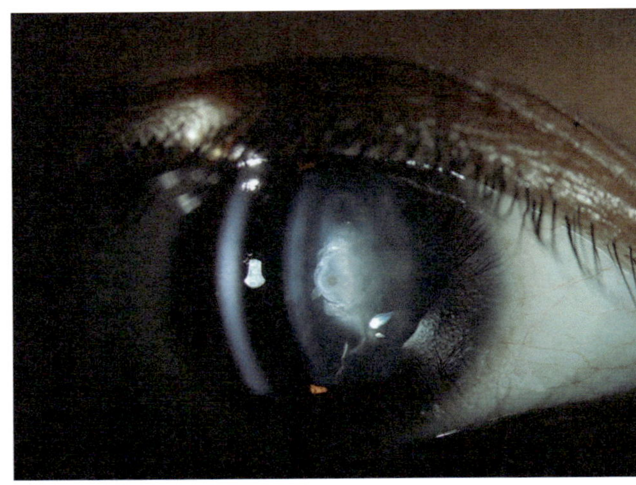

Fig. 1.36 Reduplicated cataract

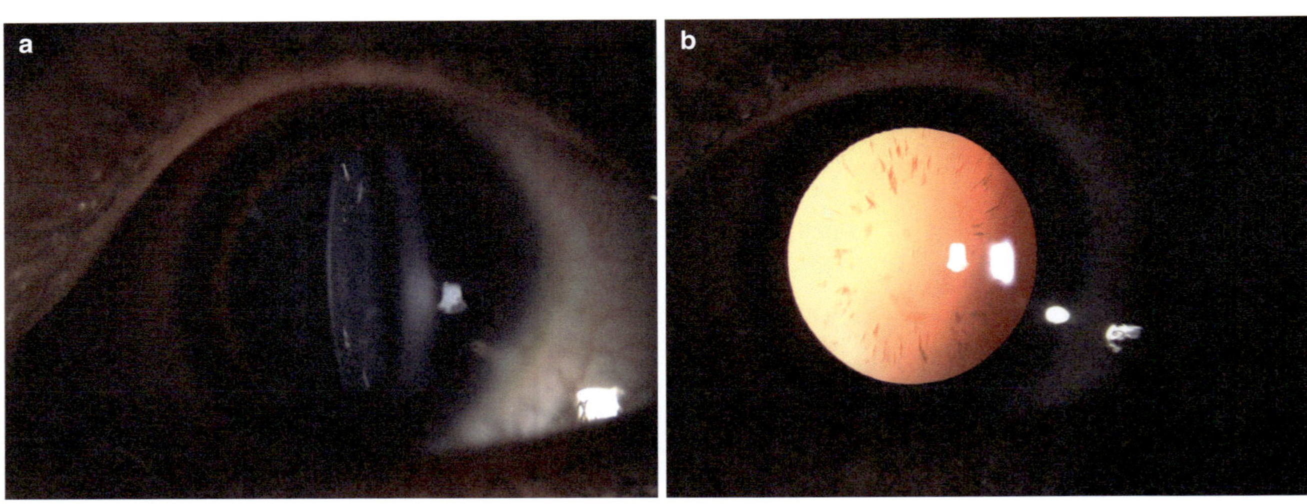

Fig. 1.37 Linear opacities or slit-like opacities. (**a**) Slit lamp examination, (**b**) retroillumination of the same

(Fig. 1.38). They may have polychromatic luster and are generally visually significant.

1.6.11 Nodular Cataract

This is a rare morphology seen as nodular calcifications in total cataract in long-standing untreated cases of congenital cataract (Fig. 1.39).

1.6.12 Stem of Cactus Cataract

In this morphology typically central cataract is associated with cortical cataract seen as buds of cactus arising from the stem (Fig. 1.40). We have seen this morphology in 8 eyes and have found an association with posterior capsular plaque or posterior capsular defect in all cases.

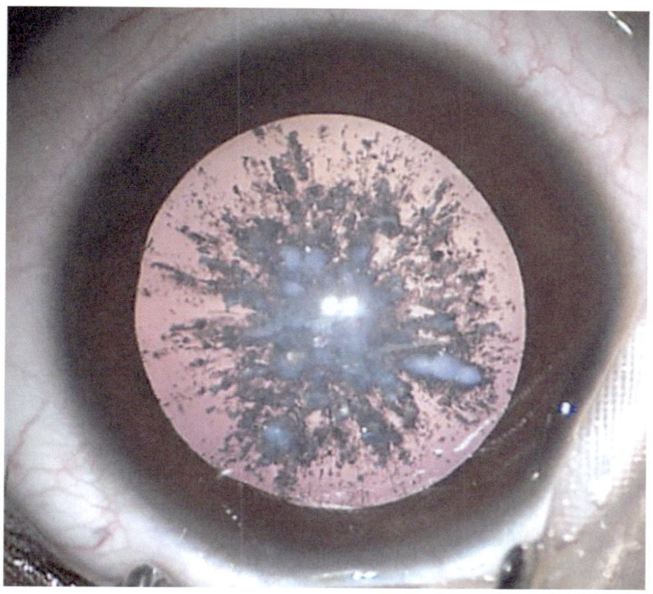

Fig. 1.38 Crystalline cataract

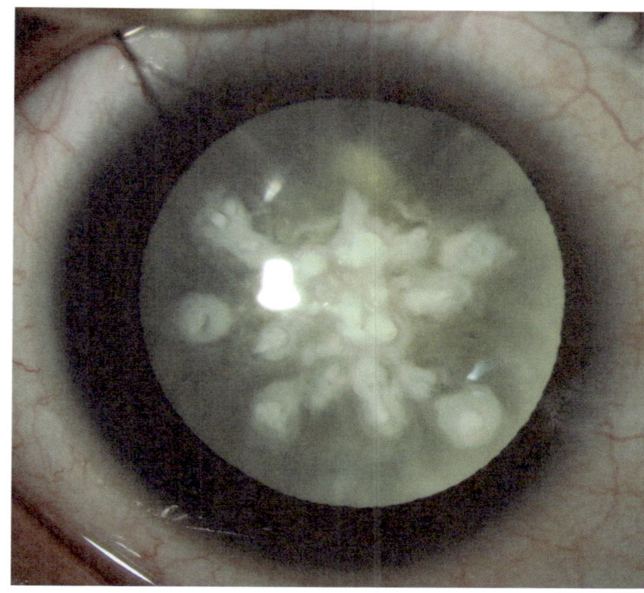

Fig. 1.39 Nodular cataracts

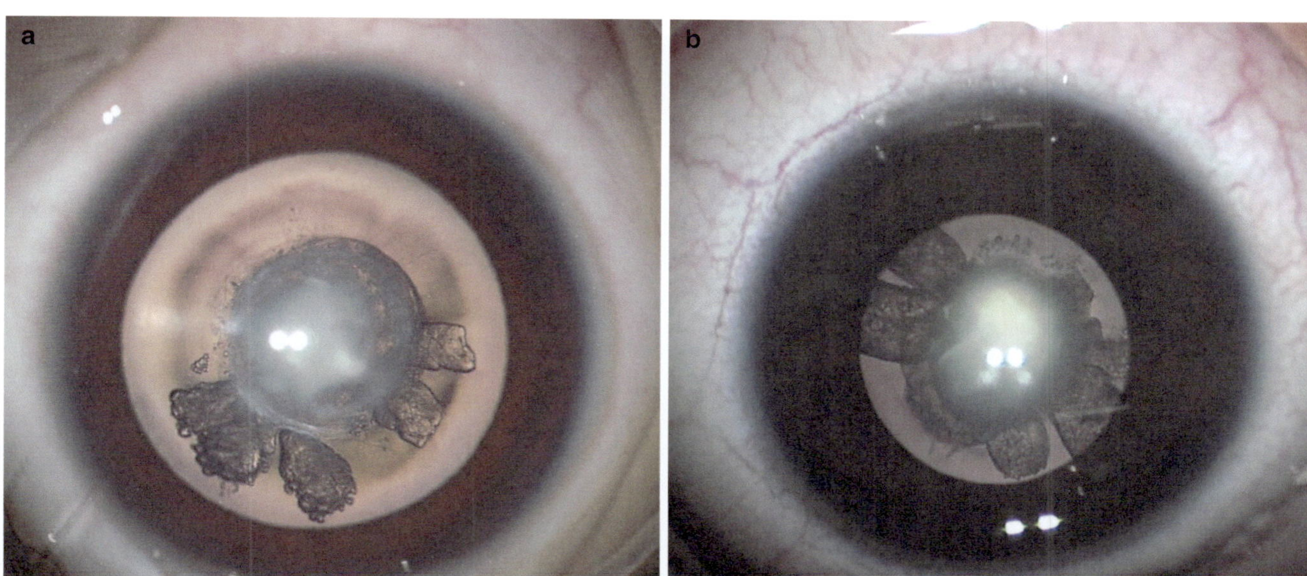

Fig. 1.40 Stem of cactus cataract—central nuclear cataract with cortical cataract with fluid vacuoles with posterior capsular plaque or defect. (**a**) Posterior capsular plaque in association with stem of cactus cataract, (**b**) prexisting posterior capsular defect plaque in association with stem of cactus cataract

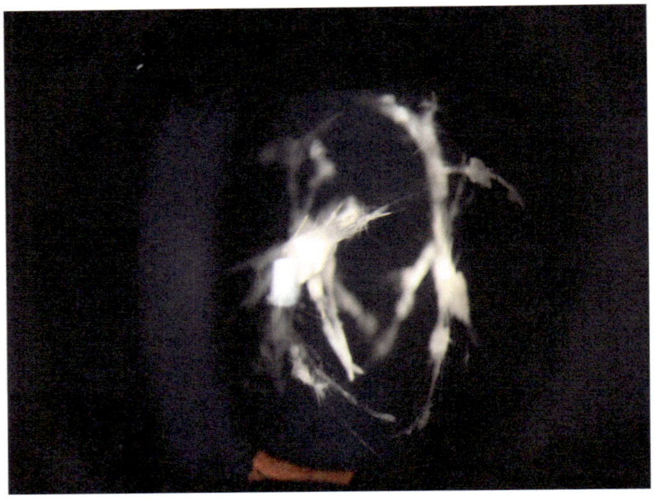

Fig. 1.41 Barbed fence wire-like cataract

1.6.13 Barbed Fence Wire-Like Cataract

It is a very unique morphology of cataract where linear wire-like lens opacities are seen in association with spicules (Fig. 1.41). We have encountered a single family with this morphology with autosomal dominant inheritance. We have described this in chapter pertaining to hereditary cataract.

References

1. Sheeladevi S, Lawrenson JG, Fielder AR, Suttle CM. Global prevalence of childhood cataract: a systematic review. Eye (Lond). 2016;30(9):1160–9.
2. Amaya L, Taylor D, Russell-Eggitt I, Nischal KK, Lengyel D. The morphology and natural history of childhood cataracts. Surv Ophthalmol. 2003;48(2):125–44.
3. Khokhar SK, Pillay G, Dhull C, Agarwal E, Mahabir M, Aggarwal P. Pediatric cataract. Indian J Ophthalmol. 2017;65:1340–9.
4. Kaya A. Preoperative usage of ultrasound biomicroscopy in pediatric cataract. Arq Bras Oftalmol. 2016;79(1):62.
5. Xiang D, Chen L, Hu L, Song S, Xie W, Long J. Image features of lens opacity in pediatric cataracts using ultrasound biomicroscopy. J AAPOS. 2016;20(6):19–522.
6. Forster JE, Abadi RV, Muldoon M, Lloyd IC. Grading infantile cataracts. Ophthalmic Physiol Opt. 2006;26:372–9.
7. Wilson ME, Hennig A, Trivedi RH, Thomas BJ, Singh SK. Clinical characteristics and early postoperative outcomes of pediatric cataract surgery with IOL implantation from Lahan, Nepal. J Pediatr Ophthalmol Strabismus. 2011;48:286–91.
8. Long E, Lin Z, Chen J, et al. Monitoring and morphologic classification of pediatric cataract using slit-lamp-adapted photography. Transl Vis Sci Technol. 2017;6(6):2.
9. Jain IS, Pillay P, Gangwar DN, et al. Congenital cataract: etiology and morphology. J Pediatr Ophthalmol Strabismus. 1983;20:238–42.
10. Lance O. Anatomy and embryology of the lens. In: Duane TD, Jaeger EA, editors. Duane's clinical ophthalmology, vol. 1. Philadelphia: JB Lippincott; 1988, Chap 71. p. 1–8.
11. Vasavada AR, Praveen MR, Dholakia SA, Trivedi RH. Preexisting posterior capsule defect progressing to white mature cataract. J AAPOS. 2007;11:192–4.
12. Bron AJ, Habgood JO. Morgagnian cataract. Trans Ophthalmol Soc U K. 1976;96:265–77.
13. Takamura Y, Oishi N. Morgagnian cataract with an isolated posterior capsular opening. Arch Ophthalmol. 2003;121:1487–8.
14. Boger WP 3rd, Petersen RA, Robb RM. Spontaneous absorption of the lens in the congenital rubella syndrome. Arch Ophthalmol. 1981;99:433–4.
15. Ehrlich LH. Spontanous absorption of congenital cataract following maternal rubella. Arch Ophthalmol. 1948;39:205–9.
16. Rathinam SR, Namperumalsamy P, Cunningham ET. Spontaneous cataract absorption in patients with leptospiral uveitis. Br J Ophthalmol. 2000;84:1135–41.
17. Wegener JK, Sogaard H. Persistent hyperplastic primary vitreous with resorption of the lens. Acta Ophthalmol. 1968;46:171–5.
18. Lambert SR, Drack AV. Infantile cataracts. Surv Ophthalmol. 1996;40:427–58.
19. Soriano JM, Funk J. Spontaneous bilateral lens resorption in a case of Hallermann-Streiff syndrome. Klin Monatsbl Augenheilkd. 1991;199:195–8.
20. Tripathi RC, Cibis GW, Tripathi BJ. Pathogenesis of cataracts in patients with Lowe's syndrome. Ophthalmology. 1986;93:1046–51.
21. Brown N, Bron AJ. Lens disorders. Oxford: Butterworth-Heinemann Ltd; 1996. p. 133–93.
22. Khokhar S, Gupta Y, Dhull C, Surve A, Mahabir M. Cortical riders of zonular cataracts as "reverse cuneiform" cataracts: a hypothesis. Med Hypotheses. 2018;121:49–50.
23. Duke-Elder S. System of Ophthalmology, vol. 14. London: H. Kimpton; 1972. p. 352.
24. Nettleship E, Ogilvie FM. A peculiar form of hereditary congenital cataract. Trans Ophthalmol Soc U K. 1906;26:191–207.
25. Rosen E. Coppock cataract and cataracta pulverulenta centralis. Br J Ophthalmol. 1945;29:641–4.
26. Schroder HD, Nissen SH. Ant-egg cataract. An electron microscopic study. Acta Ophthalmol. 1979;57:435–42.
27. Clemmensen K, Enghild JJ, Ivarsen A, et al. "Ant-egg" cataract revisited. Graefes Arch Clin Exp Ophthalmol. 2017;255:119.
28. Vogt A. Die Spezifität angeborener und erworbener Starformen für die einzelnen Linsenzonen. Graefes Arch Ophthalmol. 1922;108:219–28.
29. Ionides A, Francis P, Berry V, et al. Clinical and genetic heterogeneity in autosomal dominant cataract. Br J Ophthalmol. 1999;83:802–8.
30. Bouzas AG. Anterior polar congenital cataract and corneal astigmatism. J Pediatr Ophthalmol Strabismus. 2000;29:210–2.
31. Khokhar S, Sinha G, Sharma R, Patil B, Mahabir M, Nayak B. Anterior pyramidal cataract a rare association. JAMA Ophthalmol. 2015;133(4):e144626. https://doi.org/10.1001/jamaophthalmol.2014.4626.
32. Govan JA. Ocular manifestations of Alports syndrome: a hereditary disorder of basement membranes? Br J Ophthalmol. 1983;67:493–503.
33. Ginsberg J, Bove KE, Fogelson MH. Pathological features of the eye in the oculocerebrorenal (Lowe) syndrome. J Pediatr Ophthalmol Strabismus. 1981;18:16–24.
34. Stevens PR. Anterior lenticonus and the Waardenburg syndrome. Br J Ophthalmol. 1970;54:621–3.
35. Osher RH, Yu BC-Y, Koch DD. Posterior polar cataracts: a predisposition to intraoperative posterior capsule rupture. J Cataract Refract Surg. 1990;16:157–62.
36. Eshagian J. Human posterior subcapsular cataracts. Trans Ophthalmol Soc U K. 1982;102:364–8.

37. Khalil M, Saheb N. Posterior lenticonus. Ophthalmology. 1984;91:1429–30, 43A.
38. Crouch ER Jr, Parks MM. Management of posterior lenticonus complicated by unilateral cataract. Am J Ophthalmol. 1978;85:503–8.
39. Kilty LA, Hiles DA. Unilateral posterior lenticonus with persistent hyaloid artery remnant. Am J Ophthalmol. 1993;116:104–6.
40. Khokhar S, Dhull C, Mahalingam K, Agarwal P. Posterior lenticonus with persistent fetal vasculature. Indian J Ophthalmol. 2018;66(9):1335–6.
41. Happle R, Kuchle HJ. Sectorial cataract: a possible example of lyonisation. Lancet. 1983;2:919–20.
42. Seery CM, Pruett RC, Liberfarb RM, Cohen BZ. Distinctive cataract in the Stickler syndrome. Am J Ophthalmol. 1990;110:143–8.
43. Beigi B, OKeefe M, Bowell R, et al. Ophthalmic findings in classical galactosaemia—prospective study. Br J Ophthalmol. 1993;77:162–4.
44. Bruck E, Rapoport S. Galactosemia in an infant with cataracts: clinical observations and carbohydrate studies. Am J Dis Child. 1945;70:267.
45. Guyot-Sionnest P. Coralliform cataracts. Bull Soc Ophtalmol Fr. 1972;72:881–7.
46. Koby FE. Cataracte familiale d'un type particulier apparament suivant le mode dominant. Arch Ophthalmol. 1923;38:492–501.
47. Sihota R, Tandon R. Parsons' diseases of the eye, vol. 18. 21st ed. New Delhi: Elsevier; 2011. p. 266.
48. Gunn RM. Peculiar coralliform cataract with crystals of cholesterine in the lens. Trans Ophthalmol Soc U K. 1895;15:119.

Hereditary Cataracts

2

Yogita Gupta, Chirakshi Dhull, and Sudarshan Kumar Khokhar

2.1 Introduction

Inheritance is observed in congenital cataracts in 8.3–25% [1, 2] of cases, with most common mode of inheritance pattern being autosomal dominant [2]. Hence, the importance of recording family history and screening family members of cases of congenital cataract presenting to an ophthalmologist. Embryological development of the lens is an interplay of many genes functioning simultaneously to bring about a well-controlled sequence of events. Almost 40 genetic loci are known, which could be affected to cause congenital cataracts. [3]

2.2 Genetics of Congenital Cataract: Lens Embryology and Its Regulation

At approximately day 25 of gestation, two lateral evaginations develop from the developing forebrain or prosencephalon, called the optic vesicle (Fig. 2.1). These then approximate to the surface ectoderm constituted by a single layer of epithelial cells. The ectodermal cells overlying the optic vesicle change to columnar cells and form the lens placode by day 27. At day 29, an indentation or lens pit appears in the center of lens placode. The lens pit continues to invaginate and the ectodermal cells separate from the surface ectoderm to form lens vesicle by day 30. The cells in the posterior layer of lens vesicle begin to elongate and form primary lens fibers that fill the lumen of optic vesicle and form the embryonic nucleus by day 40. The equatorial cells of anterior lens epithelial cells then elongate to form secondary lens fibers to form the fetal nucleus from second to eighth month of gestation. The ends of secondary lens fibers interdigitate as an anterior erect Y and posterior inverted Y sutures, evident by 8 weeks of gestation. As the lens fibers continue to grow, nearly 12 or more sutures appear in the adult lens.

Lens development and differentiation is tightly regulated by many factors like fibroblast growth factor (FGF), bone morphogenetic protein (BMP), and Pax6 homeobox genes. Most commonly, the inherited cataracts show autosomal dominant transmission and occur as a result of mutations in the genes encoding for crystallins, membrane transport, and cytoskeletal proteins [3–6].

We have studied role of α-crystallin (CRYAB), γ-crystallin (CRYGC and CRYGD), and Connexin 50 (Cx-50 or GJA8) and identified two non-synonymous novel mutations, p. R48H(4/30) and p.L281C(1/30) in CRYGC and GJA8, respectively [6, 7]. In another study, we looked for contribution of gene mutations in childhood cataract in Indian population, specifically mutations in Crystallin, alpha A (CRYAA), CRYAB, CRYGs, CRYBA1, CRYBA4, CRYBB1, CRYBB2, CRYBB3, beaded filament structural protein 1 (BFSP1), gap function protein, alpha 3 (GJA3), GJA8, and heat shock transcription factor 4 gene genes were looked into [7, 8]. We confirmed the role of mutation in crystallin beta cluster to play a major role in cataract formation [7, 8].

2.3 Mendelian Inheritance Patterns

Inheritance of childhood cataract is most commonly autosomal dominant. Inheritance patterns in addition to morphology of cataract and clinical features may give a clue to diagnosis (Table 2.1). Pedigree chart is an easy tool for identification of inheritance pattern (Fig. 2.2). Families may present with similar morphology of cataract with some variation. We encountered a family with very unique morphology of cataract resembling barbed fence wire. Pedigree of the patient suggested autosomal dominant mutation (Fig. 2.3), unique morphology in multiple members (Fig. 2.4) and genetic testing revealed novel mutation (Fig. 2.5).

Y. Gupta · C. Dhull · S. K. Khokhar (✉)
Dr. Rajendra Prasad Centre for Ophthalmic Sciences, All India Institute of Medical Sciences, New Delhi, India

S. K. Khokhar, C. Dhull (eds.), *Atlas of Pediatric Cataract*, https://doi.org/10.1007/978-981-13-6939-1_2

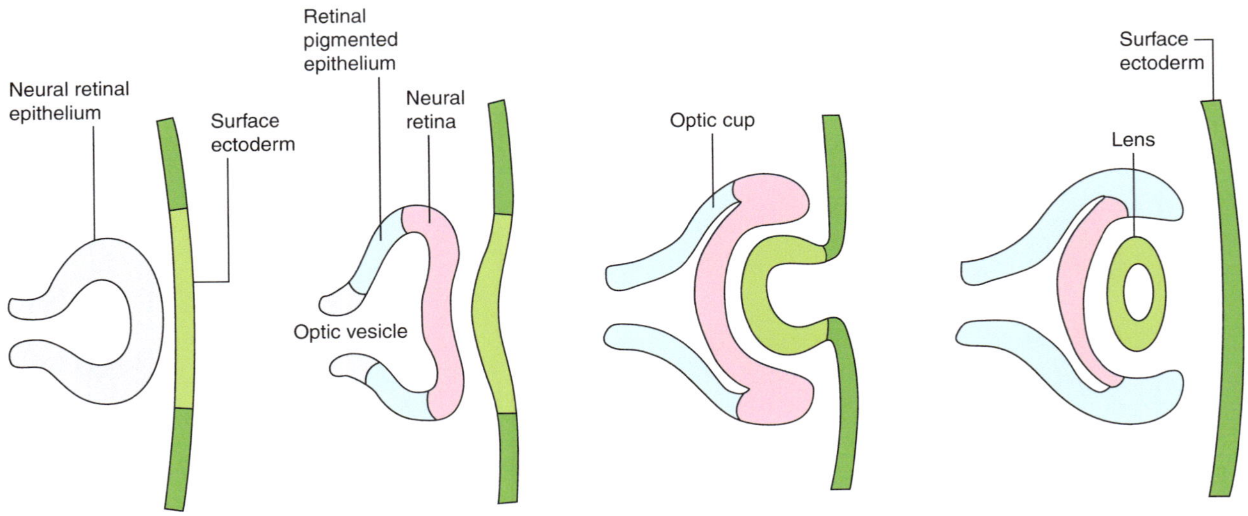

Fig. 2.1 Embryological development of lens showing formation of lens vesicle and optic cup

Table 2.1 Inheritance patterns and associated conditions

Autosomal dominant	Autosomal recessive	X-linked recessive	X-linked dominant
Hyperferritinemia cataract syndrome Coppock-like cataracts Posterior polar cataract Zonular pulverulent cataract Anterior polar cataract Cerulean type cataract Volkmann type congenital cataracts	Congenital cataracts, facial dysmorphism and neuropathy (CCFDN) Warburg micro syndrome Martsolf syndrome Hallermann–Streiff syndrome Smith–Lemli–Opitz syndrome	Norrie disease Nance–Horan syndrome	Hünermann–Conradi syndrome

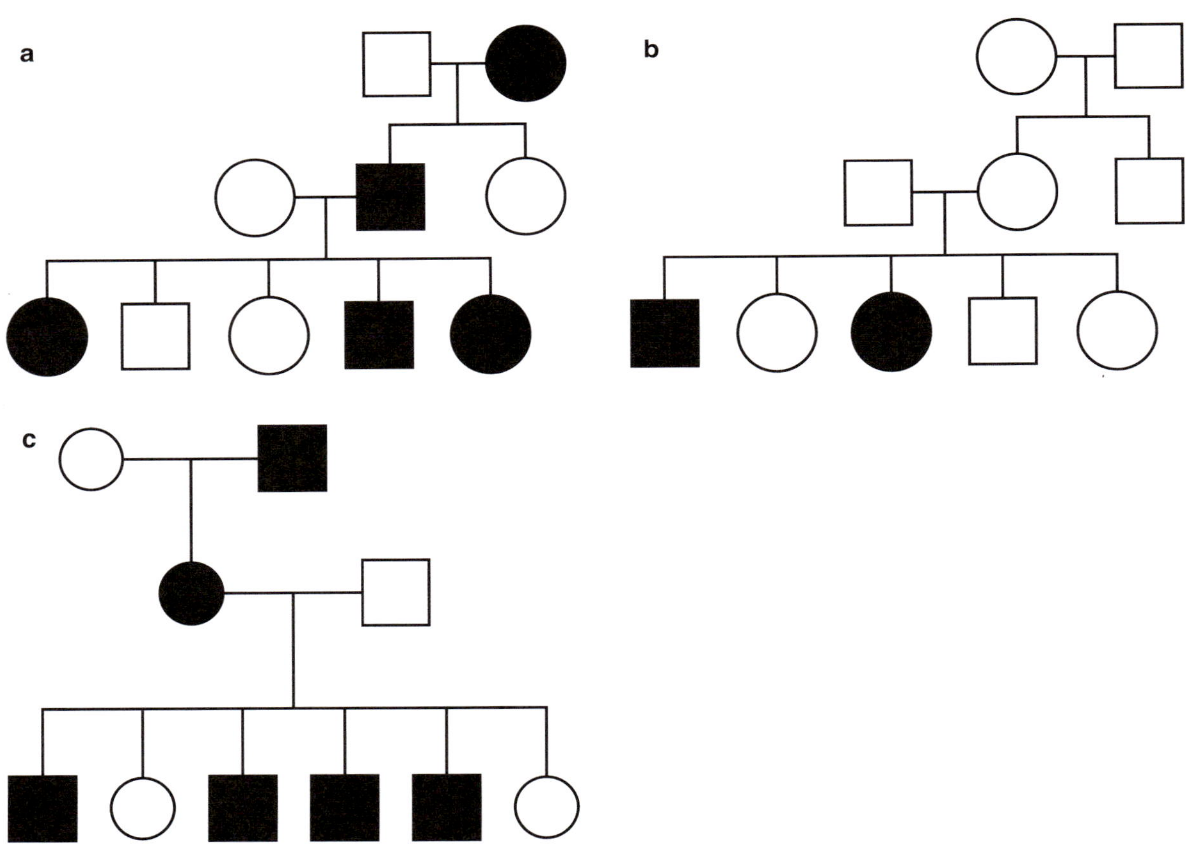

Fig. 2.2 Pedigree charts showing (**a**) autosomal dominant, (**b**) autosomal recessive, and (**c**) X-linked recessive pattern of inheritance

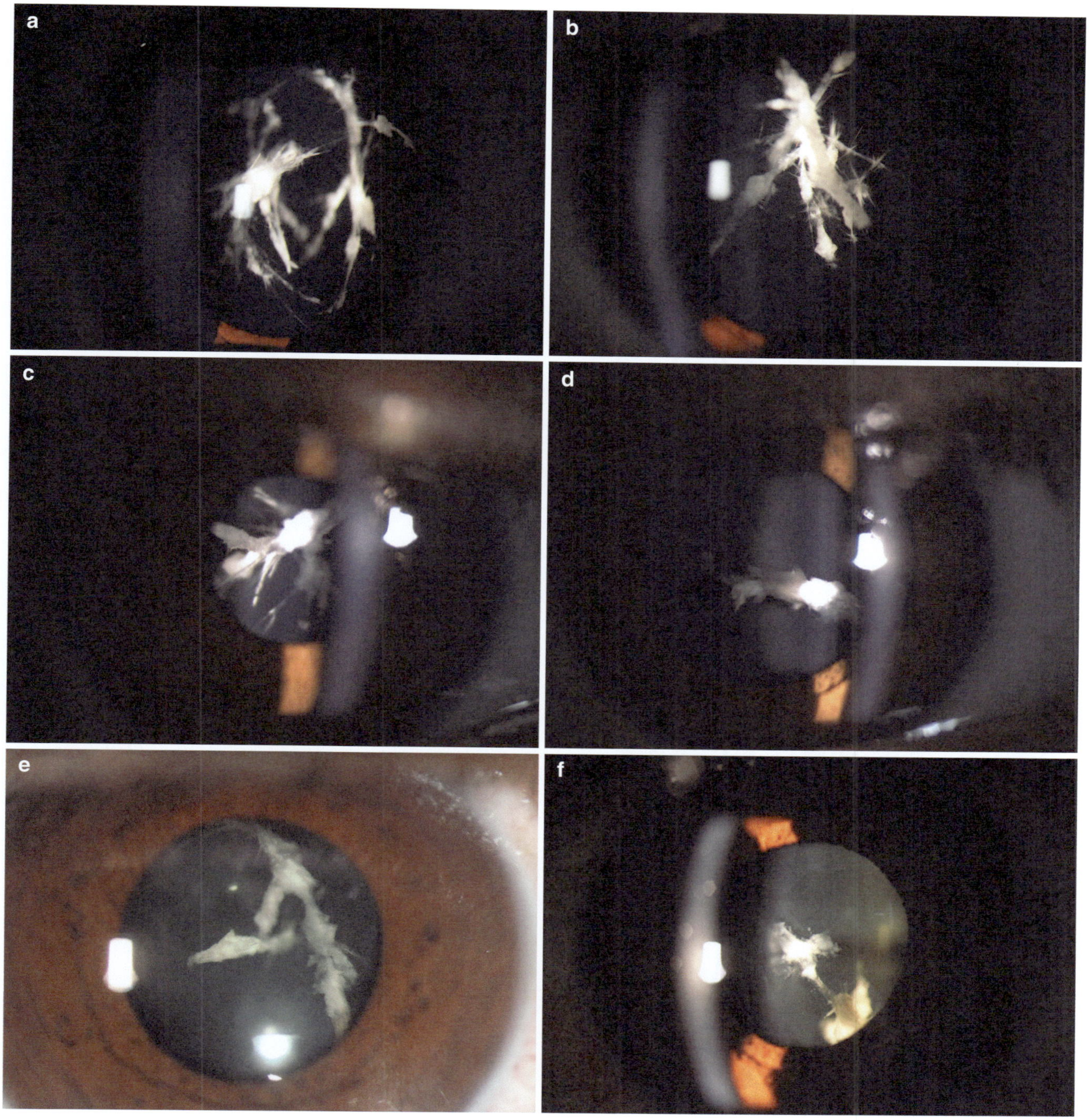

Fig. 2.3 Slit lamp photographs of an autosomal dominant congenital cataract studied in two generations of a family. Note cataracts in third generation [index case OD (**a**) OS (**b**); cousin sister 'A11' OD (**c**) OS (**d**); brother 'A7' OD (**e**), OS (**f**)

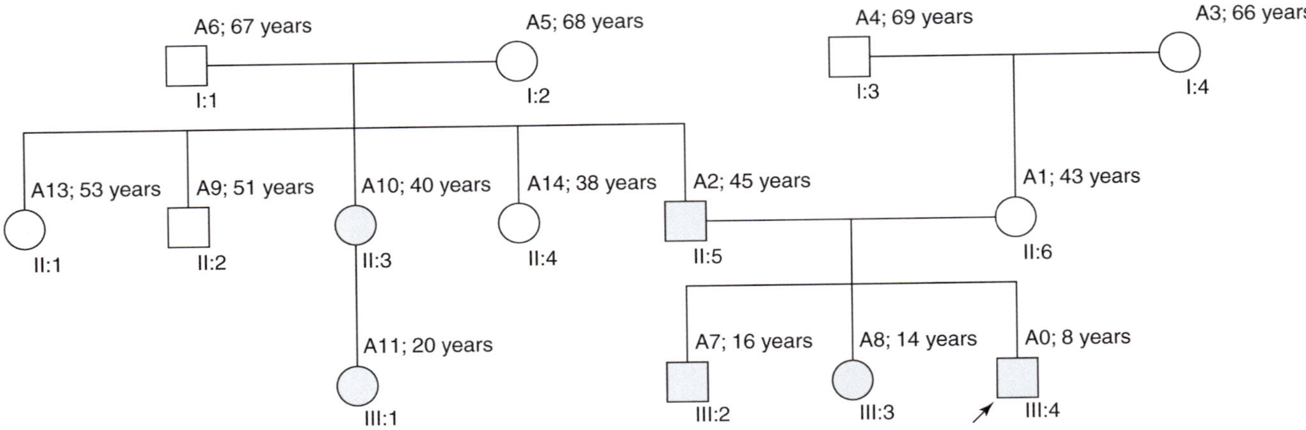

Fig. 2.4 Pedigree chart of the family shown in Fig. 2.3 suggested an autosomal dominant inheritance pattern

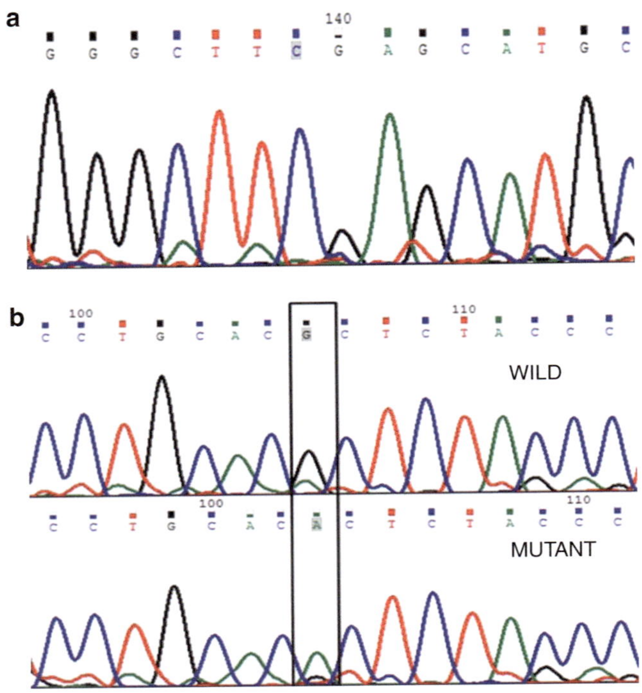

Fig. 2.5 DNA sequence of the studied family showed nucleotide variations in the involved family members showing CRYBA4: rs5761637T>A change (**a**) and rs4276A>G change (**b**)

2.4 Systemic Disorders/Syndromes Involving Pediatric Lenses

Various systemic disorders are known to be associated with pediatric cataract. Common disorders are listed in the table below (Table 2.2).

Table 2.2 Syndromes associated with congenital cataract

Syndrome	Genetic loci	Inheritance pattern	Phenotypic features
Autosomal recessive congenital infection-like syndrome (pseudo-TORCH syndrome) [9]	USP18—22q11.21	AR	Microcephaly, intracranial calcification, **congenital cataracts**, clinical course resembles congenital TORCH infection
Cerebro-oculo-facio-skeletal syndrome (COFS) [10]	ERCC6—10q11.23	AR	Microcephaly, **congenital cataracts**, microphthalmia, arthrogryposis (congenital joint contractures), rocker-bottom feet, severe developmental delay, growth failure, dysmorphism with prominent nasal root and overhanging upper lip
Rhizomelic chondrodysplasia punctata type 1 [11]	PEX7, 6q23.3	AR	Systemic shortening of proximal limb bones (i.e., rhizomelia), seizures, recurrent respiratory tract infections, **congenital cataracts**
Conradi–Hünermann–Happle syndrome (X-linked dominant chondrodysplasia punctata type 2) [11] (Figs. 2.6, 2.7, 2.8, and 2.9)	Emopamil-binding protein (EBP) gene—Xp11.23-p11.22	XLD	Chondrodysplasia (rhizomelic type), growth retardation, frontal bossing, flat nasal bridge, down-slanting space between eyelids, **cataracts (mostly sectoral)**, antimongoloid slant, asymmetrically short limbs, macrocephaly, patchy alopecia, scaly/flaky skin, ichthyosis, flexion deformities or spasms of interphalangeal joint, kyphosis or scoliosis, calcaneus valgus
Craniosynostosis-cataract syndrome [12]	–	–	Severe craniosynostosis, **bilateral nuclear cataracts,** bifid nose-tip in the female offspring of non-consanguineous parents
Cri-du-chat (cat cry) syndrome [13]	5p deletion	Most commonly, sporadic, isolated cases	High shrill cry (cat cry), microcephaly, **cataract**, hypertelorism, round face, mental retardation, antimongoloid slant of palpebral fissures, epicanthic folds, anteverted pinnae, preauricular skin tags, prominent nasal bridge, micrognathia, muscular hypotony, congenital heart, and genitourinary defects
Czeizel Lowry syndrome [14]/ CAMFAK (congenital cataracts, microcephaly, failure to thrive, and kyphoscoliosis)/CAMAK (cataract, microcephaly, arthrogryposis, and kyphosis) syndrome	–	AR	Microcephaly (with changes seen on CT scan of head), **bilateral infantile cataracts**, mental retardation and Perthes disease-like hip deformities, kyphoscoliosis, bird-like face
Down's syndrome (Figs. 2.10 and 2.11) [15]	21q22.3	Isolated cases	Flat occiput, flat facies, brachycephaly, epicanthal fold, flat nasal bridge, upslanting palpebral fissure, Brushfield spots, protruding tongue, small nose and mouth, diastasis recti, generous nuchal skin, short fifth finger with clinodactyly, single transverse palmar crease, sandal gap (wide space between first two toes), short, broad hands, short fifth middle phalanx, joint hyperflexibility, hypotonia, premature aging, dry skin, congenital heart defects, **congenital or infantile cataracts (particularly cerulean blue dot cataract)**
Early onset Cockayne syndrome [16]	ERCC8 gene, 5q12.1	AR	**Early cataracts**, microcephaly, joint contractures, kyphosis, mental retardation, large ears, enophthalmos, prominent nasal bridge
Edwards syndrome	Trisomy 18	Isolated cases	Aniridia, **cataracts**, microcephaly, microphthalmos, choanal atresia, small jaw, bullous nose
Hallermann–Streiff–Francois (oculomandibulofacial or Aubrey syndrome or Francois dyscephalic syndrome) [17]	6q22.31, GJA1 gene	Autosomal recessive	Essential seven features: Craniofacial malformations and bird-like facies, abnormal dentition, hypotrichosis, skin atrophy (esp. on nose), microphthalmia, **congenital cataract**, proportionate dwarfism
HEC syndrome [18] (Hydrocephalus, endocardial fibroelastosis, and cataract)	–	–	Communicating hydrocephalus, endocardial fibroelastosis and **congenital cataracts**

(continued)

Table 2.2 (continued)

Syndrome	Genetic loci	Inheritance pattern	Phenotypic features
Hyperferritinemia-cataract syndrome	19q13.33, FTL gene	AD	Congenital **nuclear cataract** [19] (autosomal dominant inheritance), elevated serum ferritin levels
Lowes/oculo-cerebro-renal syndrome [19] (Fig. 2.12a–c)	OCRL gene, Xq26.1	XLR	Triad of: **congenital cataracts (can be posterior or anterior lenticonus or even other morphologies)**, neonatal/infantile hypotonia with mental retardation and renal tubular dysfunction. Other features: ocular keloid, rickets, osteopenia, osteomalacia, glaucoma, joint swelling, arthritis, tenosynovitis, growth parameters like weight and length fall below third percentile by 1–3 year age, delayed teeth eruption, teeth crowding, hypoplastic enamel, constricted palate. Carrier females may have snowflake-like opacities [19]
Majewski syndrome [20] (short rib polydactyly syndrome)	NEK1 gene, 4q23	AR	Lethal syndrome includes neonatal dwarfism, short ribs, polydactyly, cleft lip, epiglottic anomalies, oval-shaped tibia, ambiguous genitalia, **cataracts**, hypertelorism, colobomata, microphthalmos
Marinesco–Sjogren syndrome [19]	5q31.2, SIL1 gene	AR	Cerebellar ataxia, **m**ental retardation, short stature, congenital **cataracts, m**uscle weakness, inability to chew food, thin brittle fingernails and sparse hair, hypergonadotropic hypogonadism, delayed psychomotor development, skeletal deformities
Martsolf syndrome [19]	1q41, RAB3GAP2 gene	AR	**M**ental retardation, **m**icrocephaly, hypogonadism in siblings of consanguineous parents, **cataracts**
Menkes syndrome [19]	Xq21.1, ATP7A gene	XLR	Kinky hair (Menkes kinky hair), severe mental retardation, bone and connective tissue lesions, pronounced cupid's bow to upper lip, hypothermia, **cataracts**
Nance–Horan syndrome [19] (Mesiodens-cataract syndrome, NHS) (Figs. 2.13 and 2.14)	Xp22Xp22.2.13-Xp22.1, NHS gene	XLD	**Congenital cataract** in almost 100% cases (bilateral, dense, mostly total), microcornea, microphthalmos, dental anomalies (Hutchinsonian teeth, supernumerary teeth with impacted teeth), facial dysmorphism (long, narrow, often rectangular face, long chin, prognathism, large nose, narrow nasal bridge, large protruding ears), mental retardation (in 30%). Cataracts: **bilateral, asymmetrical and predominantly posterior lens opacities**. Carrier females (heterozygous) have posterior Y-**sutural cataracts** with small corneas
Norrie disease [19]	Xp11.3, NDP gene	XLR	Early childhood blindness, retinal dysplasia, mental disorder, sensorineural deafness, **cataracts**
Pollitt syndrome [19] (Trichothiodystrophy 1—Sulfur-deficient hair)	ERCC2 gene, 19q13.32	AR	Sparse brittle body hair, ichthyosis, developmental delay, growth retardation, dysplastic nails, photosensitivity, xeroderma pigmentosum, eczema, microcephaly, recurrent infections, receding chin, protruding ears, conjunctivitis, nystagmus, hypoplastic genitalia, **bilateral central nuclear cataracts**
Smith–Lemli–Opitz (SLO) syndrome [19]/RSH syndrome	11q13.4, DHCR7 gene	AR	Microcephaly, broad nasal tip with anteverted nostrils, micrognathia, ptosis of eyelids, epicanthal folds, **cataracts**, broad maxillary alveolar ridges, slanted or low set ears, syndactyly of second and third toes, cleft palate, cardiac defects, cryptorchidism in males

Highlight cataract and morphology in bold in phenotypic features

Key: *AD* autosomal dominant, *AR* autosomal recessive, *XLD* X-linked dominant, *XLR* X-linked recessive; Source: From OMIM—Online mendelian inheritance in man. http://www.omim.org [9]

2.5 Syndromic Features As Aid in Diagnosis of Congenital Cataract (Table 2.3)

Table 2.3 List of systemic and facial features giving clue to syndromes of congenital cataract

Facial dysmorphism	Down's syndrome Hallermann–Streiff–Francois syndrome Lowe's oculocerebrorenal syndrome Nance–Horan syndrome Smith–Lemli–Opitz syndrome Martsolf syndrome
Short stature	Chondrodysplasiapunctata (Conradi–Hünermann syndrome) Marinesco–Sjogren syndrome Pollitt syndrome Martsolf syndrome
Microcephaly	COFS AR congenital infection-like syndrome Early onset Cockayne syndrome Cri-du-chat syndrome Czeizel Lowry syndrome Edwards syndrome Martsolf syndrome
Digital abnormalities	Majewski syndrome Smith–Lemli–Opitz syndrome
Dermatological issues	Conradi–Hünermann syndrome Pollitt syndrome Menkes syndrome
Hydrocephalus or skull deformities	HEC syndrome Craniosynostosis Martsolf syndrome

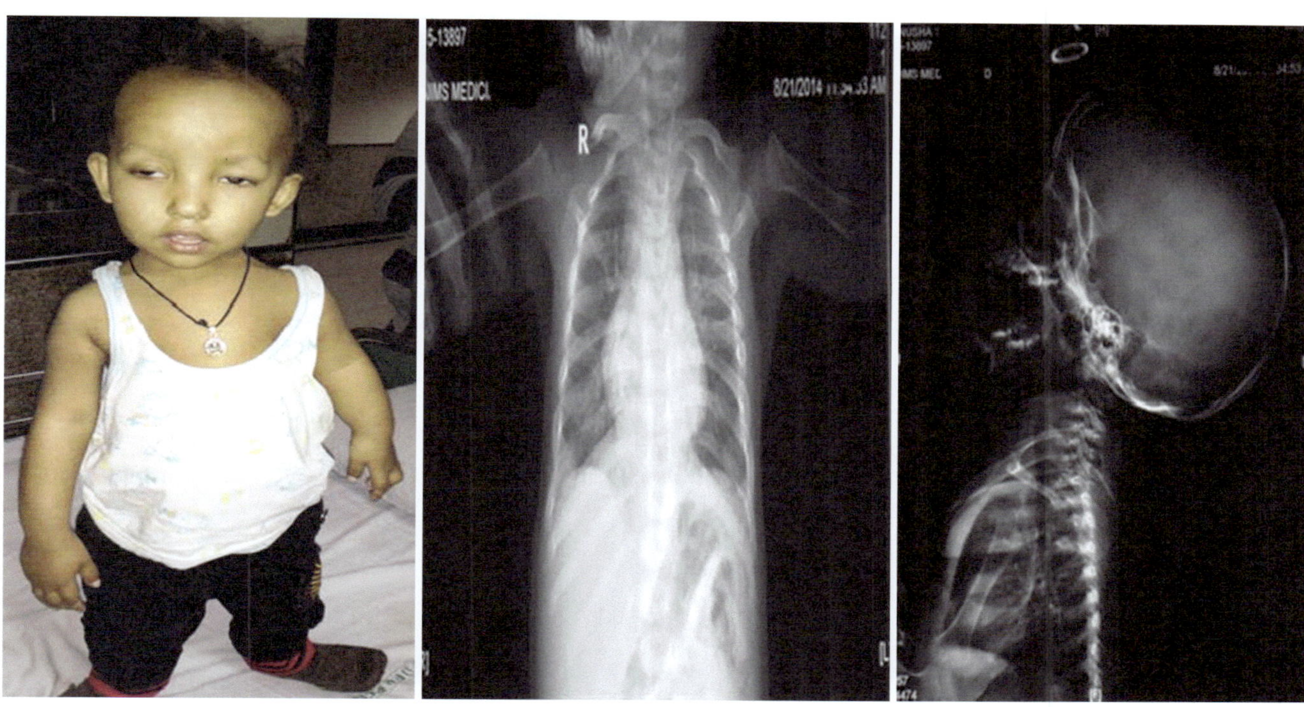

Fig. 2.6 Frontal bossing, flat nasal bridge, anti mongoloid slant, asymmetrical limbs, large head in a case of Conradi–Hünermann syndrome (Courtesy Dr Ganesh)

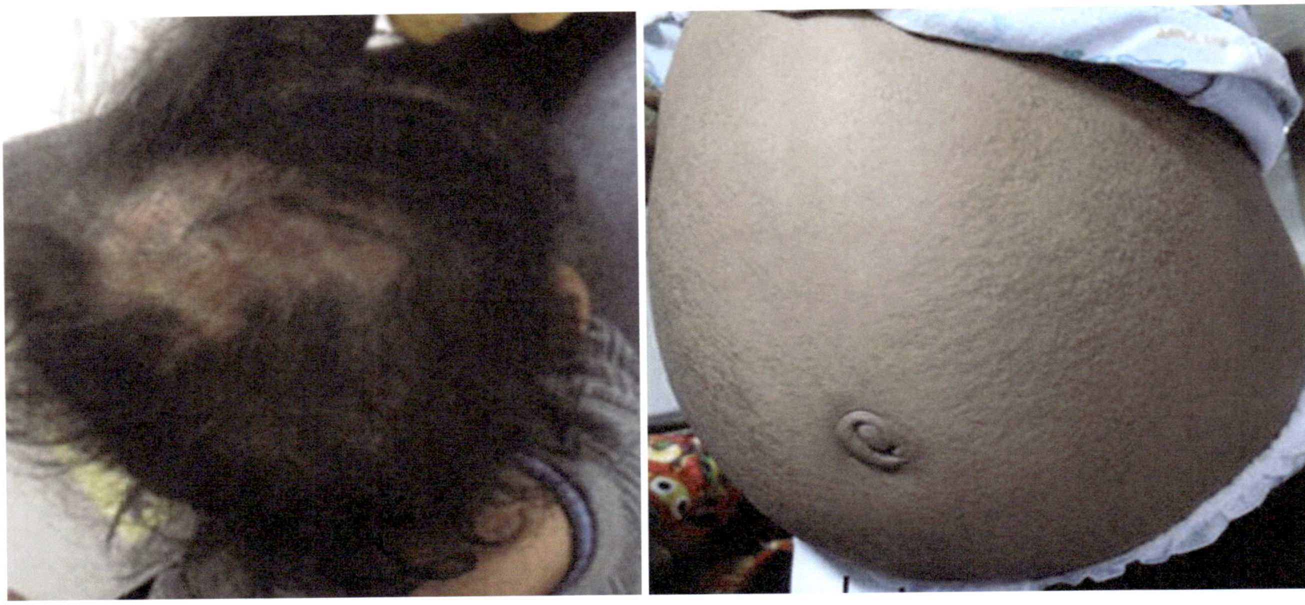

Fig. 2.7 Patchy alopecia and sparse thin hair over scalp, dry scaly skin over abdomen in a case of Conradi–Hünermann syndrome (Courtesy Dr Ganesh)

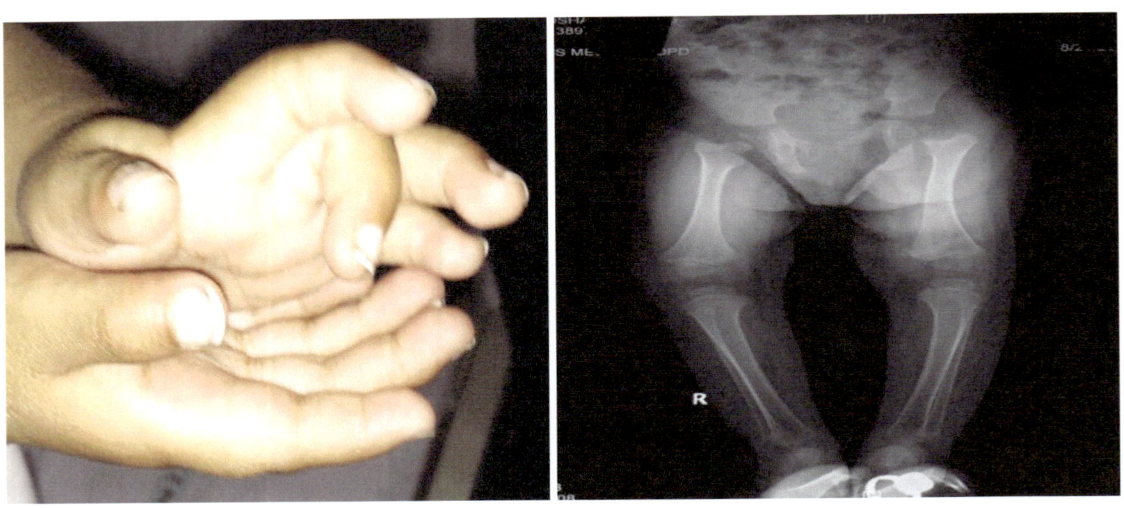

Fig. 2.8 Flexion deformity of middle finger, calcaneus valgus deformity of both feet in a case of Conradi–Hünermann syndrome

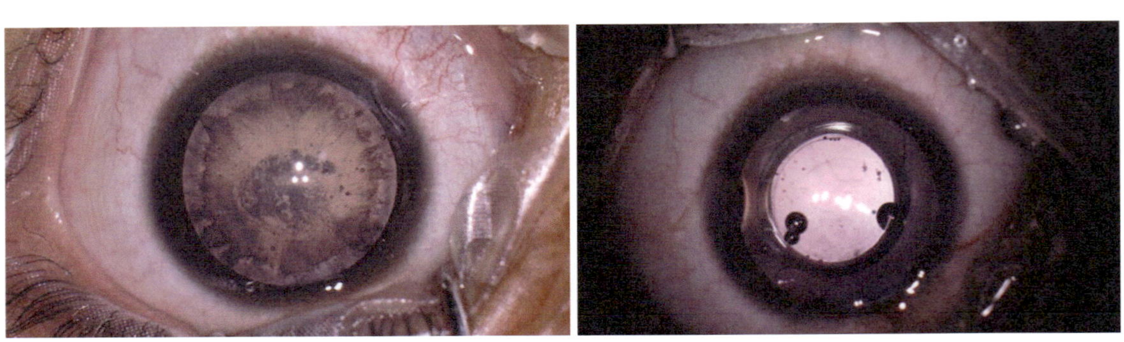

Fig. 2.9 Preoperative and postoperative photographs of cataract surgery in a case of Conradi–Hünermann syndrome

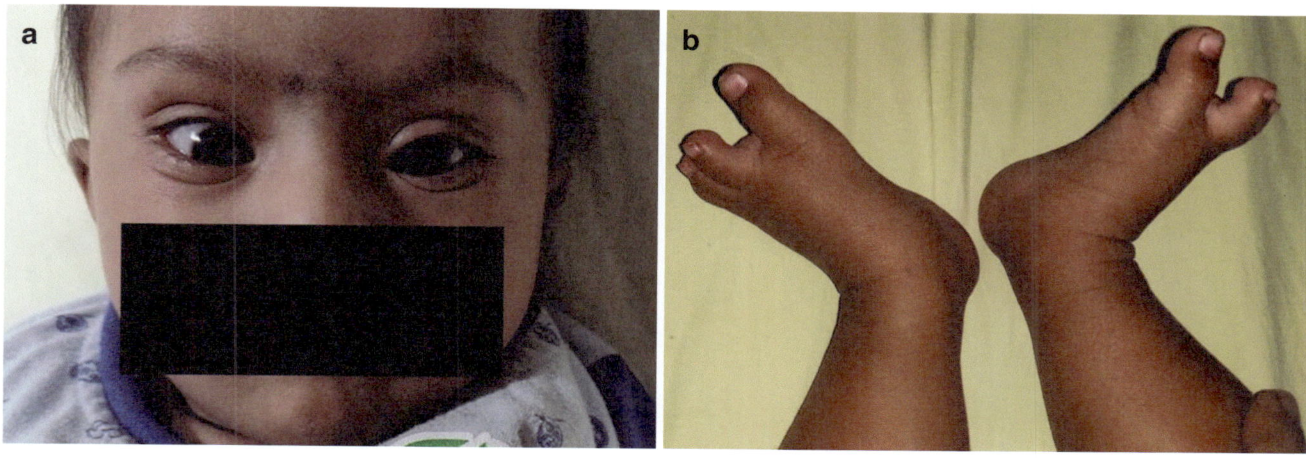

Fig. 2.10 A case of 1-year-old Down's syndrome depicting (**a**) Down's facies with mongoloid slant, broad flat face, epicanthic folds and short nose and (**b**) Sandal gap in feet

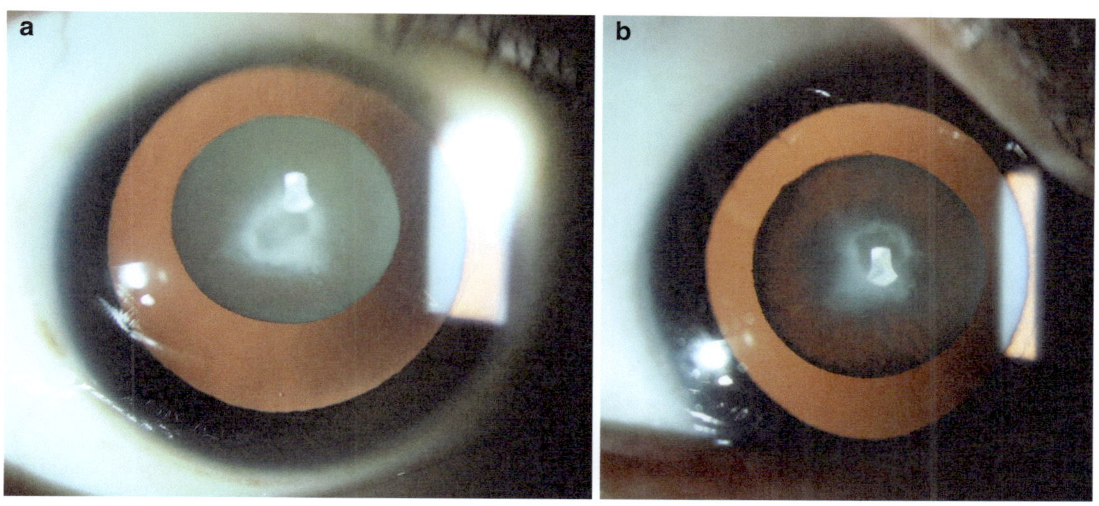

Fig. 2.11 Cataract in a 7-year-old patient of Down's syndrome (**a**, **b**)

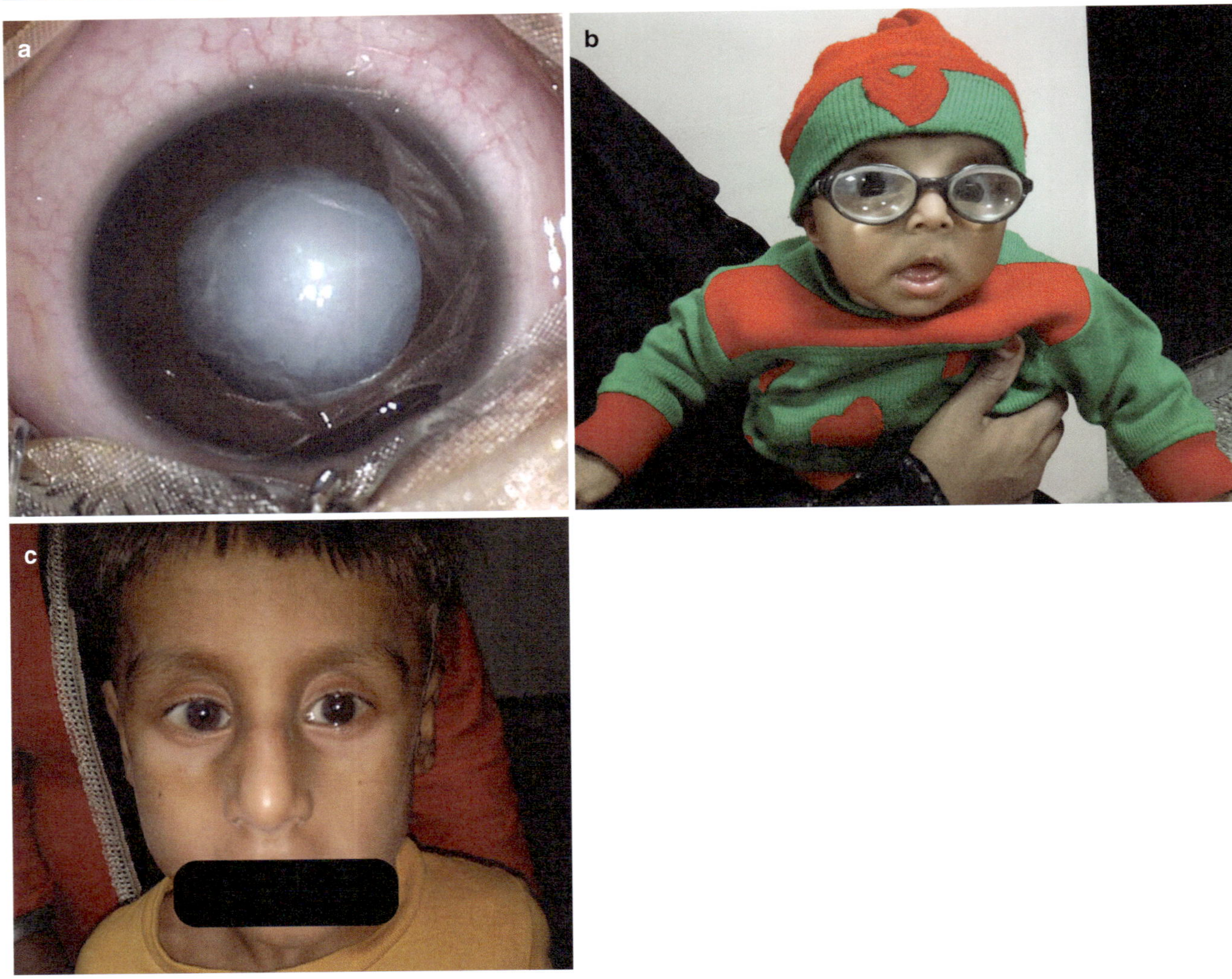

Fig. 2.12 Cataracts in a 11-month-old case of Lowe's oculocerebrorenal syndrome showing (**a**) preoperative photograph, (**b**) postop picture of child with aphakic glasses. Photograph of another 7-year-old case shows (**c**) typical facies of Lowe's syndrome. Mental retardation was also present in this case

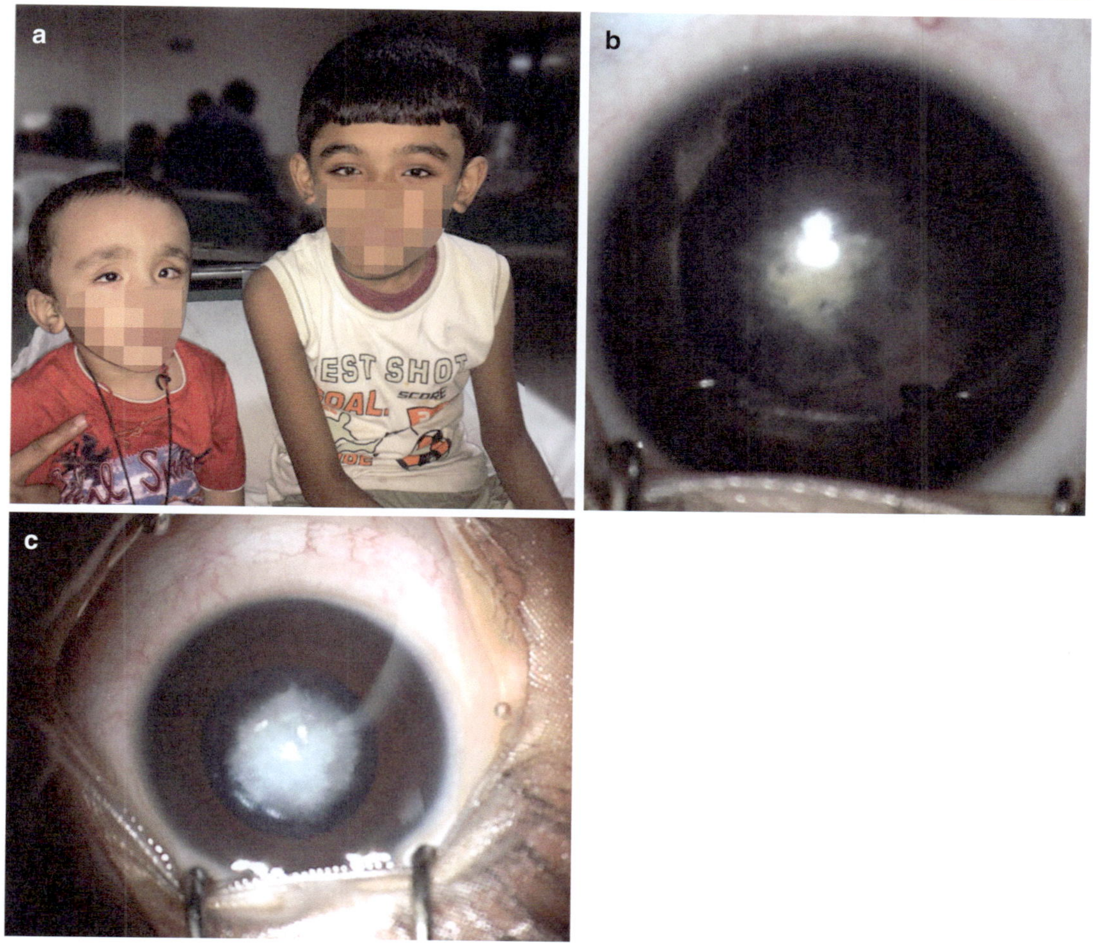

Fig. 2.13 Nance–Horan syndrome in same family. Pictures of two male siblings (**a**) with both having facial features like long, narrow, often rectangular face, long chin, prognathism, large nose, narrow nasal bridge, large protruding ears and impacted teeth and ocular features like microcornea and bilateral membranous cataracts (**b**, **c**)

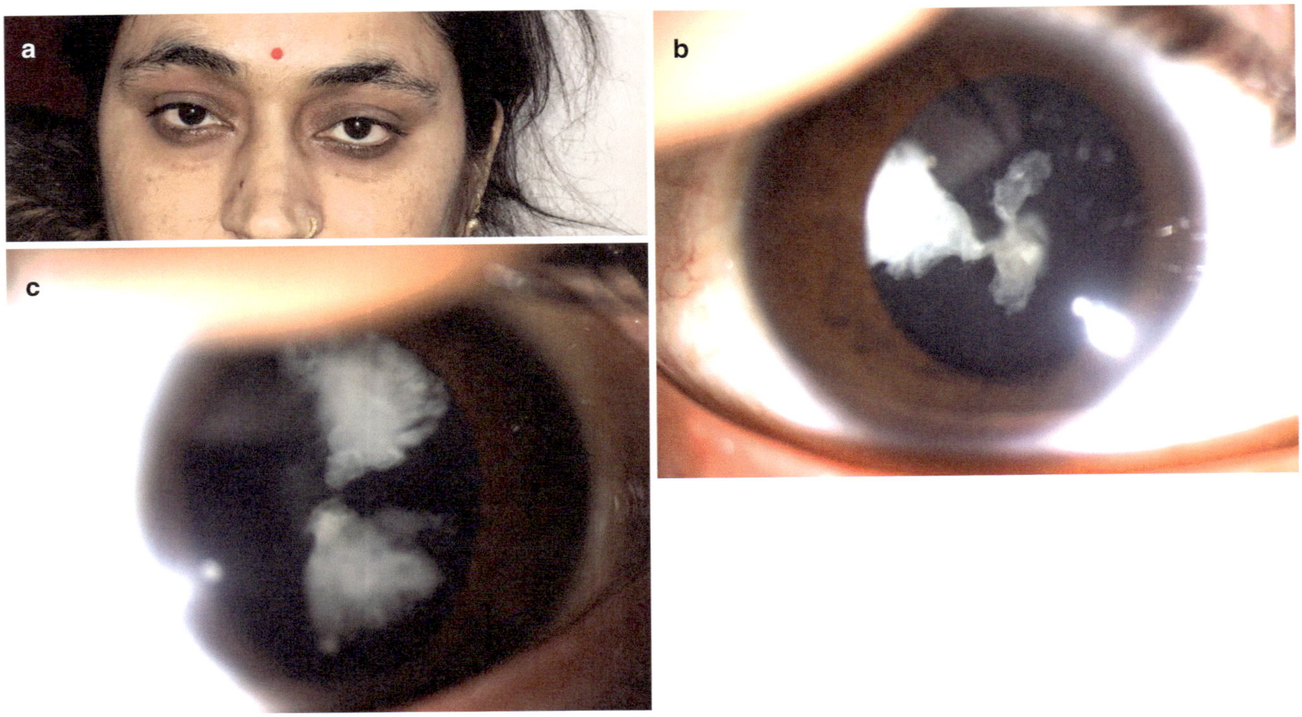

Fig. 2.14 Mother of the Nance–Horan syndrome cases in Fig. 2.13 showed bilateral microcornea (**a**) and cortical cataract in OD (**b**) and OS (**c**). Carries of Nance–Horan syndrome often have sutural cataracts

2.6 Miscellaneous

A syndrome may not be identified in all cases of congenital cataract who present with unique systemic features. We encountered a 12 month old male child who presented with bilateral dense posterior subcapsular cataract and nystagmus. He had aphalangia along with Xray showing sphondyloepiphyseal dysplasia. (Fig. 2.15a–c). There was no significant family history and no syndrome could be identified. Simply paying attension and performing a basic physical examination can help in detecting systemic associations. In conslusion, we recommended detailed family history and complete physical examinations along with necessary investigations for all children presented with bilateral congenital cataract.

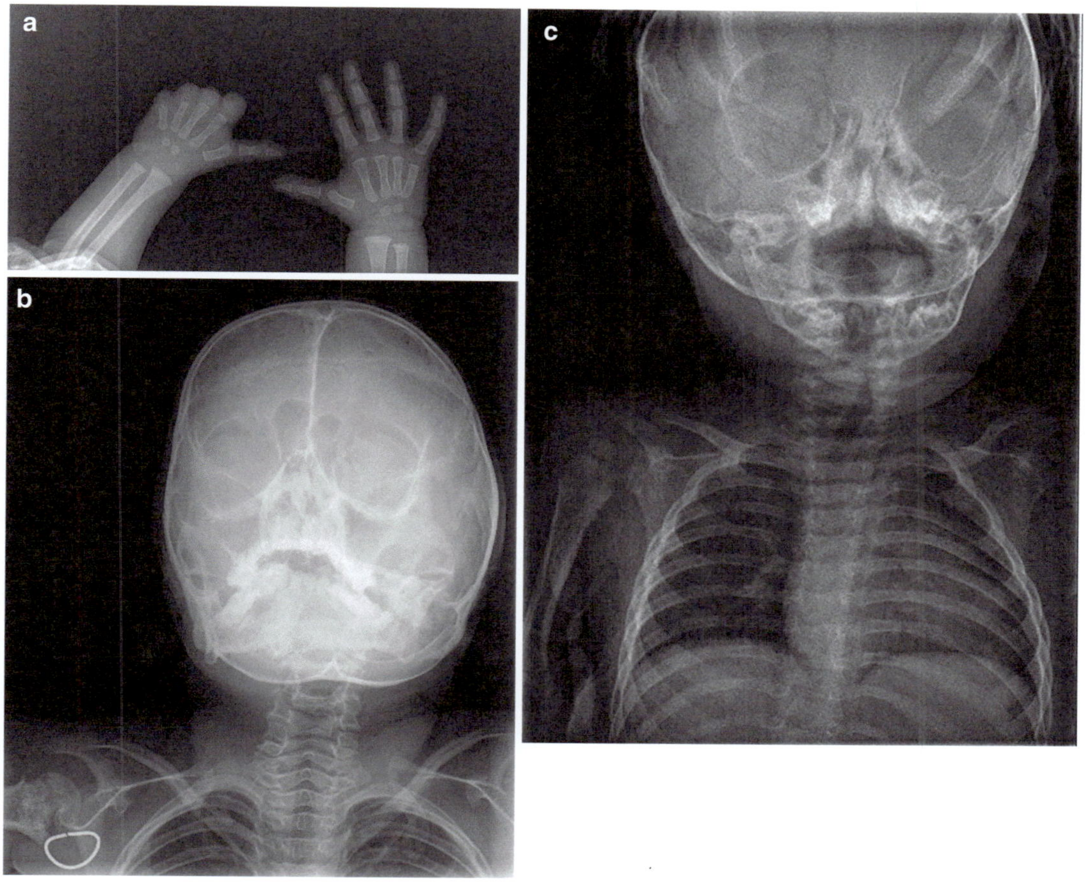

Fig. 2.15 (**a–c**) A X ray hand and wrist showing unilateral aphalangia (**b**, **c**) X ray head, neck, spine and chest showing spondyloepiphysial dysplasia

References

1. Haargaard B, Wohlfahrt J, Fledelius HC, Rosenberg T, Melbye M. A nationwide Danish study of 1027 cases of congenital/infantile cataracts: etiological and clinical classifications. Ophthalmology. 2004;111(12):2292–8.
2. Hejtmancik JF. Congenital cataracts and their molecular genetics. Semin Cell Dev Biol. 2008;19(2):134–49.
3. Churchill A, Graw J. Clinical and experimental advances in congenital and paediatric cataracts. Philos Trans R Soc Lond Ser B Biol Sci. 2011;366(1568):1234–49.
4. Liu Y, et al. A novel αB-crystallin mutation associated with autosomal dominant congenital lamellar cataract. Invest Ophthalmol Vis Sci. 2006;47:1069–75.
5. Huang B, He W. Molecular characteristics of inherited congenital cataracts. Eur J Med Genet. 2010;53:347–57.
6. Reddy MA, Francis PJ, Berry V, et al. Molecular genetic basis of inherited cataract and associated phenotypes. Surv Ophthalmol. 2004;49:300–15.
7. Kumar M, Agarwal T, Khokhar S, et al. Mutation screening and genotype phenotype correlation of α-crystallin, γ-crystallin and GJA8 gene in congenital cataract. Mol Vis. 2011;17:693–707.
8. Kumar M, Agarwal T, Kaur P, Kumar M, Khokhar S, Dada R. Molecular and structural analysis of genetic variations in congenital cataract. Mol Vis. 2013;19:2436–50.
9. Wieczorek D, Gillessen-Kaesbach G, Passarge E. A nine-month-old boy with microcephaly, cataracts, intracerebral calcifications and dysmorphic signs: an additional observation of an autosomal recessive congenital infection-like syndrome? Genet Couns. 1995;6(4):297–302; Review
10. OMIM—Online mendelian inheritance in man. http://www.omim.org/. Accessed 6 Nov 2018.
11. Spranger JW, Opitz JM, Bidder U. Heterogeneity of chondrodysplasia punctata. Humangenetik. 1971;11:190–212.
12. Orphanet. Orphanet. https://www.orpha.net/consor/cgi-bin/OC_Exp.php?lng=EN&Expert=1530.
13. Lejeune J, Lafourcade J, Berger R, Vialatta J, Boeswillwald M, Seringe P, Turpin R. Trois ca de deletion partielle du bras court d'un chromosome 5. C R Acad Sci (Paris). 1963;257:3098.
14. Czeizel A, Lowry RB. Syndrome of cataract, mild microcephaly, mental retardation and Perthes-like changes in sibs. Acta Paediatr Hung. 1990;30:343–9.
15. Haargaard B, Fledelius HC. Down's syndrome and early cataract. Br J Ophthalmol. 2006;90(8):1024–7.
16. Traboulsi EI, De Becker I, Maumenee IH. Ocular findings in Cockayne syndrome. Am J Ophthalmol. 1992;114:579–83.
17. Gorlin R, Cohen M, Levin S. Hallermann-Streiff syndrome. Syndromes of the head and neck. 3rd ed. New York: Oxford Univiversity Press; 1990. p. 306–8.
18. Devi AS, Eisenfeld L, Uphoff D, Greenstein R. New syndrome of hydrocephalus, endocardial fibroelastosis, and cataracts (HEC syndrome). Am J Med Genet. 1995;56:62–6.
19. Stambolian D, Lewis RA, Buetow K, Bond A, Nussbaum R. Nance-Horan syndrome: localization within the region Xp21.1-Xp22.3 by linkage analysis. Am J Hum Genet. 1990;47:13–9.
20. Chess J, Albert DM. Ocular pathology of the Majewski syndrome. Br J Ophthalmol. 1982 Nov;66(11):736–41.

Metabolic Cataract

3

Abhidnya Surve, Chirakshi Dhull,
and Sudarshan Kumar Khokhar

Metabolic cataract is loss of lens transparency caused by an insult to the nuclear or lenticular fibres due to an underlying metabolic disorder. They may present as an isolated condition or as a part of a particular syndrome. Most of the times being considered as a part of a congenital syndrome, the exact incidence of this cataract is unknown. Screening for underlying metabolic disorders in children with bilateral cataract can lead to their early detection and avoidance of consequences with timely initiation of treatment [1, 2]. The metabolic disorders have been divided according to the age of appearance of cataract (Table 3.1). This may be helpful in the differential diagnosis of inborn errors of metabolism presenting with cataracts. Also, specific lens changes seen in different disorders provides diagnostic clues [1–3]. Few of these disorders are described here in detail.

Table 3.1 Metabolic cataract according to the age of their appearance

Birth	• Sorbitol dehydrogenase deficiency. • Zellweger syndrome. • Lowe's syndrome.
Newborn	• Galactosaemia (Gal-l-P uridyl transferase deficiency). • UDP galactose-4-epimerase deficiency. • Marginal maternal galactokinase deficiency. • Hyperglycinuria.
Infant	• Mannosidosis. • Hypoglycaemia. • Galactokinase deficiency. • Partial galactokinase deficiency. • Marginal maternal galactokinase deficiency. • Galactitol or sorbitol accumulation of unknown origin.
Young age group	• Diabetes mellitus. • Wilson's disease. • Hypoparathyroidism. • Pseudohypoparathyroidism. • Alport's syndrome.

3.1 Galactosaemia

Galactosaemia is an autosomal recessive metabolic disorder. It is caused by the deficiency of one of the three enzymes involved in the metabolism of galactose. These include galactokinase, galactose-l-phosphate uridylyltransferase (GALT) or uridine diphosphate galactose-4-epimerase. This results in accumulation of galactitol leading to cataract. Classical galactosaemia occurs due to deficiency of GALT involving chromosome 9. The typical cataract appearance seen in this disorder is "Oil-droplet central opacity" (Fig. 3.1). Galactokinase deficiency involves mutation of GALK1 gene on chromosome 17q24 and is known to present with cataract and rarely pseudotumor cerebri. The cataract may have a typical lamellar shape in infancy (Fig. 3.2) [2, 4].

In galactosaemia, patients may have food intolerance, hypoglycaemia, hepatomegaly, liver failure, muscle hypotonia or sepsis. The early recognition of this disorder by an ophthalmologist forms a crucial role in the early diagnosis and initiation of treatment. Diagnosis can be made by screening of urine for reducing substances. The ocular involvement, systemic involvement, the severity of involvement, enzyme assay and genetic linkage helps in further differentiating the enzyme deficiency involved. The galactose-free diet in these individuals can lead to reversal of lenticular opacities [2, 3, 5].

3.2 Mannosidosis

Mannosidosis is an uncommon disorder affecting glycoprotein metabolism due to lysosomal accumulation of mannose-rich substrates. These are normal at birth and typically develop distinctive coarse facies and dysostosis multiplex by 2 years of age. Mental retardation, hearing loss, and recurrent infection is seen [6]. Lens involvement is seen in alpha-mannosidosis in early infancy and maybe nuclear, capsular or total (Fig. 3.3) [7]. A progressively developing wheel-like cataract and optic disc pallor have been described in man-

A. Surve · C. Dhull (✉) · S. K. Khokhar
Dr. Rajendra Prasad Centre for Ophthalmic Sciences, All India Institute of Medical Sciences, New Delhi, India

S. K. Khokhar, C. Dhull (eds.), *Atlas of Pediatric Cataract*, https://doi.org/10.1007/978-981-13-6939-1_3

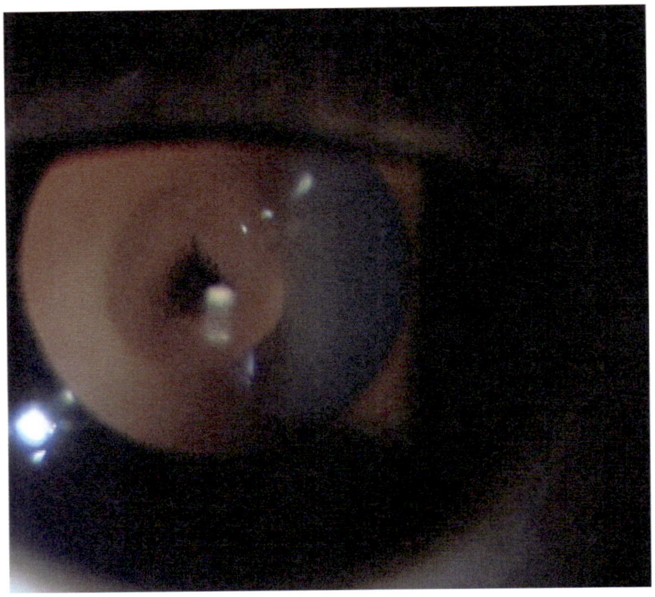

Fig. 3.1 Oil-droplet cataract in a case with classical galactosaemia

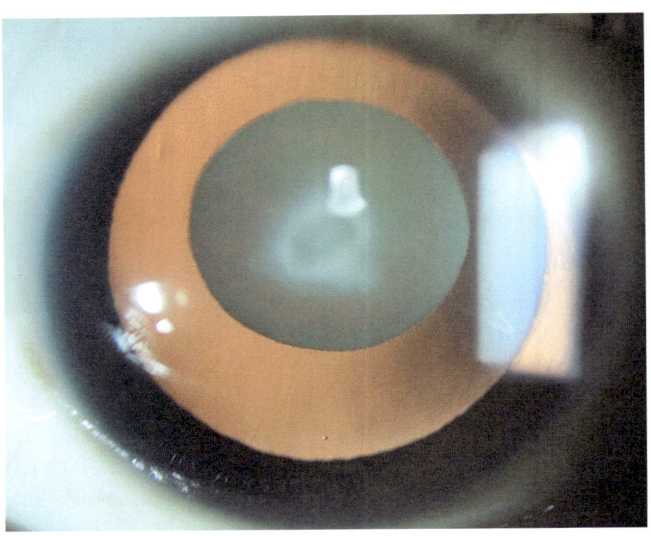

Fig. 3.2 Lamellar cataract with central opacities seen in an infant with galactokinase deficiency

nosidosis [8]. Also, it is well known that during infancy, hypoglycaemia can result in cataract formation [9].

3.3 Sorbitol Dehydrogenase Deficiency

Sorbitol dehydrogenase deficiency leads to accumulation of sorbitol in lens causing an osmotic inflow of water resulting in lenticular opacity [10]. Inhibition of this enzyme may form a potential therapeutic option.

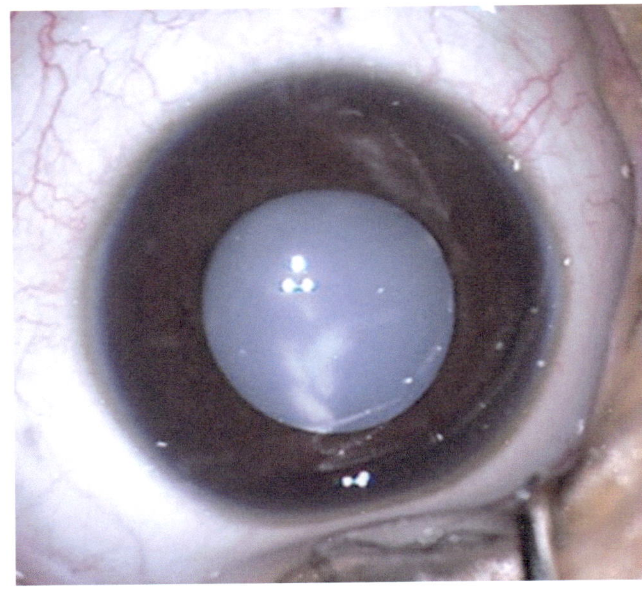

Fig. 3.3 Total cataract in a child with mannosidosis

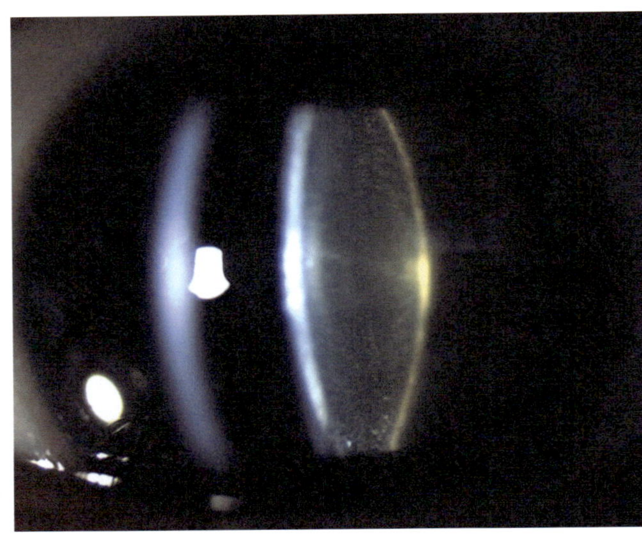

Fig. 3.4 Snowflake cataract seen in a case with diabetes mellitus

3.4 Diabetes

Cataract is seen in both insulin-dependent and insulin-independent diabetes mellitus. The various changes occurring in the lens in diabetes are refractive changes, light scattering, autofluorescence, cataract development and age-related increase in thickness and curvature. Cataract is seen more commonly in people with diabetes than in general population. Young diabetic cataract is characterised by variable morphology. It could be typical cortical "snowflake opacities" (Fig. 3.4), diffuse anterior and/or posterior subcapsular (Fig. 3.5a, b) or a combination of both

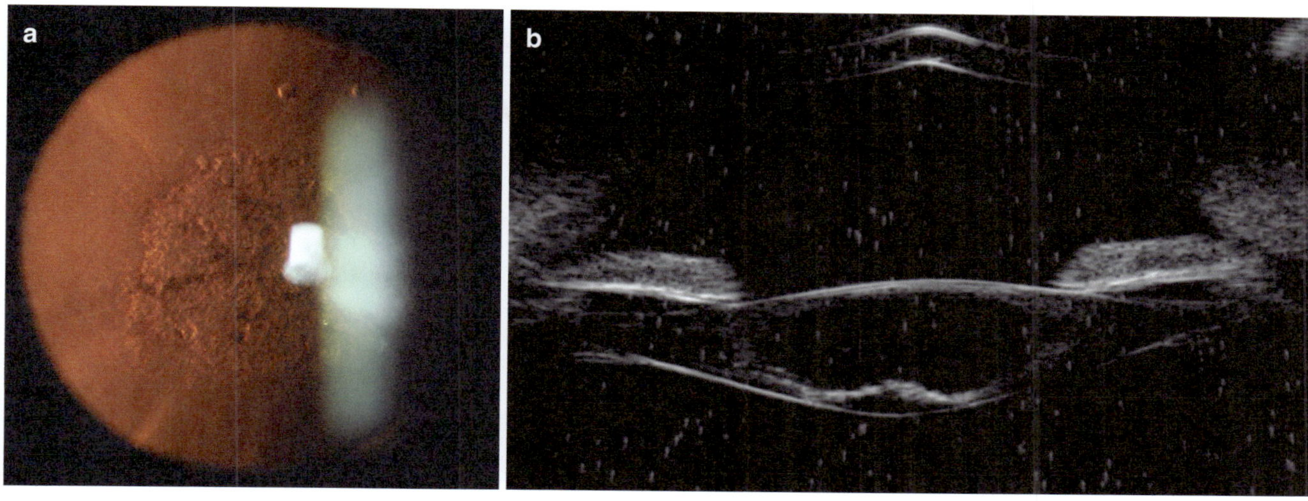

Fig. 3.5 Posterior subcapsular cataract (PSC) in a teenage patient. (**a**) Distant direct examination showing central involvement, PSC and few fluid droplets, (**b**) ultrasound biomicroscopy of the same showing posterior subcapsular involvement

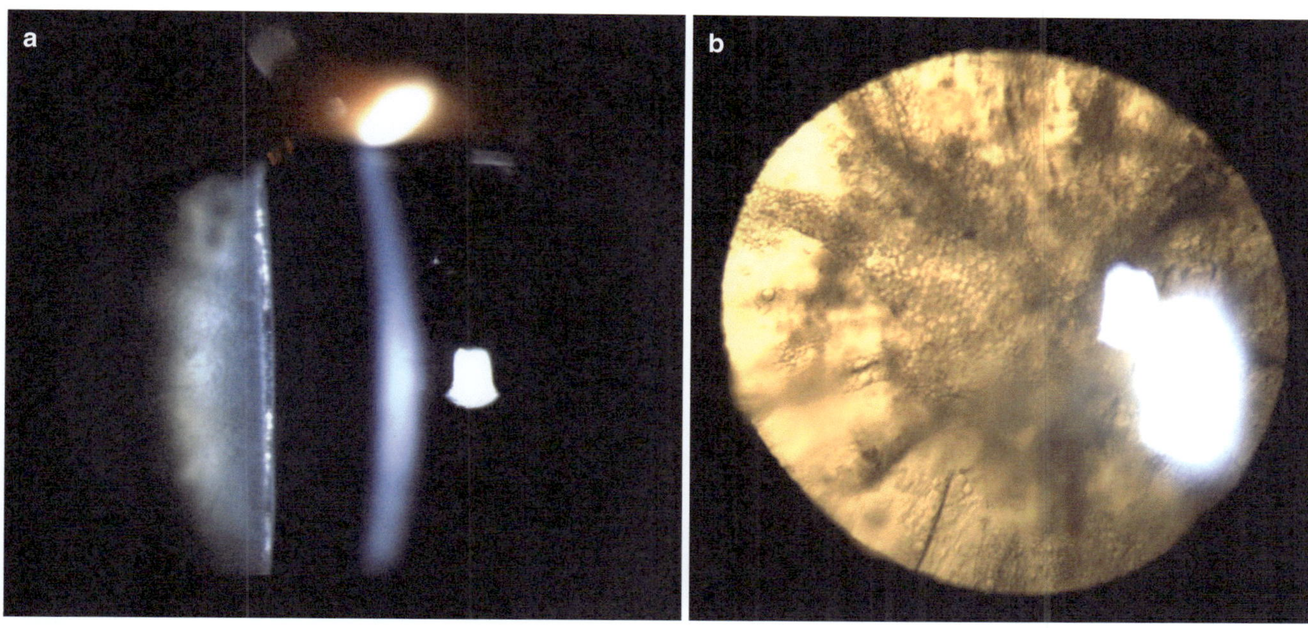

Fig. 3.6 Anterior and posterior subcapsular cataract with diffuse cataract, notice the presence of fluid pockets. (**a**) Slit lamp picture, (**b**) retroillumination picture

(Fig. 3.6a, b). Cataract with predominant fluid pockets may also be seen in such cases especially with poor metabolic control (Fig. 3.7). Such cataracts can cause disproportionate vision loss. The pathogenesis of diabetic cataract in type 1 diabetes mellitus is not clear. Uncontrolled blood sugar with consequential ketoacidosis and dehydration has been known to have an important part in the development of early diabetic cataract [11, 12]. Early stages may resolve with systemic control but in long-standing cases, it is permanent due to coagulation of lens proteins [13, 14]. They may develop acutely over weeks or over a period of several months. The polyol pathway also plays a role in the pathogenesis of cataract [15]. Fundus examination must be carried out in all these patients as they may have diabetic retinopathy.

3.5 Hypoparathyroidism

Though the mechanism is unknown, cataract is a well-known component in cases with hypoparathyroidism. The typical lenticular appearance seen maybe cuneate radial opacities with slow progression (Fig. 3.8), anterior or posterior subcapsular cataract or diffuse dense cataract (Fig. 3.9). Rapid development of cataract is seen in cases with altered serum calcium and phosphate levels or those with hepatic and renal failure [16].

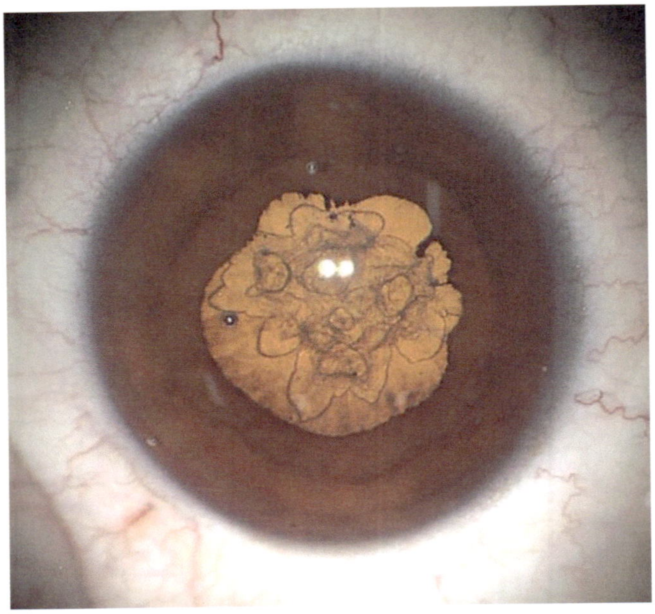

Fig. 3.7 Fluid pockets seen in retroillumination in a patient with diabetic ketoacidosis. Persistent pupillary membrane is also seen

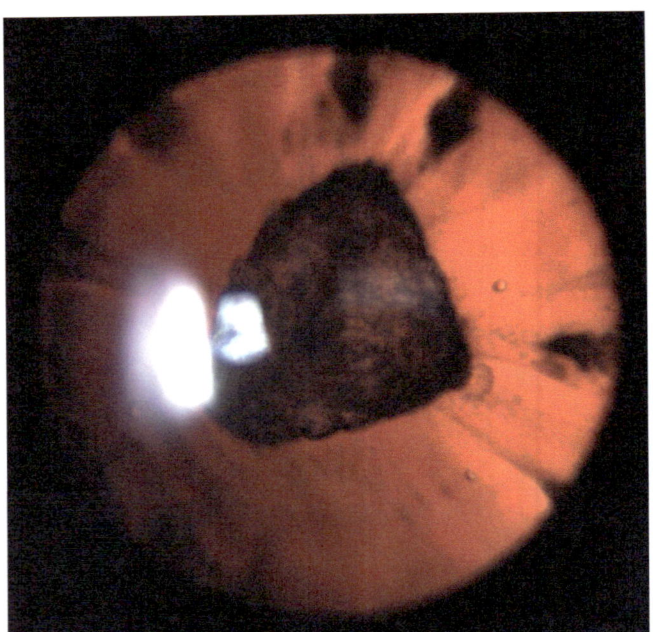

Fig. 3.8 Posterior subcapsular cataract with cuneate radial lenticular opacities in hypoparathyroidism

3.6 Fabry Disease

Fabry disease involves glycosphingolipids deposits in ocular structures progressively. The different ocular manifestations include vascular abnormalities in conjunctiva or retina and opacities in the corneal (cornea verticillata) or lens. Two types of lenticular opacities—anterior subcapsular or capsular cataract and radial-posterior subcapsular cataract can occur in Fabry disease. Anterior capsular or subcapsular opacity is usually bilateral, wedge-shaped and radially distributed with apices toward the centre of anterior capsule. The posterior subcapsular cataract comprises linear opacities in the posterior subcapsular area and have spoke-like appearance (Fig. 3.10). These are less commonly seen due to the rarity of disease but when present are pathognomic of Fabry disease and are thus called Fabry cataract [17].

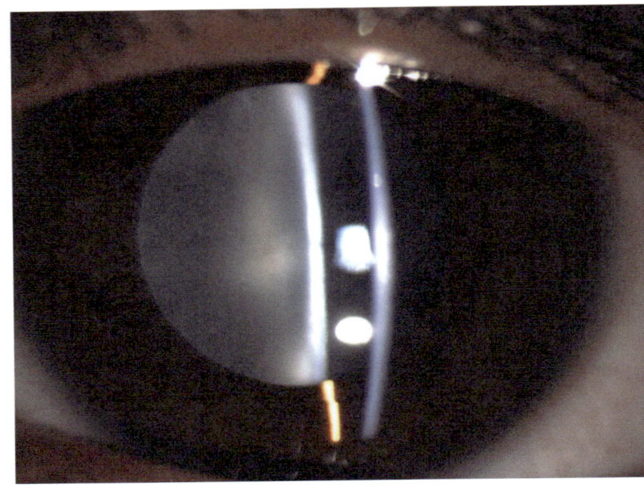

Fig. 3.9 Diffuse dense cataract in a teenage patient with long-standing hypoparathyroidism

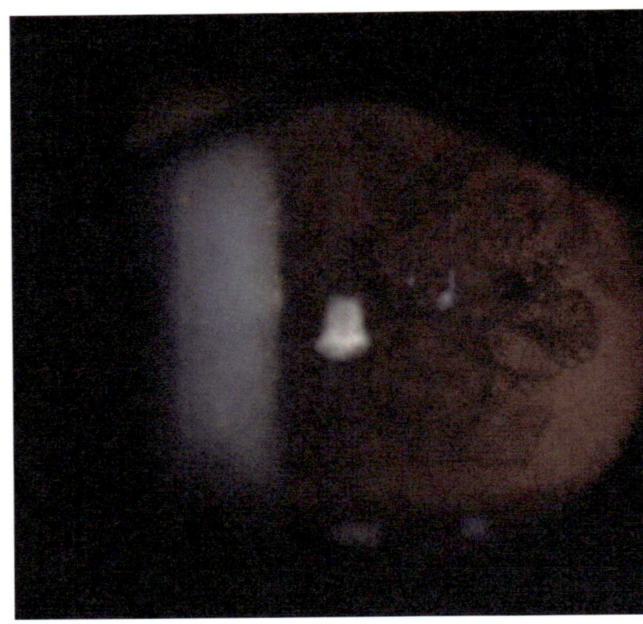

Fig. 3.10 Posterior subcapsular—spoke-like cataract in Fabry disease

3.7 Alport

Alport syndrome consists of involvement of kidney primarily manifesting as haematuria and progressive renal failure. Also, hearing loss and ocular involvement is seen. The cornea, lens and retina are involved. The lens abnormality in Alport syndrome includes anterior lenticonus and cataract. The thinnest and weakest part of the capsule allows anterior conical protrusion of the lens leading to anterior lenticonus. Thinned capsule and vertical tears have been seen on electron microscopy. It usually presents as difficulty with focusing which progresses with time. It is seen as an oil droplet reflex on direct ophthalmoscope (Fig. 3.11a) while the slit lamp examination shows anterior bulging of the lens (Fig. 3.11b). Small spontaneous ruptures can occur which on healing leads to formation of cataract. This leads to cessation of lenticonus progression. In symptomatic cases and those with cataract, lens removal and intraocular lens implantation is advised [18].

3.8 Wilson's Disease

Wilson's disease is a genetic disorder where copper metabolism is affected. In this disorder, copper accumulates in various area including brain, liver, kidney, and cornea. A characteristic finding is the presence of the Kayser–Fleischer ring, which is common, and pathognomic. It occurs due to deposition of copper in the Descemet's membrane and may vary in intensity from a faint line visible only on gonioscopy to dense deposits seen with naked eyes (Fig. 3.12a, b). Sunflower cataract is a rare finding and it is usually reversible with treatment. Sunflower cataract, typically seen in this disorder, is characterised by thin, centralised opacification under the anterior capsule with secondary opacifications in the surrounding area arranged in a ray-like structure (Fig. 3.13). This pattern with a large central disc surrounded by petals mimics a sunflower [19].

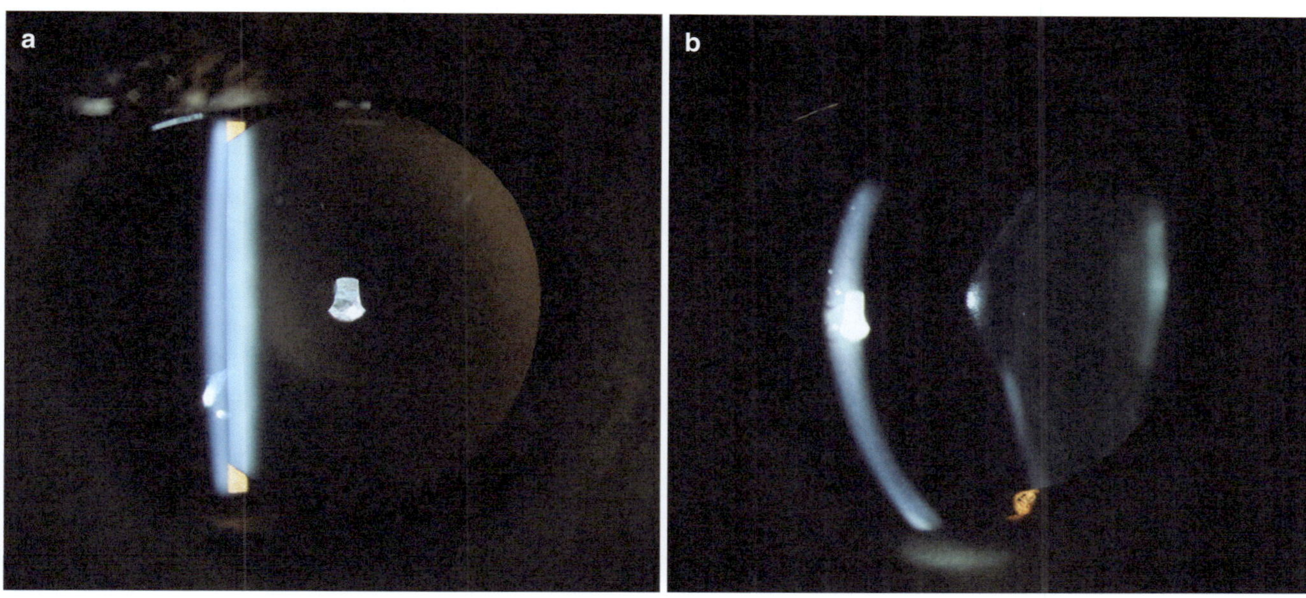

Fig. 3.11 Anterior lenticonus in Alport syndrome. (**a**) Retroillumination image showing oil droplet reflex. (**b**) Slit lamp image showing bulging of anterior capsule

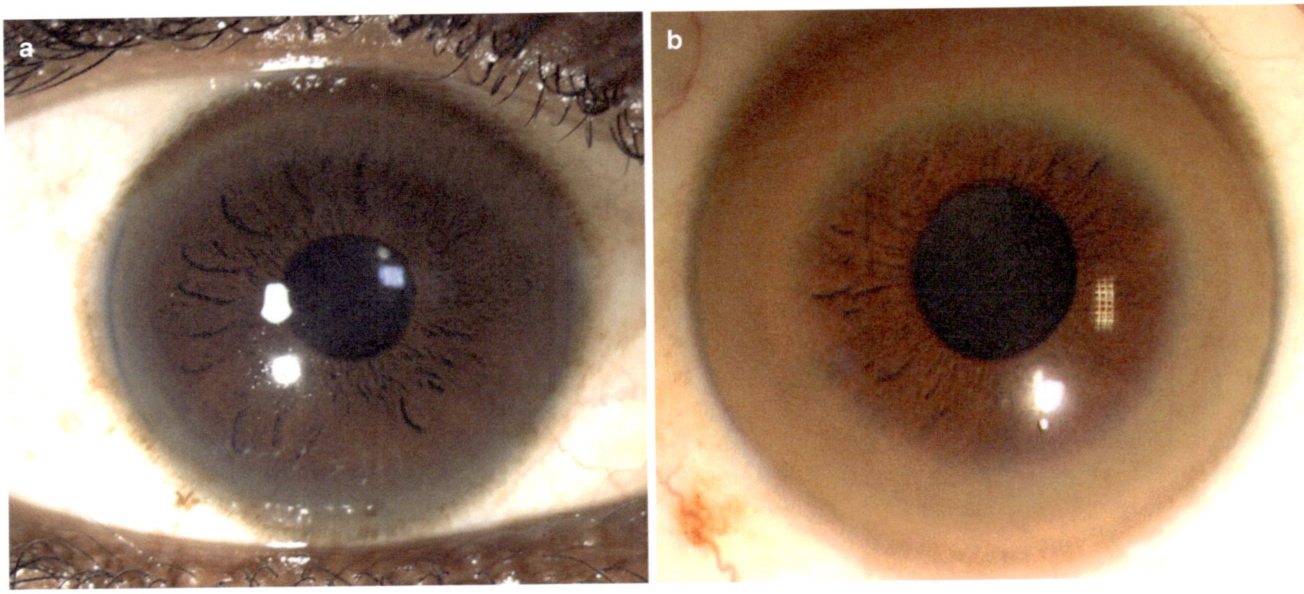

Fig. 3.12 Kayser–Fleischer ring in two patients with Wilson's disease. (**a**) Fine pigmented ring seen near corneal limbus, (**b**) extensive deposition of copper seen covering >3 mm ring in cornea

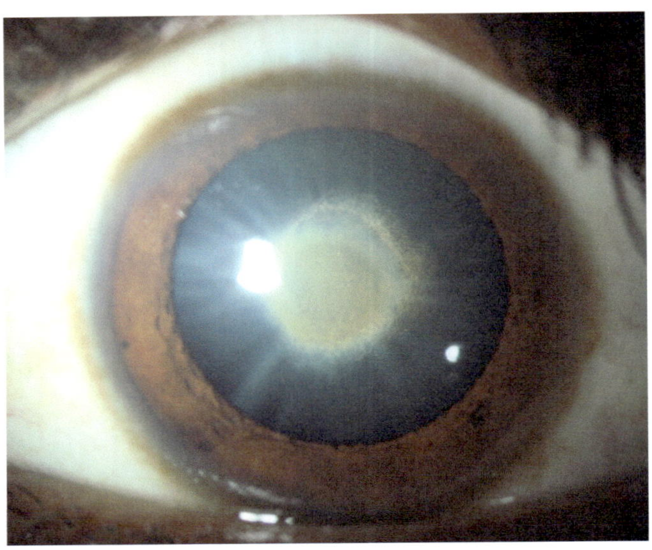

Fig. 3.13 Sunflower cataract in Wilson's disease

References

1. Wijburg MT, Wenniger-Prick LJM, Bosch AM, Visser G, Bams-Mengerink A. Bilateral cataract in childhood years: always an indication for screening on a metabolic disorder. Ned Tijdschr Geneeskd. 2008;152(11):632–6.
2. Cavallini GM, Forlini M, Masini C, et al. Dismetabolic cataracts: clinicopathologic overview and surgical management with B-MICS technique. J Genet Syndr Gene Ther. 2013;4(7):165.
3. Endres W, Shin YS. Cataract and metabolic disease. J Inherit Metab Dis. 1990;13(4):509–16.
4. Bosch AM, Bakker HD, van Gennip AH, van Kempen JV, Wanders RJA, Wijburg FA. Clinical features of galactokinase deficiency: a review of the literature. J Inherit Metab Dis. 2002;25(8):629–34.
5. Stambolian D. Galactose and cataract. Surv Ophthalmol. 1988;32(5):333–49.
6. Yunis JJ, Lewandowski RC, Sanfilippo SJ, Tsai MY, Foni I, Bruhl HH. Clinical manifestations of mannosidosis—a longitudinal study. Am J Med. 1976;61(6):841–8.
7. Arbisser AI, Murphree AL, Garcia CA, Howell RR. Ocular findings in mannosidosis. Am J Ophthalmol. 1976;82(3):465–71.
8. Aguire G, Stamm L, Haskins M, Jezyk P. Animal models of metabolic eye diseases. Defects in glycoproteins degradation. Mannosidosis. In: Goldberg's, editor. In genetic and metabolic eye diseases, vol. 2. Boston: Little Brown and co.; 1986. p. 152–7.
9. Merin S, Crawford JS. Hypoglycemia and infantile cataract. Arch Ophthalmol. 1971 Nov;86(5):495–8.
10. Vetter V, Shin YS. Lens sorbitol dehydrogenase deficiency in a patient with congenital cataract. Eur J Pediatr. 1995;154(5):389–91.
11. Goturu A, Jain N, Lewis I. Bilateral cataracts and insulin oedema in a child with type 1 diabetes mellitus. BMJ Case Rep. 2013;2013:bcr2012008235.
12. Uspal N, Schapiro E. Cataracts as the initial manifestation of type 1 diabetes mellitus. Pediatr Emerg Care. 2011;27(2):132–4.
13. Bilginturan AN, Jackson RL, Ide CH. Transitory cataracts in children with diabetes mellitus. Pediatrics. 1977;60:106–9.
14. Santiago AP, Rosenbaum AL, Masket S. Insulin-dependent diabetes mellitus appearing as bilateral mature diabetic cataracts in a child. Arch Ophthalmol. 1997;115:422–3.
15. Bron AJ, Sparrow J, Brown NA, Harding JJ, Blakytny R. The lens in diabetes. Eye (Lond). 1993;7:260–75.
16. Haviv YS, Safadi R, Zamir E. A rapidly progressive cataract in a patient with autoimmune hypoparathyroidism and acute liver and renal failure. Am J Nephrol. 1999;19(4):523–6.
17. Sodi A, Ioannidis A, Pitz S. Ophthalmological manifestations of Fabry disease. In: Mehta A, Beck M, Sunder-Plassmann G, editors. Fabry disease: perspectives from 5 years of FOS. Oxford: Oxford PharmaGenesis; 2006.
18. Savige J, Sheth S, Leys A, Nicholson A, Mack HG, Colville D. Ocular features in Alport syndrome: pathogenesis and clinical significance. Clin J Am Soc Nephrol. 2015;10(4):703–9.
19. Langwińska-Wośko E, Litwin T, Dzieżyc K, Członkowska A. The sunflower cataract in Wilson's disease: pathognomonic sign or rare finding? Acta Neurol Belg. 2016;116:325–8.

Persistent Fetal Vasculature

4

Chirakshi Dhull and Sudarshan Kumar Khokhar

Persistent fetal vasculature (PFV) is a congenital anomaly of the eye occurring from failure of the embryological, primary vitreous, and hyaloid vasculature to regress. The previous term persistent hyperplastic primary vitreous (PHPV) [1] has been replaced by PFV, coined by Goldberg [2]. Presentation in most cases is unilateral and varies from primarily anterior, posterior, or mixed variety.

4.1 Clinical Presentation

Anterior presentation typically involves the presence of persistent pupillary membrane (PPM), Mittendorf dot, cataract, vessels over lens, enlarged ciliary processes, glaucoma, and/or retrolental membranes. Posterior presentation may contain Bergmeister papilla, stalk of PFV, falciform fold, and/or retinal detachment. Mixed variety, which contains the combination of the two, is the commonest variant (Fig. 4.1).

Persistent pupillary membrane (PPM): It is a mild variant of PFV in which anterior tunica vasculosa lentis fails to regress leaving stands of iris or regressed vessels attached to lens. In most cases, it is visually insignificant but in rare cases may be associated with posterior stalk especially when associated with cataract or retrolental membrane. Sometimes, PPM may be severe and may cause lenticular myopia (Fig. 4.2). Such cases may require surgery.

Mittendorf dot: It is seen in 0.7–2.0% of the population [3]. Typically, it is small white dot on the posterior capsule on the nasal side representing incomplete regression of the hyaloid artery from its point of attachment (Fig. 4.3).

Enlarged ciliary processes: They may be seen in association with cataract or retrolental membrane. The contraction of membrane may be responsible for elongation of the ciliary processes, which may become visible as the pupil is dilated (Fig. 4.4).

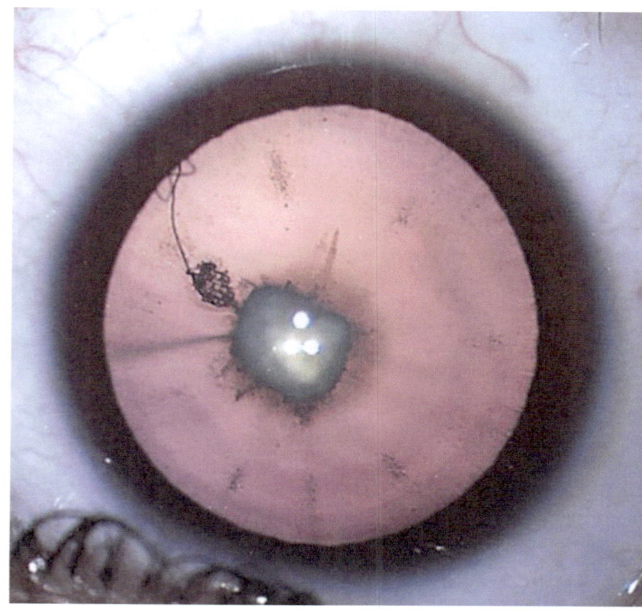

Fig. 4.1 Mixed variety of PFV with PPM, central cataract and stalk of PFV seen on the left

Fibrovascular membrane: The lens may be cataractous or partially absorbed or rarely completely absorbed. Sometimes only a part of lens is involved (Fig. 4.5). Usually, it is associated with small vessels over the fibrosed lens which may or may not bleed during surgery. They constitute a vascular connection between the posterior and the anterior tunica vasculosa lentis (Fig. 4.6).

Salmon patch sign: The lens may be associated with posterior capsular plaque where the vessels seem to have regressed. In some cases, there may be pink hue seen from the plaque which may predict the presence of PFV [4] (Fig. 4.7a–d).

C. Dhull · S. K. Khokhar (✉)
Dr. Rajendra Prasad Centre for Ophthalmic Sciences, All India Institute of Medical Sciences, New Delhi, India

S. K. Khokhar, C. Dhull (eds.), *Atlas of Pediatric Cataract*, https://doi.org/10.1007/978-981-13-6939-1_4

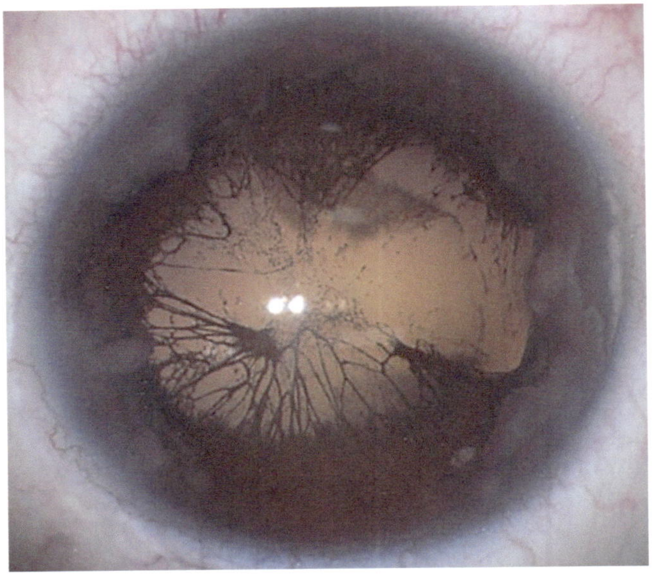

Fig. 4.2 Extensive PPM seen in association with minimal lamellar cataract

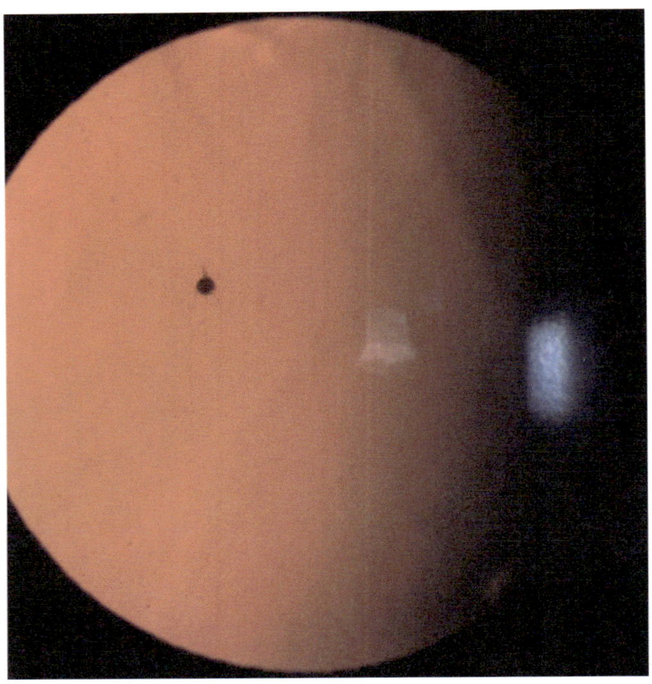

Fig. 4.3 Mittendorf dot seen in the left eye (nasal to the center)

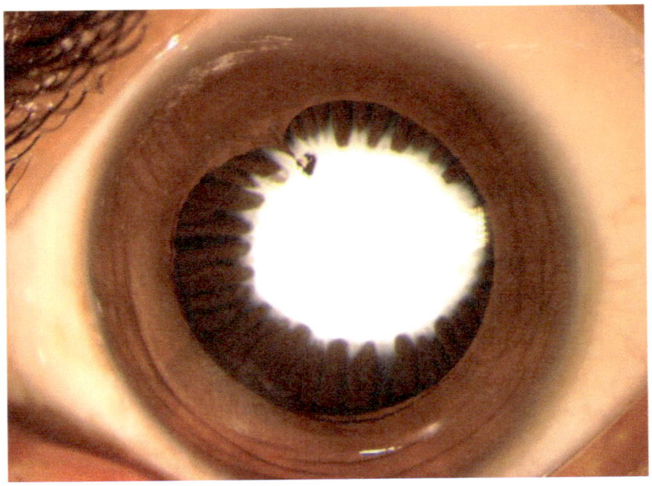

Fig. 4.4 Anterior variety of PFV with enlarged ciliary processes

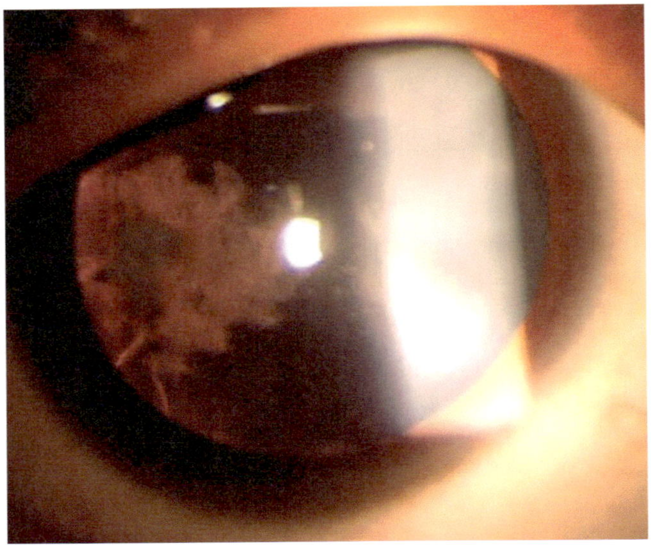

Fig. 4.5 Posterior subcapsular cataract with plaque with faint vessels seen

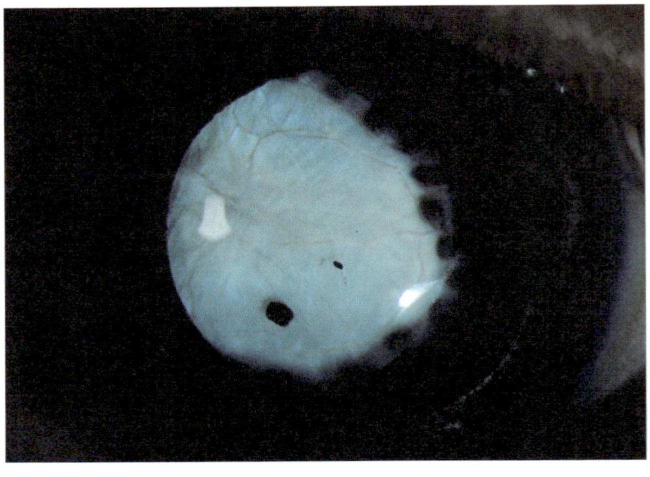

Fig. 4.6 Anterior PFV with fibrovascular membrane with visible multiple vessels crossing pupil and enlarged ciliary processes

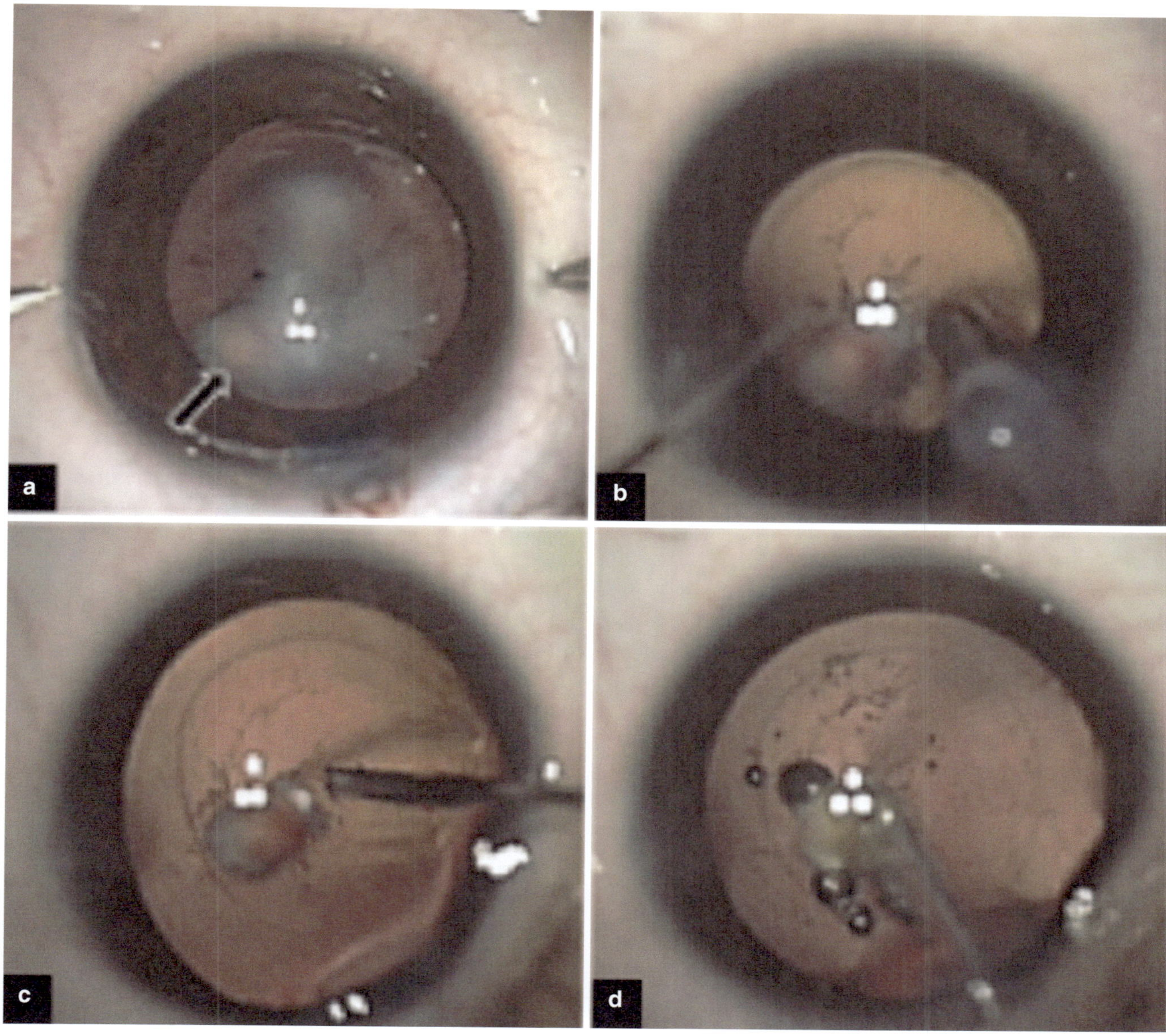

Fig. 4.7 (**a**) A congenital cataract showing the presence of an eccentric salmon pink sign intraoperatively (arrow). (**b**) Irrigation aspiration of the lens matter further enhances the pinkish hue from the retrocapsular plaque. (**c**) Posterior capsulorhexis is being performed with a bent 26 gauge needle. (**d**) The vascularized mass is coagulated with Fugo plasma blade PC. Source S Khokhar et al. [4]

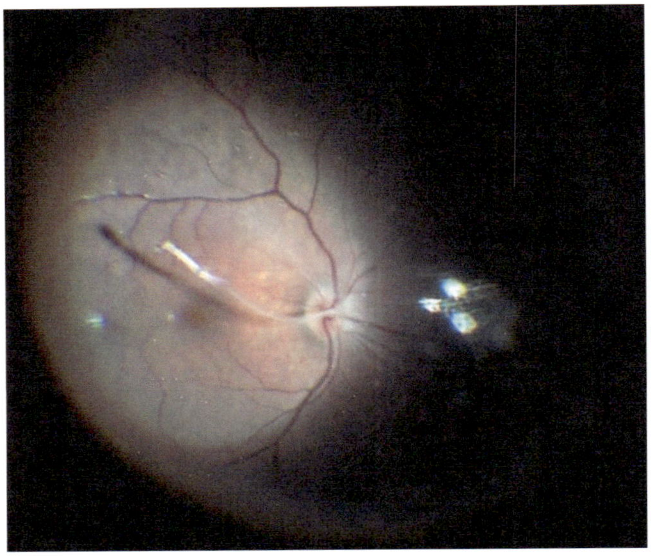

Fig. 4.8 Stalk of hyaloid artery remnant seen intraoperatively using wide angle viewing system in a case of posterior PFV

Persistent hyaloid artery: The fetal hyaloid artery lies within the Cloquet canal and regresses around the seventh month of gestation. If it persists, a stalk may be seen arising from the disc to behind the lens (Fig. 4.8).

Bergmeister papilla: Refers to remnant of hyaloid artery to disc and can be seen as fibrovascular tuft at disc. It may be associated with other disc or macular abnormalities.

4.2 Tools for Diagnosis

Despite the clinical manifestations, diagnosing PFV may sometimes be challenging. Any child with a cataract, especially unilateral, should be suspected of having PFV. The differential diagnosis includes diseases causing leukocoria, including retinoblastoma, Norrie's disease, ocular toxocariasis, retinal dysplasia, incontinentia pigmenti, uveitis, congenital cataract, coat's disease, retinopathy of prematurity, familial exudative vitreoretinopathy or endophthalmitis.

4.2.1 Ultrasonography (USG)

It is noninvasive, inexpensive tool of great use in cases of identifying PFV as well as ruling out other causes of leukocoria. Both USG and ultrasound biomicroscopy (UBM) of the anterior segment are valuable [5, 6]. USG typically shows a small globe and a stalk in vitreous extending from the posterior lens capsule to the disc area [6]. It can also reveal whether a retinal detachment is present or not. UBM may

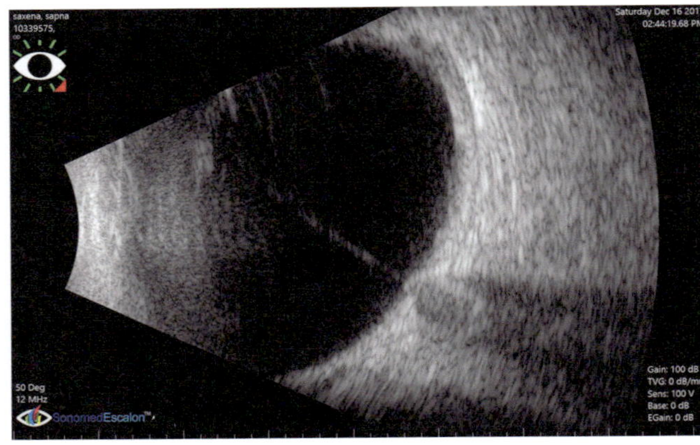

Fig. 4.9 USG picture showing hyperechoic stalk seen attached from disc to posterior surface of lens

show swollen lens with a resultant shallow anterior chamber or partially absorbed lens with enlarged ciliary processes and thickened anterior vitreous face [5]. Although effective, sensitivity ranges from 70% to 80% (Fig. 4.9).

4.2.2 Color Doppler Imaging

It detects blood flow within the stalk. It can also differentiate between arterial or venous flow (Fig. 4.10).

4.2.3 Magnetic Resonance Imaging (MRI)

MRI as well as computerized tomography (CT scan) have also been reported as excellent tool in the diagnosis of PFV [7, 8]. It helps in ruling out more severe differential diagnosis such as retinoblastoma. Sensitivity is almost 100% (Fig. 4.11).

4.2.4 Histopathology

Histopathology and electron microscopy can be used in confirming the diagnosis. It can be performed on enucleated eyes or tissue retrieved from PFV structures intraoperatively. Blood vessels associated with loose connective tissue can be identified in remnants of PFV (Fig. 4.12).

4.3 Management

Surgical is indicated in patients with visually significant cataract or fibrovascular membrane. Previously, surgery was indicated only to avoid complications and visual

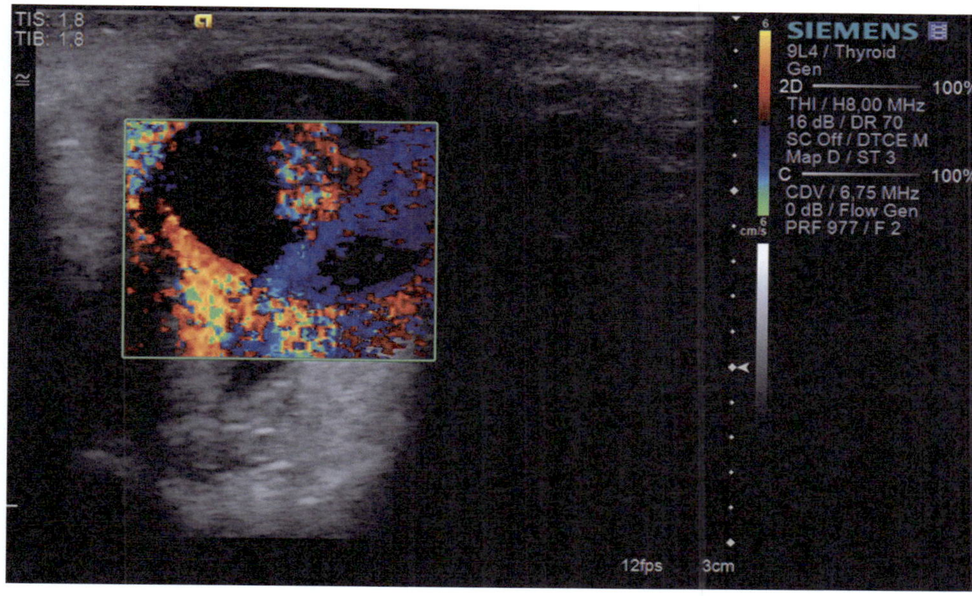

Fig. 4.10 Color Doppler of a 1-year-old child suggestive of arterial blood flow in the stalk

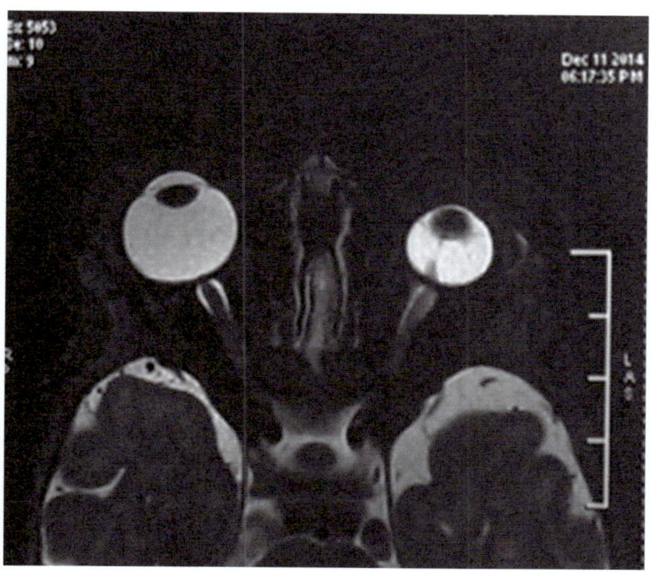

Fig. 4.11 T-2 W image of MRI of a 3-month-old baby showing left eye smaller in size with hypointense stalk attached from disc to lens confirm PFV

prognosis was very guarded [1, 9–11]. Various advances have come since then and successful management of cataract with posterior stalk has been possible [12–15]. Surgical approach can be anterior or posterior. The common steps like any congenital cataract include lensectomy along with anterior vitrectomy with management of the vascular structures. Hemostasis can be achieved by raised IOP, diathermy of vessels (Fig. 4.13), or using plasma knife [16]. The plasma knife (Fugo blade) is a radiofrequency electrosurgical incising instrument that uses electromagnetic energy to perform cutting and provides non-cauterizing hemostasis called "autostasis" [17]. The advantage of anterior approach is that IOL can be placed at the time of surgery.

Figure 4.14a–d shows the steps of surgery where after lensectomy, vascular stalk is visible. The posterior capsular plaque with attached stalk is cut using plasma knife (Fugo blade) avoiding inadvertent bleed. Afterward, the stalk is cut with microincision forceps. We can see the intact rim of sulcus for placement of IOL.

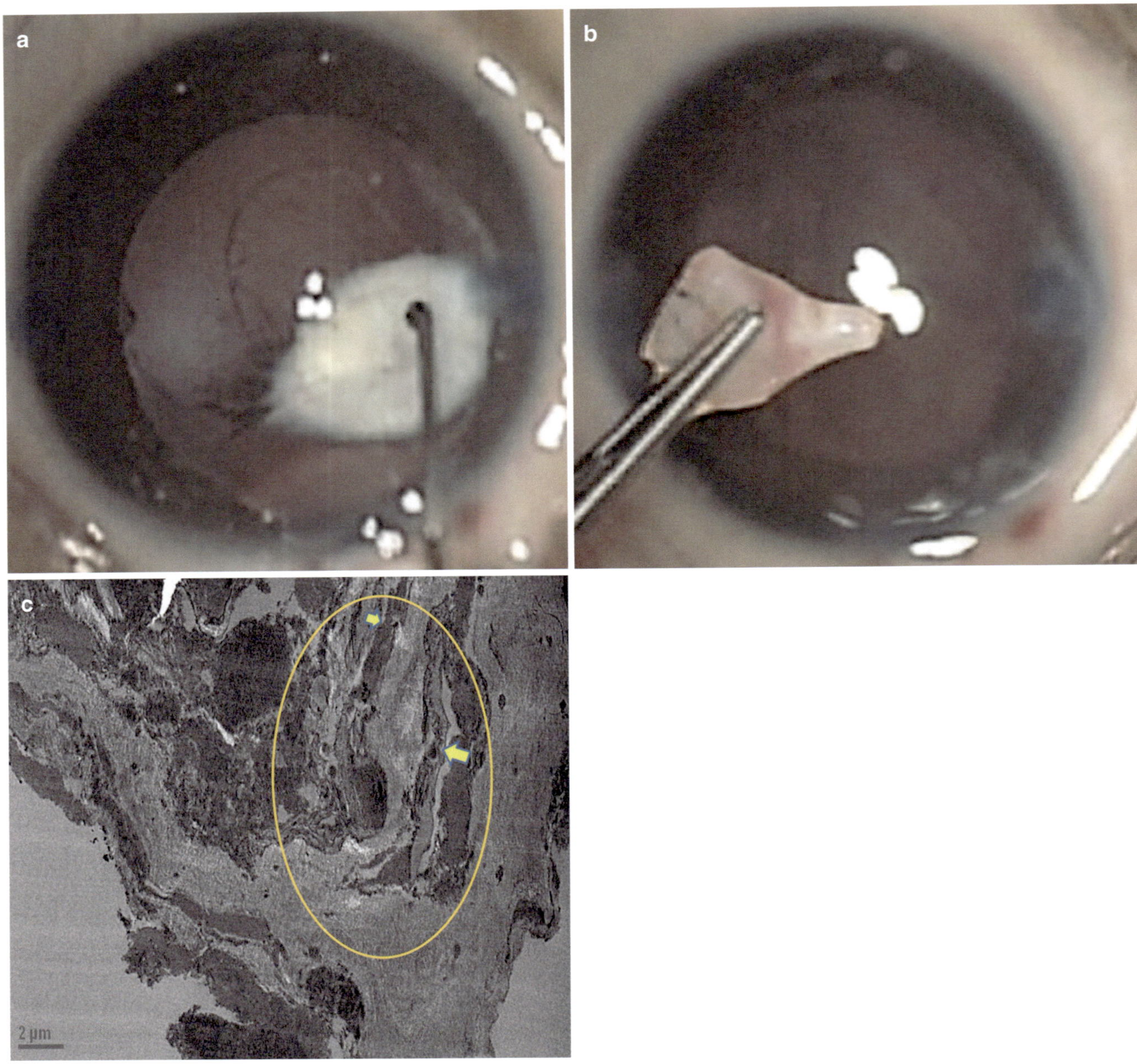

Fig. 4.12 (**a**) Intraoperative image of mixed variant of PFV after lens aspiration showing posterior capsular plaque with attached stalk. (**b**) Posterior plaque along with remnant of PFV removed. (**c**) Electron microscopy of the same showing loose elastic tissue (circle) with vessels (arrows)

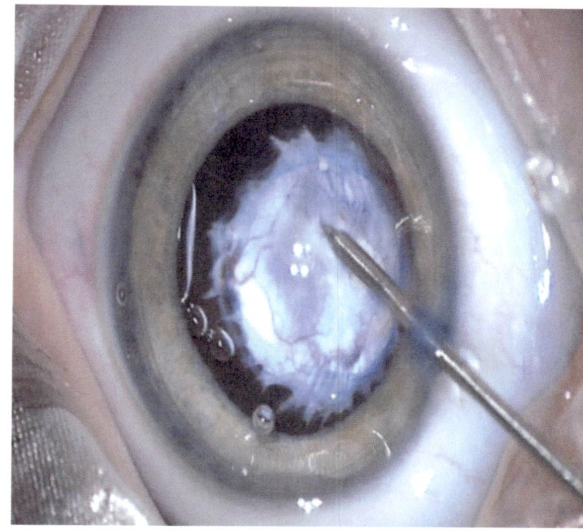

Fig. 4.13 Intraoperative image of anterior PFV where vessels are being cauterized using diathermy

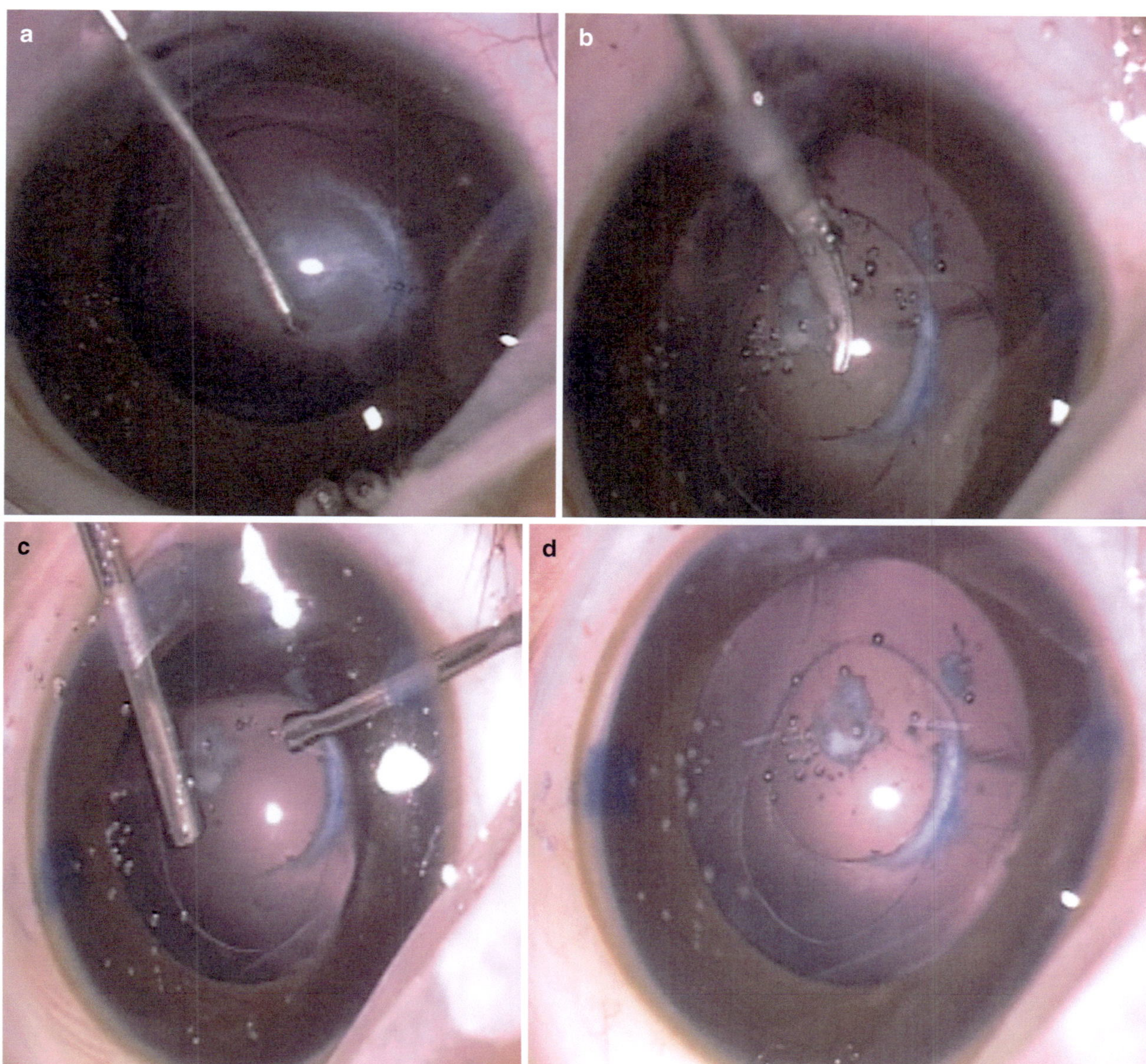

Fig. 4.14 (**a**) Fugo blade is used to cut the posterior capsule along with PFV stalk. (**b**) After hemostasis, stalk is cut with microincision forceps. (**c**) Stalk seen falling back. (**d**) After anterior vitrectomy, rim of sulcus is intact, IOL can be placed

4.4 Prognosis

Favorable outcomes may be achieved in children with PFV, irrespective of surgical approach by early intervention followed by aggressive amblyopic treatment [12–15, 18]. Still outcomes remain inferior compared to other children with unilateral cataract without PFV. It may be due to higher percentage of complications including glaucoma, visual axis opacification, vitreous hemorrhage, and retinal detachment [12, 13, 19, 20].

References

1. Reese AB. Persistent hyperplastic primary vitreous. Am J Ophthalmol. 1955;40:317–31.
2. Goldberg M. Persistent fetal vasculature (PFV): an integrated interpretation of signs and symptoms associated with persistent hyperplastic primary vitreous (PHPV). LIV Edward Jackson Memorial Lecture. Am J Ophthalmol. 1997;124:587–626.
3. Wright KW. Embryology. In: Cook CS, Sulik KK, Wright KW, editors. Pediatric ophthalmology and strabismus. St. Louis, MO: Mosby; 1995. p. 1–43.
4. Khokhar S, Gupta S, Gogia V, Nayak B. Salmon pink patch sign: diagnosing persistent fetal vasculature. Oman J Ophthalmol. 2016;9(1):68–9.
5. MacKeen LD, Nischal KK, Lam WC, et al. High-frequency ultrasonography findings in persistent hyperplastic primary vitreous. J AAPOS. 2000;4:217–24.
6. Frazier Byrne S, Green RL. Intraocular tumors. In: Fraziet Byrne S, Green RL, editors. Ultrasound of the eye and orbit. St. Louis, MO: Mosby; 1992. p. 201–4.
7. Mafee MF, Goldberg MF. Persistent hyperplastic primary vitreous (PHPV): role of computed tomography and magnetic resonance. Radiol Clin N Am. 1987;25:683–92.
8. Potter PD, Shields CL, Shields JA, et al. The role of magnetic resonance imaging in children with intraocular tumors and simulating lesions. Ophthalmology. 1996;103:1774–83.
9. Haddad R, Font RL, Reeser F. Persistent hyperplastic primary vitreous. A clinicopathologic study of 62 cases and review of the literature. Surv Ophthalmol. 1978;23:123–34.
10. Jensen OA. Persistent hyperplastic primary vitreous. Cases in Denmark. Acta Ophthalmol. 1968;46:418–29.
11. Olsen J, Moller PM. Persistent primary hyperplastic vitreous. Acta Ophthalmol. 1968;46:412–7.
12. Anteby I, Cohen E, Karshai I, et al. Unilateral persistent hyperplastic primary vitreous: course and outcome. J AAPOS. 2002;6:92–9.
13. Alexandrakis G, Scott IU, Flynn HW Jr, et al. Visual acuity outcomes with and without surgery in patients with persistent fetal vasculature. Ophthalmology. 2000;107:1068–72.
14. Dass AB, Trese MT. Surgical results of persistent hyperplastic primary vitreous. Ophthalmology. 1999;106:280–4.
15. Mittra RA, Huynh LT, Ruttum MS, et al. Visual outcomes following lensectomy and vitrectomy for combined anterior and posterior persistent hyperplastic primary vitreous. Arch Ophthalmol. 1998;116:1190–4.
16. Khokhar S, Tejwani LK, Kumar G, Kushmesh R. Approach to cataract with persistent hyperplastic primary vitreous. J Cataract Refract Surg. 2011;37:1382–5.
17. Fugo RJ, Delcampo DM. The Fugo Blade: The next step after capsulorhexis. Ann Ophthalmol. 2001;33:13–20.
18. Lambert SR, Buckley EG, Drews-Botsch C, et al. A randomized clinical trial comparing contact lens with intraocular lens correction of monocular aphakia during infancy: grating acuity and adverse events at age 1 year. Arch Ophthalmol. 2010;128:810–8.
19. BenEzra D. The surgical approaches to pediatric cataract. Eur J Implant Refract Surg. 1990;2:241–4.
20. BenEzra D, Cohen E. Posterior capsulectomy in pediatric cataract surgery: the necessity of a choice. Ophthalmology. 1997;104:2168–74.

Preexisting Posterior Capsular Defect

5

Chirakshi Dhull, Barkha Gupta, and Sudarshan Kumar Khokhar

Congenital cataract with preexisting posterior capsular defect (PCD) is a rare condition and can pose as a surgical challenge. Preexisting PCD is described as lens abnormality manifesting in infants and small children as a congenital cataract where there is a defect in the posterior capsule [1]. Incidence of the condition ranges from 2% to 6.7% [2, 3]. PCD can also be seen in cases of trauma [4, 5] but they are excluded from the terminology of preexisting PCD.

PCD has been hypothesized to begin as posterior lenticonus [6] which later progresses to full thickness defect. There may be a causal association of posterior lenticonus with persistent fetal vasculature in unilateral or bilateral cases [7, 8]. Breaks may form in posterior capsule secondary to traction or progressive thinning of capsule. Once the posterior capsule is breached, lens matter comes in contact with outside fluid and opacification of the lens is seen. This may range from dense posterior, cortical, nuclear, or total cataract. These cataracts make identification of PCD more difficult especially in children who are not cooperative for examination.

5.1 Clinical Presentation

Children with PCD present with total or subtotal grayish to white cataract. Defect may not be seen directly but may be picked up by associated signs (Fig. 5.1). The following should be looked for carefully to diagnose PCD clinically in a fully dilated pupil:

- Deep anterior chamber (AC) with flattened or concave anterior capsule.
- Presence of white dots on the posterior capsule and/or in the anterior vitreous—"white dot sign" [2].

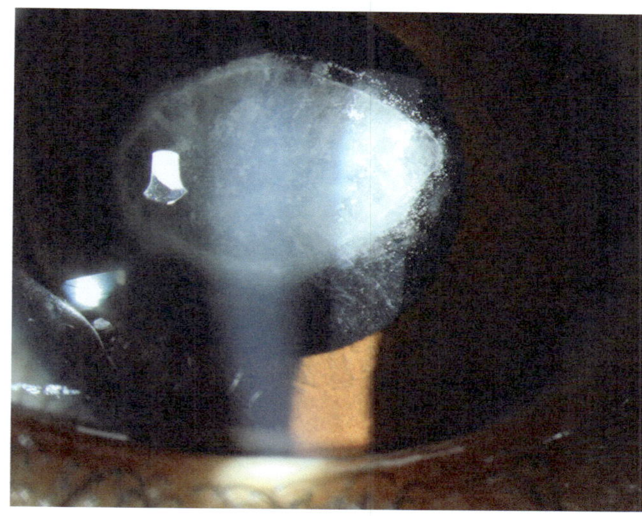

Fig. 5.1 Congenital cataract with telltale signs of PCD. Deep AC, white dot sign is seen along with well-defined spindle-shaped PCD

- Fish tail sign—as seen in cases of posterior polar cataract and PCD is indicative of breach in posterior capsule [2].
- Well-defined defect in posterior capsule, could be any shape but spindle shape is the commonest in our experience.
- Presence of vacuoles in the vicinity of cataract.

Congenital cataract with PCD can present in various forms. Cataract may be total (Fig. 5.2) or localized with predominant posterior component (Figs. 5.3 and 5.4). Posterior polar cataracts may also be associated with PCD [9]. Lens thickness is generally reduced [10] and most of the lens matter lies posterior to posterior capsule. In some cases, lens may be partially absorbed leaving posterior capsular plaque which is seen commonly in developing countries.

We have divided the defect in posterior capsule into three types. This classifications helps in better surgical planning and management.

C. Dhull · B. Gupta · S. K. Khokhar (✉)
Dr. Rajendra Prasad Centre for Ophthalmic Sciences, All India Institute of Medical Sciences, New Delhi, India

S. K. Khokhar, C. Dhull (eds.), *Atlas of Pediatric Cataract*, https://doi.org/10.1007/978-981-13-6939-1_5

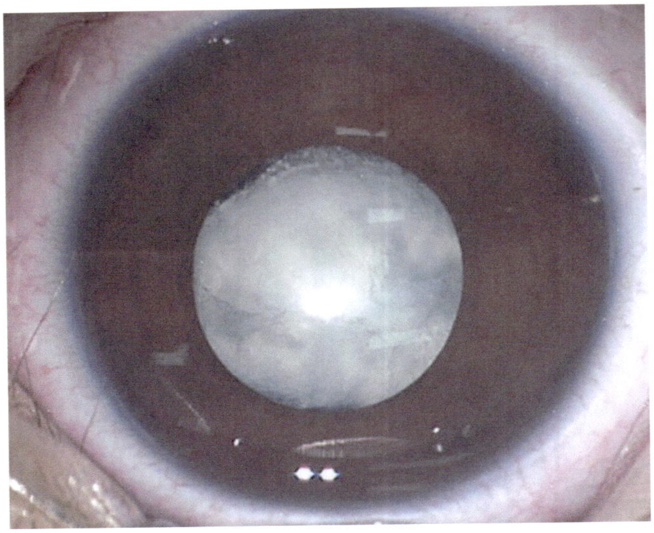

Fig. 5.2 Total white cataract with PCD. Carefully notice white dots at superior pupillary border and margin of PCD

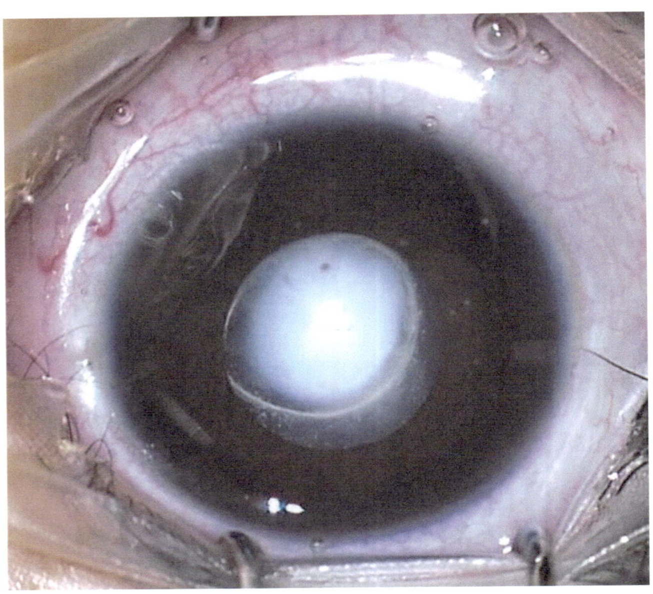

Fig. 5.3 Subtotal cataract, with predominantly lens matter behind the posterior capsular defect

- Type 1: Well-defined defect, with sharp edges and minimal fibrosis (Fig. 5.5a, b).
- Type 2: Circular or regular defect with fibrosis (Fig. 5.6).
- Type 3: Posterior capsular plaque where the defect is sealed (Fig. 5.7).

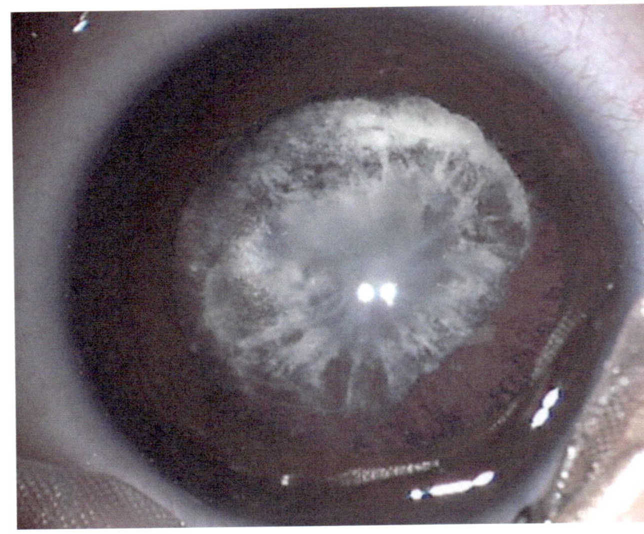

Fig. 5.4 Posterior opacification of lens with periphery spared. Few fluid vacuoles are seen in the periphery

5.2 Investigations

In cases of diagnostic difficulty, ultrasound biomicroscopy (UBM) with 35 MHz should be performed for confirmation. Signs of PCD are enhanced and discontinuity in posterior capsule is generally visible (Fig. 5.8a, b). In addition, biometric parameters such as lens thickness and anterior chamber depth may help in prediction of PCD (Fig. 9a, b) [10].

5.3 Surgical Management

Surgery is recommended in visually significant cataracts. Mild cataracts should be followed up as they are likely to progress over time.

Apart from the usual the standard surgical steps for pediatric cataract surgery, certain precautions should be taken. Anterior chamber should be maintained throughout surgery. Small incisions (1 mm) can be used for manual capsulorhexis. Anterior chamber is generally deep and longer microincision forceps provides better chamber stability. Hydrodissection is avoided to prevent PCD extension and lens matter drop in vitreous cavity. Bimanual aspiration is the preferred method. Low flow rate and low IOP settings are recommended. We prefer using 23 Gauge anterior vitrector in Irrigation Aspiration mode for lens aspiration as it can be used for anterior vitrectomy in vitrectomy mode without need for changing instruments. This reduces chances of PCD extension and vitreous prolapse.

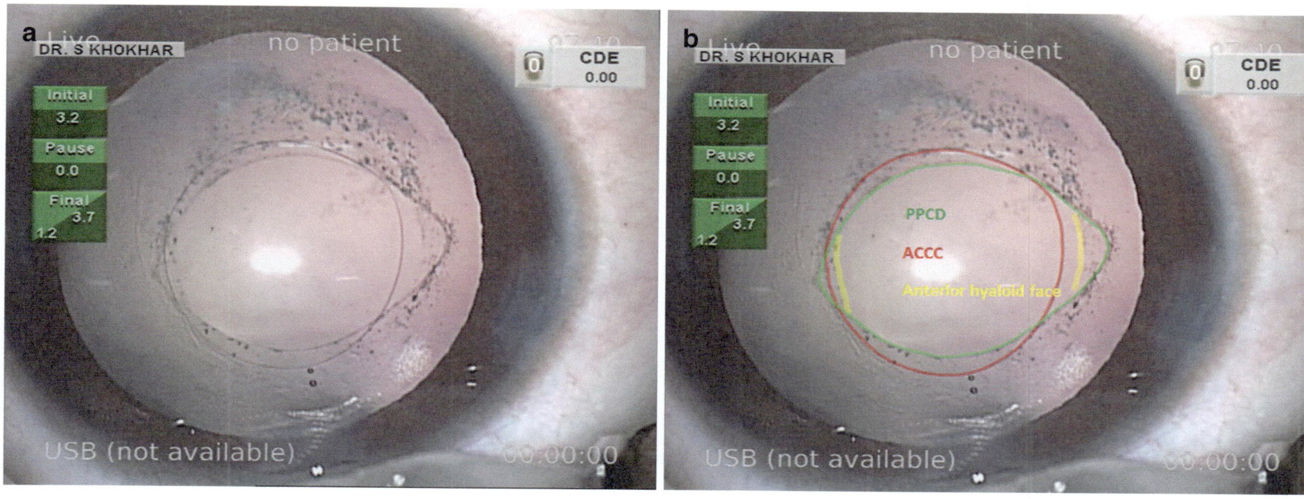

Fig. 5.5 (**a**) Intraoperative picture of type 1 PCD, notice the spindle shape, sharp edges, and lack of fibrosis. (**b**) Marked anterior capsulorhexis (ACCC), preexisting PCD (PPCD), and anterior hyloid face in the same (**a**)

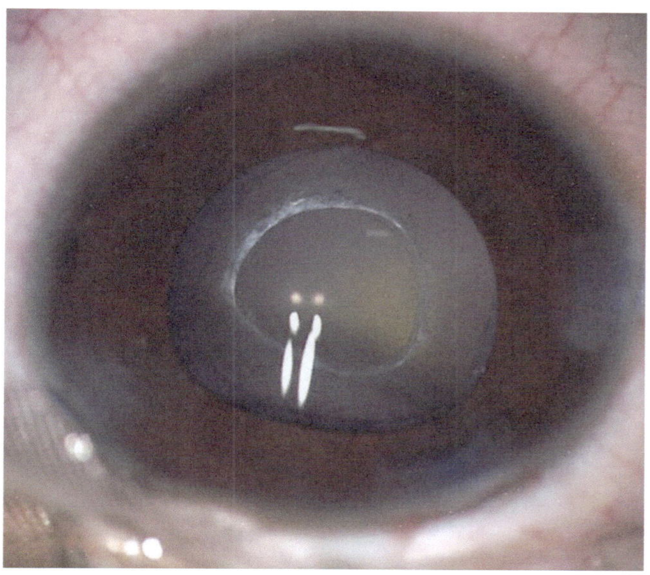

Fig. 5.6 Type 2 PCD with fibrosed margins

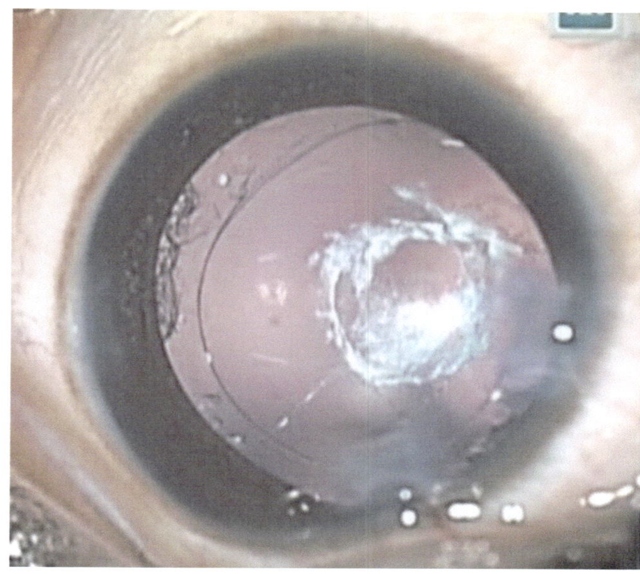

Fig. 5.7 Type 3 PCD with posterior capsular plaque

Posterior capsule management depends on type of PCD. In type 1, PCD (if small) can be converted to posterior capsulorhexis (PCCC) (Fig. 5.10a). While performing PCCC, anterior chamber should be formed, without filling the bag. PCD can be held with microincision forceps and pulled in fashion to create PCCC. Intraocular lens can be placed in the bag using safe technique where IOL is implanted under the anterior capsule [11]. In cases of large type 1 defect, PCCC may not be possible. Hence, PCIOL can be placed in sulcus with or without capture (Fig. 5.10b). In type 2 PCD, IOL can be placed in the bag using similar technique (Fig. 5.11). In type 3 PCD, posterior capsular plaque can be first peeled using a sinskey hook followed by removal with microincision forceps (Fig. 5.12). After removal of plaque, manual PCCC and IOL insertion in bag can be performed. Alternately where peeling of plaque is not possible, PCCC can be done with vitrector followed by IOL insertion in bag.

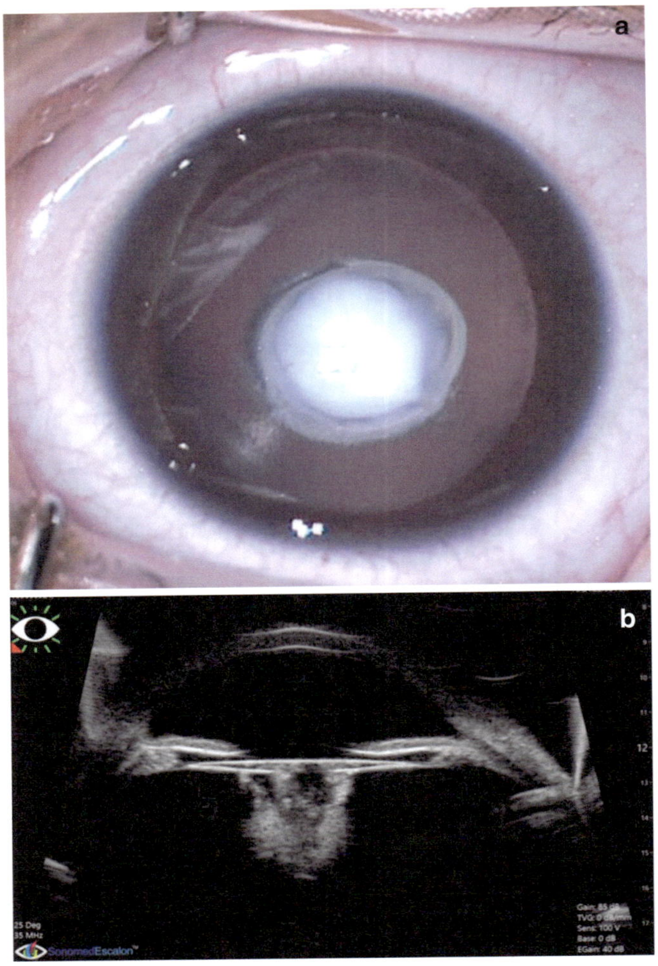

Fig. 5.8 (**a**) Clinical picture of PCD with central cataract. (**b**) UBM showing deep anterior chamber, flat anterior capsule, discontinuity in posterior capsule, and lens matter in anterior vitreous

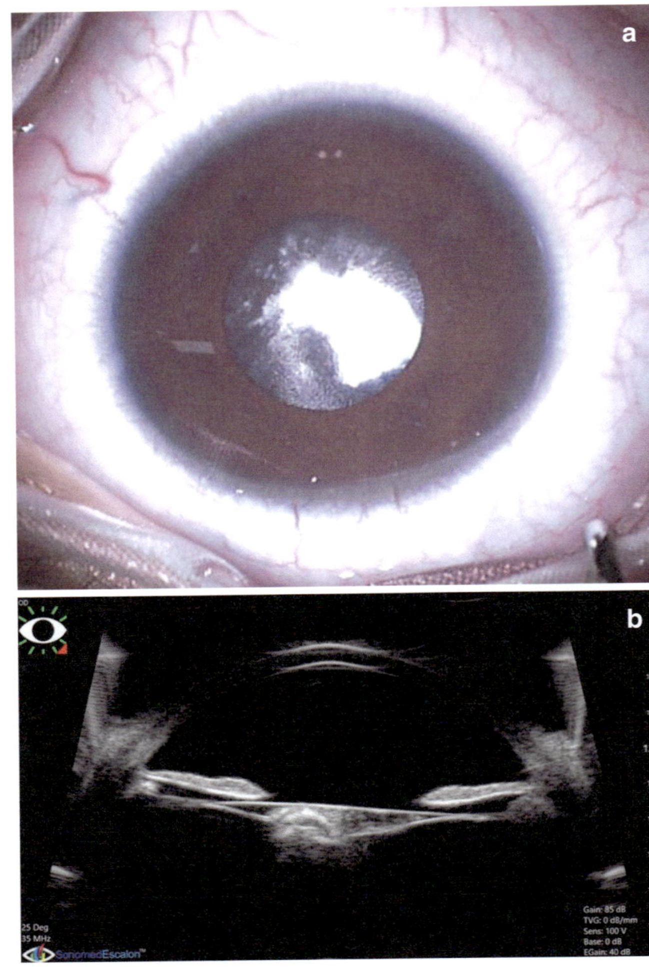

Fig. 5.9 (**a**) Clinical picture of congenital cataract, partially absorbed cataract with central opacity. No definitive PCD seen. (**b**) UBM of the same showing PCD with lens matter in anterior vitreous

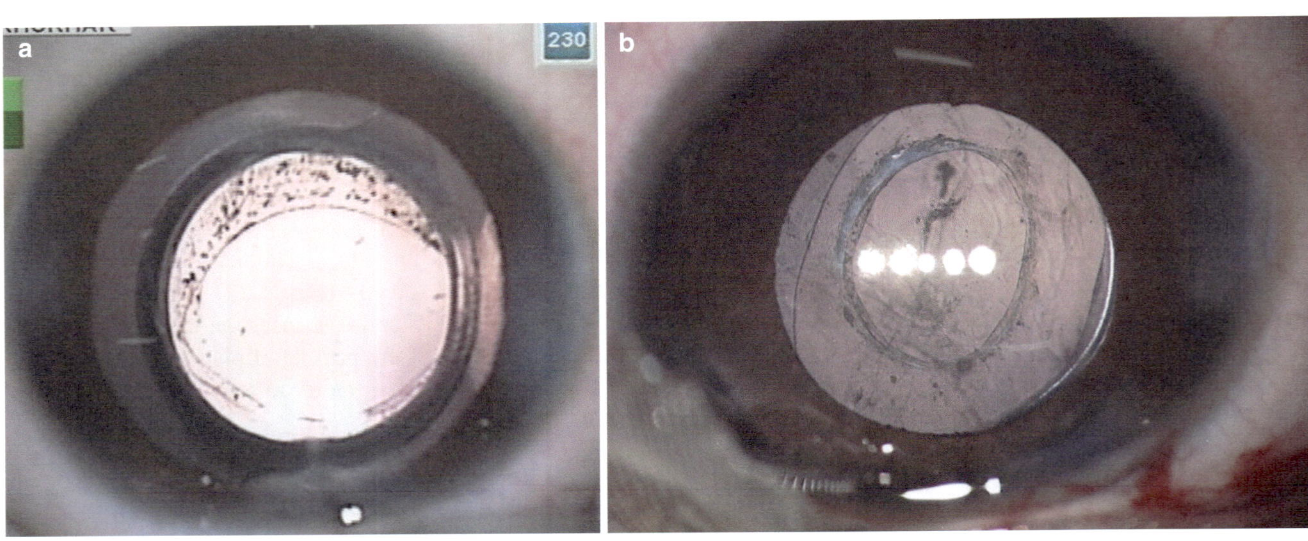

Fig. 5.10 (**a**) Postoperative picture of type 1 PCD with PCIOL in bag. (**b**) Intraoperative picture of large type 1 PCD, PCIOL in sulcus with multipiece with optic capture done

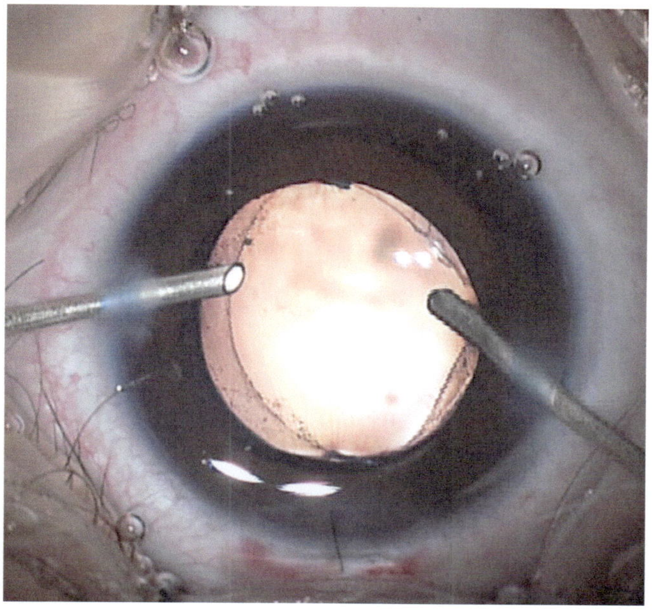

Fig. 5.11 Postoperative picture of type 2 PCD with fibrosed PCD and PCIOL in bag

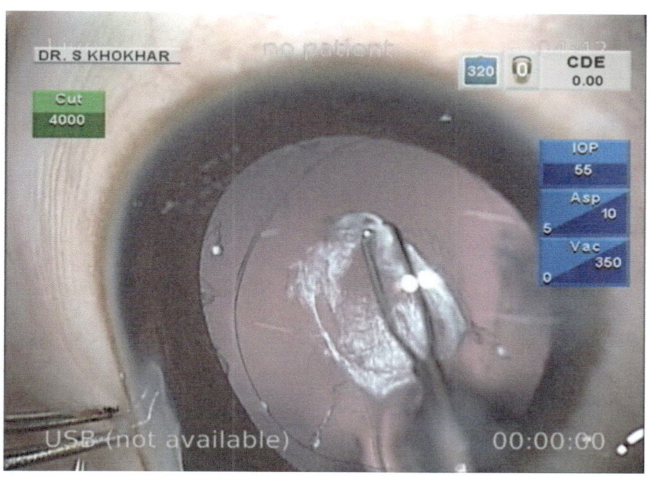

Fig. 5.12 Intraoperative picture of posterior capsular plaque, removal of plaque is done using microincision forceps

Most cases are associated with anatomical and good outcomes [2, 3, 10].

In conclusion, congenital cataracts associated with preexisting PCD are surgically challenging. Preoperative diagnosis can be made with the help of specific clinical signs. Ultrasound biomicroscopy can help in cases with diagnostic difficulty. Careful surgery can help in preventing inadvertent complications and attaining good outcomes.

References

1. Vajpayee RB, Sandramouli S. Bilateral congenital posterior-capsular defects: a case report. Ophthalmic Surg. 1992;23:295–6.
2. Vasavada AR, Praveen MR, Nath V, Dave K. Diagnosis and management of congenital cataract with preexisting posterior capsule defect. J Cataract Refract Surg. 2004;30:403–8.
3. Wilson ME, Trivedi RH. Intraocular lens implantation in pediatric eyes with posterior lentiglobus. Trans Am Ophthalmol Soc. 2006;104:176–82.
4. Krishnamachary M, Rathi V, Gupta S. Management of traumatic cataract in children. J Cataract Refract Surg. 1997;23:681–7.
5. Vajpayee RB, Angra SK, Honavar SG, et al. Pre-existing posterior capsule breaks from perforating ocular injuries. J Cataract Refract Surg. 1994;20:291–4.
6. Wilson ME, Trivedi RH, Pandey SK. Pediatric cataract surgery: techniques, complications, and management. Philadelphia, PA: Lippincott Williams & Wilkins; 2005.
7. Kilty LA, Hiles DA. Unilateral posterior lenticonus with persistent hyaloid artery remnant [letter]. Am J Ophthalmol. 1993;116:104–5.
8. Khokhar S, Dhull C, Mahalingam K, Agarwal P. Posterior lenticonus with persistent fetal vasculature. Indian J Ophthalmol. 2018;66(9):1335–6.
9. Osher RH, Yu BC-Y, Koch DD. Posterior polar cataracts: a predisposition to intraoperative posterior capsule rupture. J Cataract Refract Surg. 1990;16:157–62.
10. Li Z, et al. Morphological and biometric features of preexisting posterior capsule defect in congenital cataract. J Cataract Refract Surg. 2018;44(7):871–7.
11. Khokhar S, Sharma R, Patil B, Sinha G, Nayak B, Kinkhabwala RA. A safe technique for in-the-bag intraocular lens implantation in pediatric cataract surgery. Eur J Ophthalmol. 2015;25(1):57–9.

Lenticular Subluxation

6

Sudarshan Kumar Khokhar, Pulak Agarwal, Abhidnya Surve, and Chirakshi Dhull

Subluxated lens is partial displacement or malposition of the natural crystalline lens from its normal position in the patellar fossa (Fig. 6.1). Though subluxated lens and ectopia lentis are used interchangeably, it is preferable to use latter for lens subluxation due to hereditary causes. The term "Ectopia lentis" was coined by Stellwag in 1856. Term "Ectopia" is a Latin word which means "outside." It signifies compromised zonular fibers and is caused by different congenital, developmental, metabolic, or systemic disorders. Acquired subluxation may occur with trauma or intraocular surgery [1, 2] (Table 6.1).

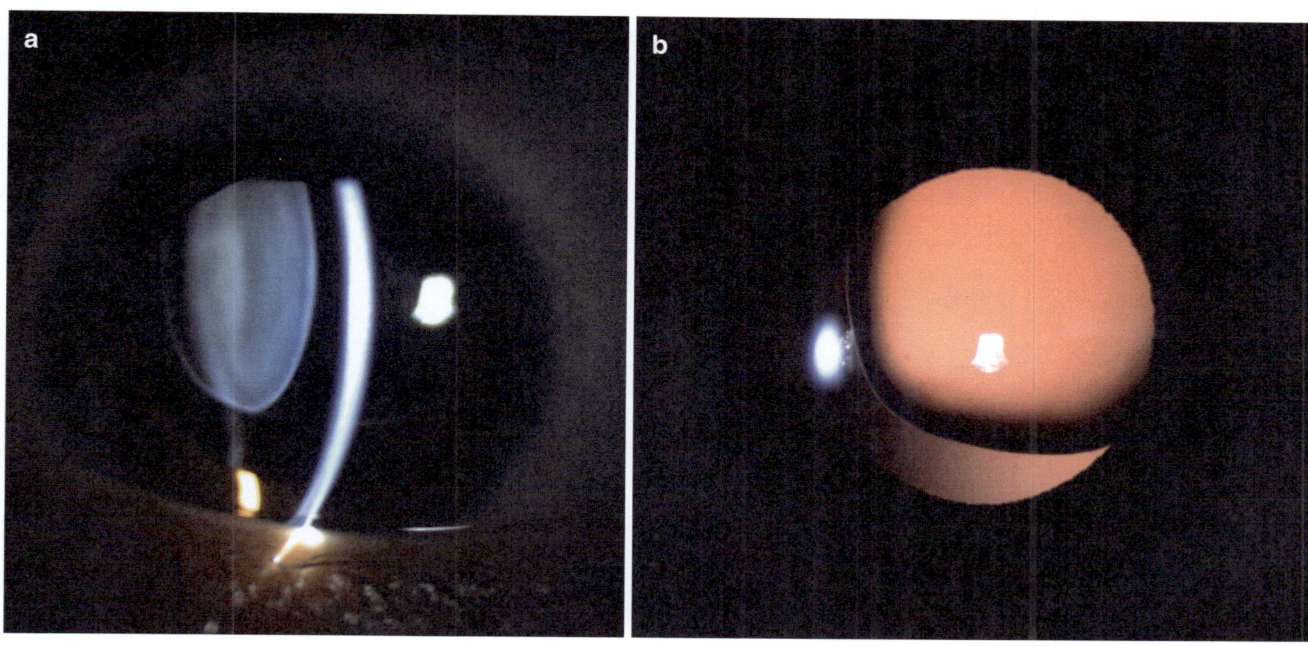

Fig. 6.1 Lenticular subluxation. (**a**) Slit examination and (**b**) retroillumination image of supero-temporally subluxated clear lens

S. K. Khokhar · P. Agarwal · A. Surve · C. Dhull (✉)
Dr. Rajendra Prasad Centre for Ophthalmic Sciences, All India Institute of Medical Sciences, New Delhi, India

S. K. Khokhar, C. Dhull (eds.), *Atlas of Pediatric Cataract*, https://doi.org/10.1007/978-981-13-6939-1_6

Table 6.1 Etiology of subluxated lens

Isolated ocular abnormality	Associated with systemic syndromes	Associated with metabolic syndromes	Associated with other ocular conditions	Other
• Simple ectopia lens • Simple Microspherophakia	• Marfan's syndrome • Weil–Marchesani syndrome • Ehler Danlos syndrome • Rieger's syndrome • Sturge Weber syndrome • Pflander's syndrome • Crouzon's syndrome • Chondrodysplastic dwarfism • Oxycephaly	• Homocystinuria • Hyperlysinemia • Sulfite oxidase deficiency • Lysyl hydroxyl deficiency	• Congenital aniridia • Ectopia lentis et pupillae • High myopia • Hypermature cataract • Pseudoexfoliation syndrome • Congenital glaucoma • Buphthalmos • Megalocornea • Staphyloma • Uveal coloboma • Cornea plana • Uveitis • Retinitis pigmentosa	• Traumatic • Surgical trauma

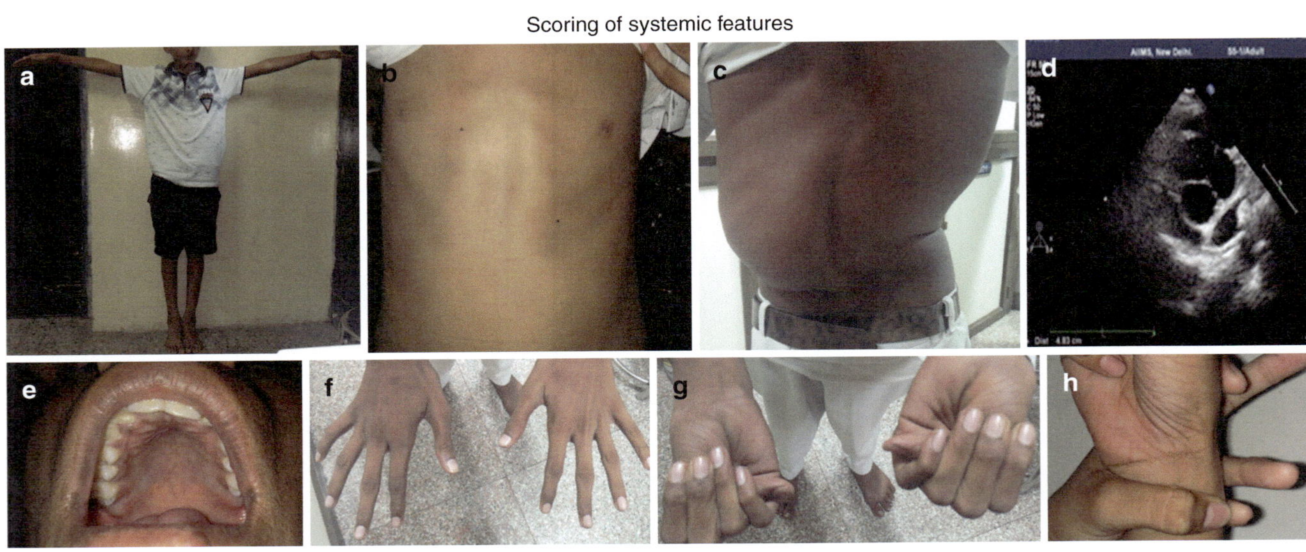

Fig. 6.2 Marfan's syndrome (**a**) Increased arm span, increased upper segment to lower segment ratio, (**b**) Pectus carinatum, (**c**) kyphoscoliosis, (**d**) echocardiogram with aortic root regurgitation, (**e**) high arched palate, (**f**) arachnodactylyl, (**g**) positive thumb sign, (**h**) positive wrist sign

6.1 Symptoms and Signs

Subluxation of lens can occur at any age. Even congenital cases may manifest later in life due to progressive changes associated with the disease. Patient may present with decreased or fluctuating vision due to lenticular astigmatism or refractive error, monocular diplopia, impaired accommodation, photophobia, or glare. Complications like pupillary block and angle closure may develop due to dislocation into the anterior chamber or pupil. These patients may present with pain, redness, watering, nausea, vomiting, blurred vision, and colored haloes. Obvious signs include phacodonesis, vitreous prolapse, iridodonesis, and lens subluxation. It is also important to detect subtle signs such as the visibility of lens equator during eccentric gaze, decentered nucleus in primary position, iridolenticular gap, changes in contour of lens periphery, and focal iridodonesis.

6.2 Workup

History: Appropriate history should include the onset and severity of visual symptoms, relevant trauma, and treatment received. Due to association of many metabolic and systemic syndromes with ectopia lentis, it is crucial to assess the family history and perform complete physical examination to detect other associated anomalies.

Systemic evaluation: A detailed systemic examination of skeletal, cardiovascular, neurological, respiratory, and genitourinary system helps us to identify the syndromic diagnosis and also allows an early referral to pediatrician or physician to prevent morbidity and mortality due to disease.

Cases of **Marfan syndrome** are diagnosed based on modified Ghent's criteria and have features such as increased arm span, arachnodactyly, high arched palate, aortic root dilation, and mitral valve prolapse (Fig. 6.2) [3, 4]. It's a

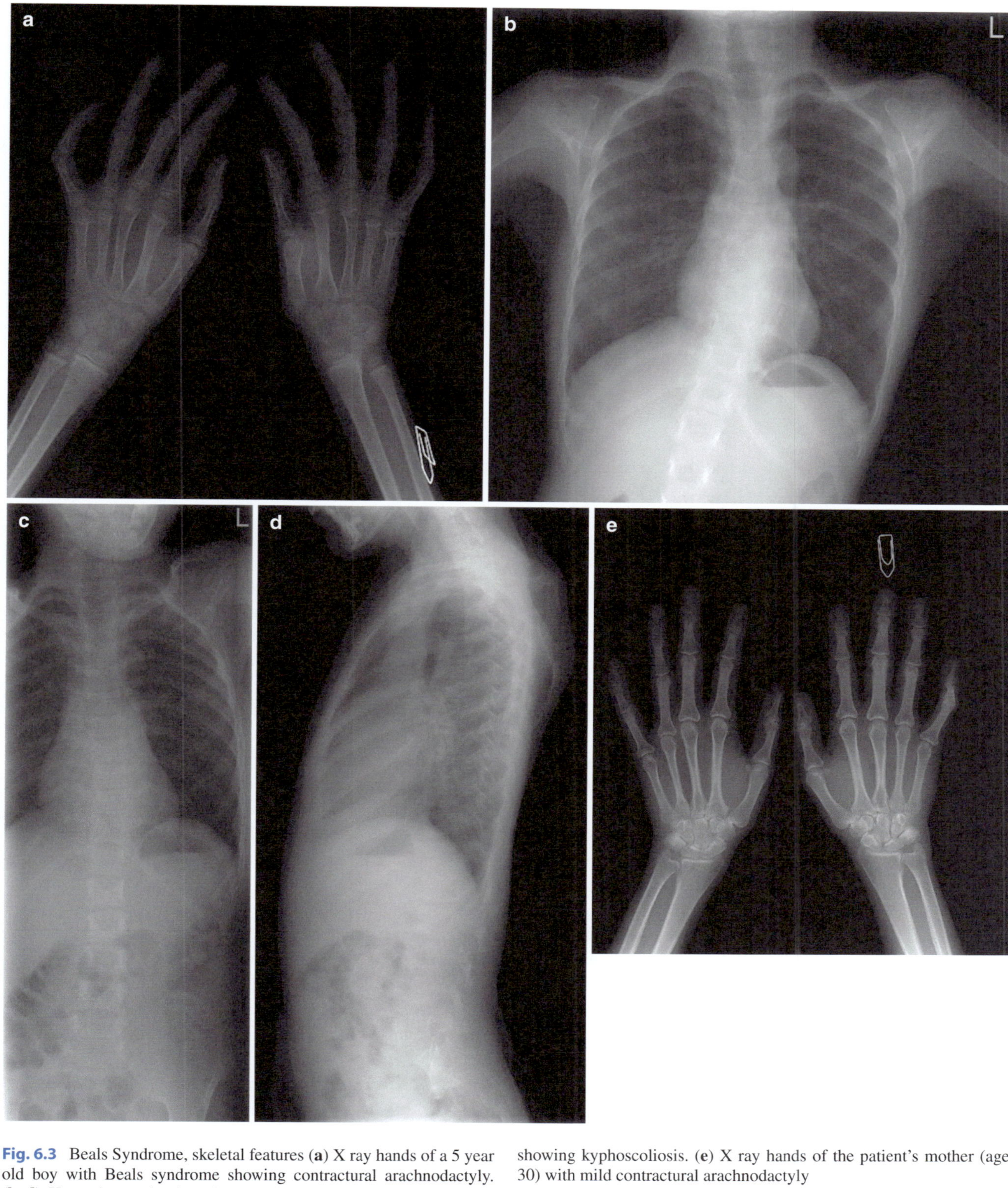

Fig. 6.3 Beals Syndrome, skeletal features (**a**) X ray hands of a 5 year old boy with Beals syndrome showing contractural arachnodactyly. (**b–d**) X ray chest, spine Anterio-posterior and lateral view respectively showing kyphoscoliosis. (**e**) X ray hands of the patient's mother (age 30) with mild contractural arachnodactyly

genetic condition caused due to Fibrillin-1 gene (FBN1) mutation. It has an autosomal dominant inheritance. Other ocular manifestations like high myopia, retinal detachment, premature cataracts, strabismus, and megalocorneas can also be associated. In rare cases, subluxation is noted with associated marfanoid phenotype who donot fit in modified Ghent's criteria. Such cases may turn out to be cases of Beals syndrome (Fig. 6.3a–e). Fibrillin -2 (FBN 2) gene mutation is noted in these cases. Also known as Congenital contractural arachnodactyly (CCA), it has some similarities with Marfan's

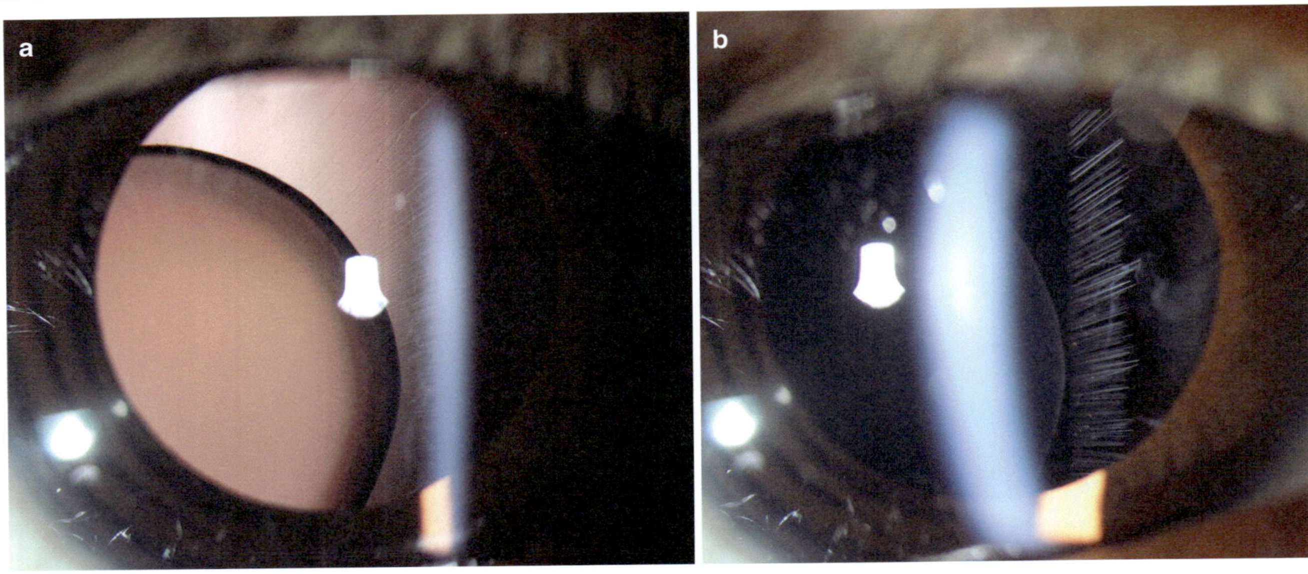

Fig. 6.4 Subluxated clear lens with stretched intact zonules in (**a**) retroillumination, (**b**) slit examination

syndrome such as skeletal marfanoid habitus, arachnodactyly, camptodactyly and kyphoscoliosis [5]. However, they have congenital contractures and do not typically have the cardiovascular complications seen in Marfan's syndrome. Subluxation of lens is also not as common as Marfan's syndrome.

Weill–Marchesani syndrome cases show features such as short stature, brachydactyly, and joint stiffness [6].

Homocystinuria is a metabolic condition due to cystathionine beta-synthase deficiency (Chr. 12). It is an autosomal recessive disorder. Prominent systemic features can be ADHD, developmental delay, mental retardation, increased chances of thromboembolic phenomenon, etc. Myopia and lens subluxation are prominent ocular features. Serum homocysteine level helps in diagnosing homocysteinemia and also an assessment of the steps to be taken to prevent thrombophilia [7, 8]. Genetic testing is done in cases where family history is present.

Ophthalmic examination: Visual acuity (both distant and near), external ocular examination, slit lamp examination, retinoscopic refraction (through phakic and aphakic areas), intraocular pressure, and dilated fundus examination must be done in all cases. The slit lamp examination must be performed under maximum mydriasis and attention must be given to the following details:

- Direction of subluxation.
- Number of clock hours involved.
- Status of zonules: stretched or absent [9] (Fig. 6.4).
- Clear or cataractous lens (Fig. 6.5).
- Degree of phacodonesis.
- Presence or absence of any vitreous in anterior chamber.
- Presence of any lens coloboma along with subluxation (Fig. 6.6). Lens coloboma in isolation is a rare entity (Fig. 6.7).
- Pupillary ectopia.
- **Ectopia lentis et pupillae** (Fig. 6.8): It is a rare congenital inherited disorder characterized by lenticular and pupillary ectopia. It has been postulated that a neuroectodermal defect results in hypoplasia or absence of the posterior pigment epithelium layer and dilator muscle of the iris which allows the pupil to be drawn to the opposite meridian, resulting in pupillary ectopia and poor dilatation. Marked stretching of the iris and deficiency of the posterior pigmented layer may cause transillumination effect. The localized iris abnormality coexists with a corresponding zonular defect which results in ectopia lentis in the opposite direction.
- Other prominent features are iridodonesis, iris transillumination, enlarged corneal diameter, microspherophakia, persistent pupillary membranes, iridohyaloid adhesions, anterior uveitis, elevated intraocular pressure, cataract, and retinal detachment. These ocular conditions are discussed in respective chapters.
- Examination for signs of trauma (corneal/scleral injury, iris hole, iridodialysis, lens capsule integrity, capsular fibrosis) and gonioscopy for angle recession. Traumatic subluxation is discussed in detail in the respective chapter.

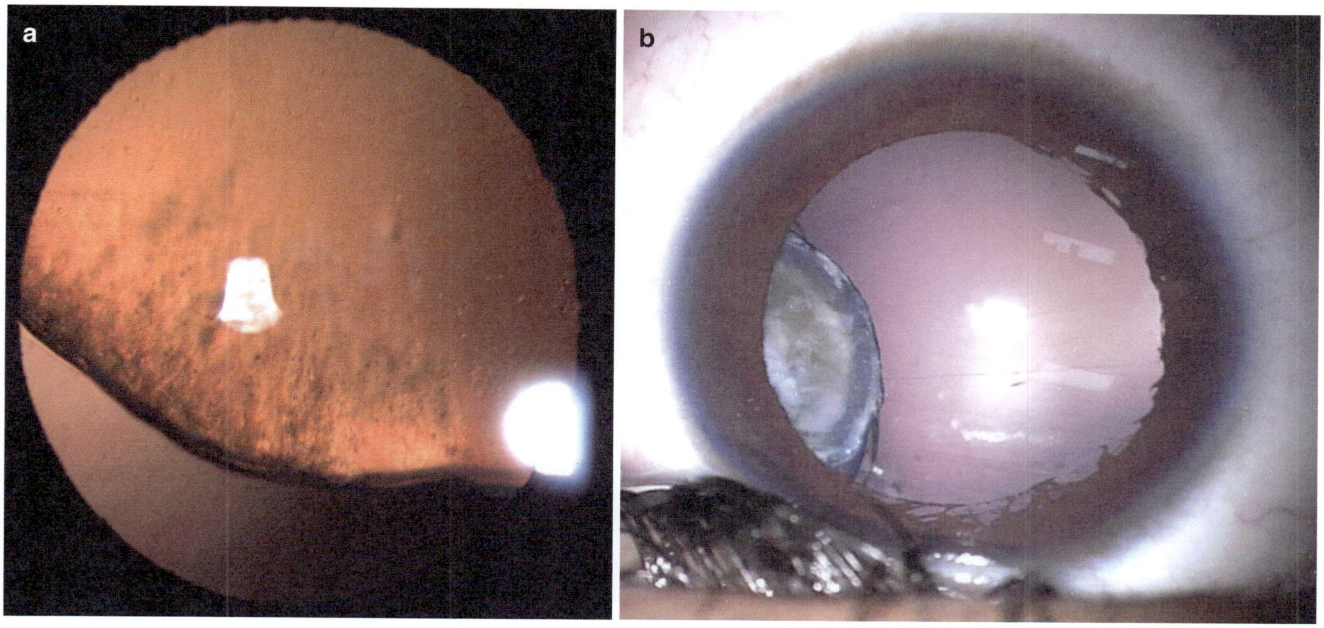

Fig. 6.5 Subluxated cataractous lens. (**a**) Posterior subcapsular cataract, (**b**) calcified sclerotic cataract seen in children with extreme subluxation

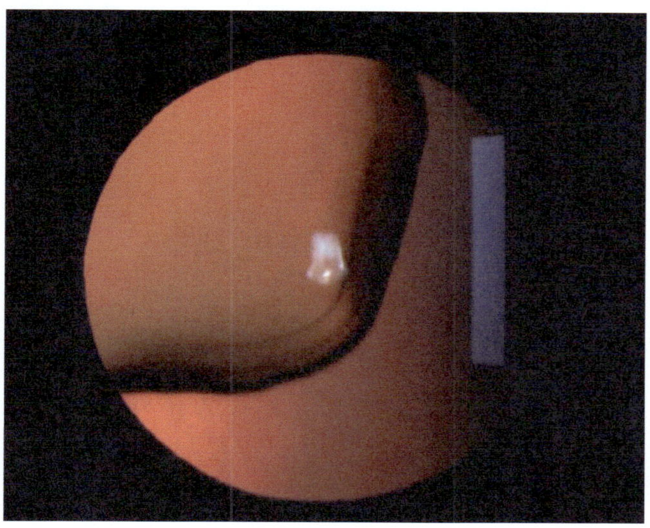

Fig. 6.6 Subluxated clear lens with lens coloboma, note the notch in lens due to broken zonules

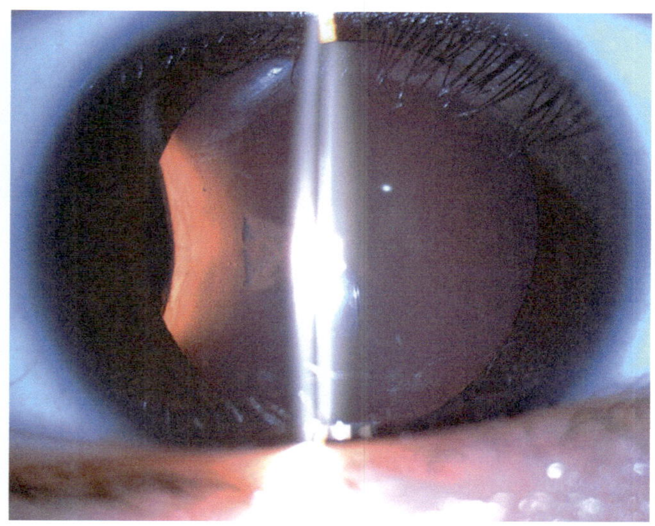

Fig. 6.7 Isolated coloboma of lens without subluxation, with visually insignificant cataract

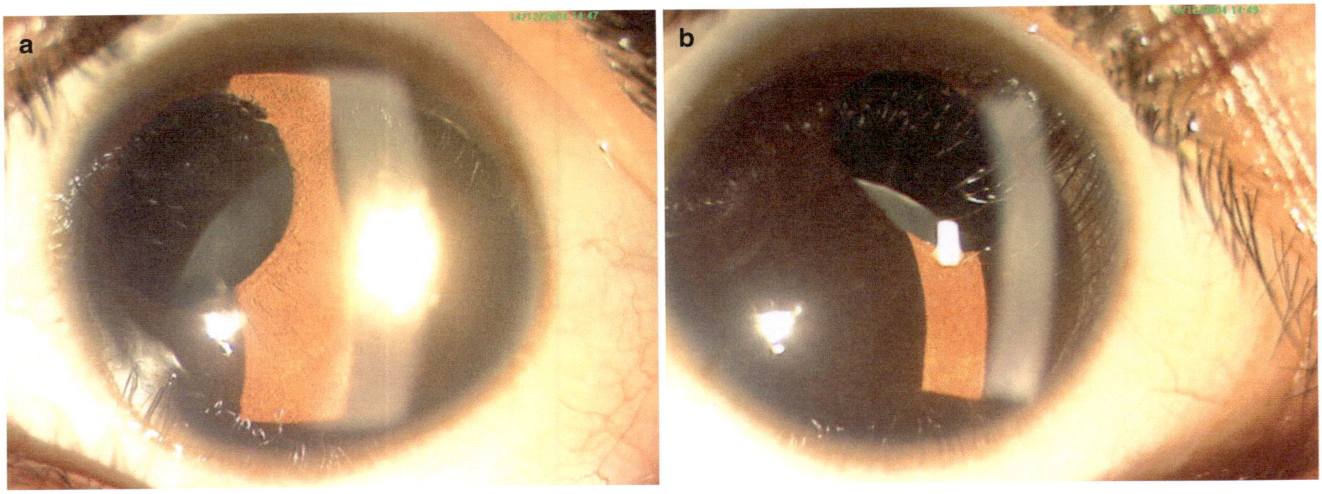

Fig. 6.8 (**a, b**) OD&OS, respectively, showing ectopia lentis et pupillae. Subluxation is seen in direction opposite to pupil

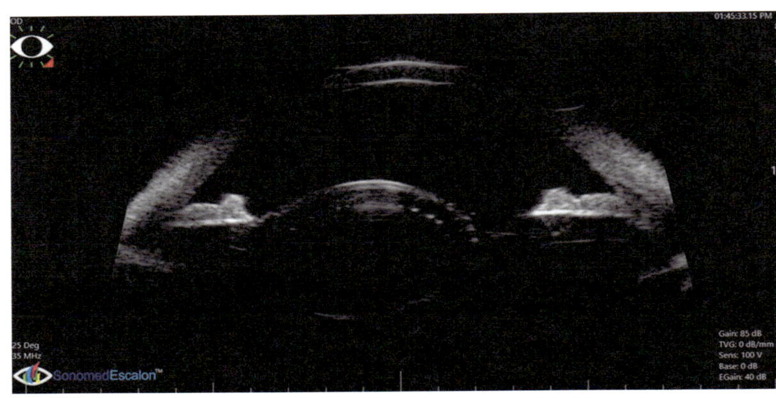

Fig. 6.9 Ultrasound biomicroscopy of subluxated lens showing no tilt, stretched zonules, and minimal opacification of lens

6.3 Investigations

In case of non-visualization of fundus, ultrasonography should be performed to assess the posterior segment status. Ultrasound biomicroscopy (UBM) can detect the area and extent of zonular dehiscence or stretching (Fig. 6.9).

Further increased lenticular sphericity, ciliary body flattening, and increased lens–ciliary body distance are indirect signs of zonular defects. Also, it allows the assessment of the lens in the supine position which is also the surgical position as subluxated lens is known to show variation with posture [10]. The endothelial count is documented as cases with pseudoexfoliation or aniridia may have preoperative low endothelial count and these surgeries are known to be difficult further lowering the endothelial count. With knowledge of these, extra precautions can be taken to avoid the endothelial loss.

6.4 Classification and Grading of Subluxation

6.4.1 Clarke gave one of them which goes as follows:

Clarke classification of congenital dislocation of lens [2].

Simple	There is a defective zonule and ciliary body, and apart from the dislocation of the lens, the eye is grossly normal
Associated with anomalies of ocular dimension	E.g., ectopia with axial myopia, microphthalmos or buphthalmos
Associated with anomalies of ocular structure	E.g., persistent pupillary membrane, corectopia, aniridia, polycoria, coloboma of iris, choroid, or lens, and megalocornea
Associated with congenital anomalies elsewhere in the body	E.g., dwarfism or arachnodactyly

6.4.2 Classification Based on Degree of Subluxation

Hoffman [10] classified degree of subluxation based on slit lamp examination under dilated pupil conditions (Fig. 6.10a–c):

Minimal to mild	The lens edge uncovers 0–25% of the dilated pupil
Moderate	The lens edge uncovers 25–50% of the dilated pupil
Severe	The lens edge uncovers greater than 50% of the dilated pupil

6.4.3 Another Classification Proposed

Another classification proposed, based on the lens displacement in relation to the undilated pupil, also allowed postoperative outcome prediction [11]. Using red field illumination, the subluxated lens was graded as: grade 1—lens seen on the pupillary area, grade 2—lens seen on 2/3 of the pupillary area, grade 3—lens seen on 1/2 of the pupillary area, or grade 4—lens absent from the pupillary area.

6.5 Management

6.5.1 Conservative Management

The management of subluxated lens depends on multiple factors including age of the patient, uncorrected and best corrected visual acuity, correction of refractive error achieved, visual discomfort to the patient, and the degree of lens subluxation [12]. Optimal correction of refractive error with glasses or contact lens should be the first line of management [13]. In mildly subluxated lens with lens in the pupillary axis or markedly subluxated lens with clear pupillary axis, patient may benefit with phakic or aphakic refractive correction, respectively. Other conservative methods like minimizing diplopia with the use of miotics or enlarging the phakic zone with the use of mydriatics are rarely used nowadays.

6.5.2 Surgical Treatment

Surgery is indicated in the following conditions:

- Significant refractive error in older children and adults, not corrected by conventional means like glasses or contact lens or patient unable to wear glasses and contact lens intolerant.
- Significant risk of amblyopia or amblyopia progression in younger children where no improvement is observed with optimal refractive correction and patching.
- Significant diplopia caused by subluxated lens bisecting the pupillary axis.
- Significant progressive subluxation of lens or lens threatening to dislocate anterior or posteriorly.
- Significant cataract and angle closure glaucoma.
- Secondary glaucoma related to lens subluxation.

6.5.3 Route of Surgery

The route of lensectomy depends upon the comfort of the surgeon and case requirement. Anterior route can be used when limited anterior vitrectomy is planned along with IOL implantation. Pars plana route can be used for more extensive vitrectomy especially when IOL implantation is not to be done, or in cases with severe lens subluxation posteriorly into the vitreous cavity in the supine position [14].

6.5.4 Surgical Techniques

Cataract surgery in subluxated lenses requires good technique. The type of surgery and the requirement of use of endocapsular support devices depends on the nature of disease and the degree of subluxation. (Table 6.2) It is safer to make incision opposite to the direction of subluxation as it allows for counteraction against the strongest zonular area and prevents any sudden loss of viscoelastic to cause vitreous prolapse in the wound area. Vitreous in the anterior chamber is first taken care of by limited vitrectomy. The vitreous can be identified by triamcinolone acetonide use [15]. However, care should be taken to avoid its excessive use. The exposed posterior hyaloid face can be covered with dispersive ophthalmic viscosurgical device (OVD) which prevents further vitreous prolapse and avoids posterior migration of the lens fragments. The anterior chamber should be maintained with OVD repeatedly during the entire surgery. The loss of OVD during surgery can cause progressive shallowing of the anterior chamber and increased lens movement which can complicate the surgery.

Capsulorhexis is a crucial step to allow phacoemulsification and bag preservation during surgery. The zonular compromise and elasticity present challenges to create a continuous circular centered capsulorhexis. The capsulorhexis must be centered on the crystalline lens and not on the pupil or corneal apex. Also, 2 mm edge must be

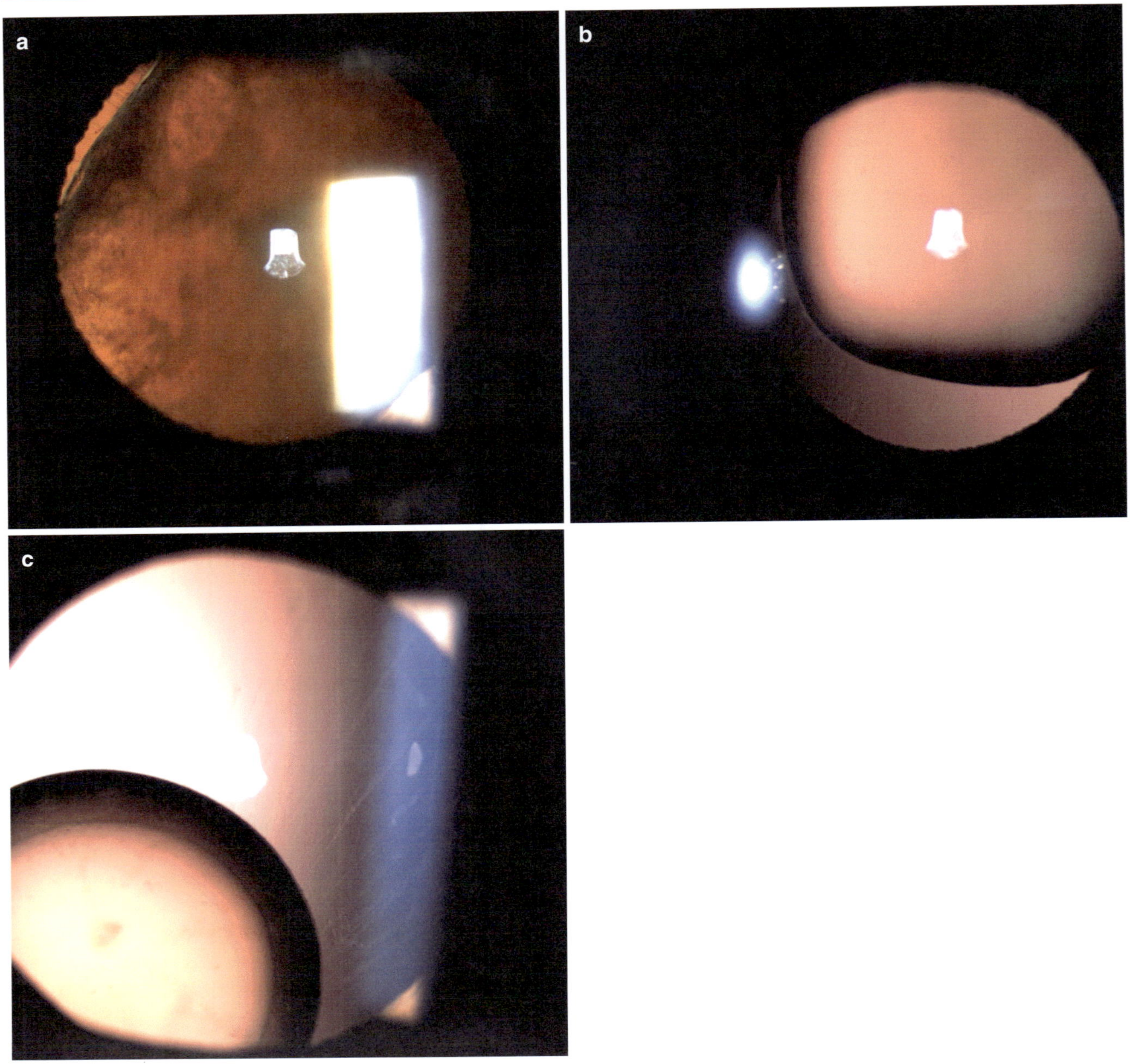

Fig. 6.10 Grading of subluxation. (**a**) Mild subluxation, (**b**) moderate subluxation, (**c**) severe subluxation

Table 6.2 Surgical management of ectopia lentis

Up to 3 clock hours	CTR(capsular tension ring) with IOL implantation Larger sized IOL can be used with haptics being used to stretch the bag
>3 to 6 clock hours	Modified CTR with single loop(Cionni) with IOL implantation
>6 to 9 clock hours	Modified CTR with double loop/Cionni or dual support—Modified CTR with CTS(capsular tension segment) with IOL implantation in the bag
>9 clock hours	ICCE or intralenticular aspiration with ACIOL or scleral fixated IOL in the same or different sitting

maintained between the capsulorhexis edge and the equator. Staining with few drops of trypan blue dye across the anterior capsule in an OVD-filled anterior chamber prevents minimal entry of dye in the vitreous to cause red reflex loss. A standard cystitome, a microvitreoretinal blade, or a straight 25-gauge needle can be used to penetrate the capsule. Vitreoretinal forceps can be used to complete capsulorhexis and allows entry through a smaller wound with decreased risk of loss of OVD from the anterior chamber as compared to capsulorhexis forceps. To support the bag, flexible iris retractors can be used to hook the capsulorhexis edge after capsulorhexis is made. Capsule hooks on contrary support the bag at its equator keeping it distended.

Hydrodissection and viscodissection are important steps as when inadequately performed they can create excessive stress on the zonule during phacoemulsification and cortical aspiration. Soft lens in younger children allows for aspiration of lens matter with irrigation/aspiration (I/A) handpieces or a cannula. A modified technique of endocapsular lens aspiration by the limbal route in severely subluxated lens has been recently described [16, 17].

6.5.5 Endocapsular Support Devices

The endocapsular support devices like capsular tension ring (CTR), Ahmed capsular tension segments (CTS), or Cionni are helpful in improving intraoperative safety and providing long-term stability of the IOL-capsule system. It also reduces postoperative capsular contraction and subsequent IOL decentration [18–20]. Although some amount of capsular phimosis is inevitable even with CTR in site (Fig. 6.11). By creating an equally distributed centrifugal force to the equator of the bag, the CTR recruits tension from stronger zonules to support the areas of weak or absent zonules. This stabilizes the entire IOL-capsule complex in mild subluxated cases but difficult to achieve recentration in severe cases [21]. In these situations, a Cionni or a CTS provides a stable long-term solution through scleral-fixation [22] (Fig. 6.12).

CTS is a partial PMMA ring segment of 120-deg arc with an anteriorly positioned fixation eyelet. Also, cases with a progressive pathology, zonular problems are expected to worsen over time and thus CTR/CTS/Cionni should be placed in these patients even if subluxation is mild. Presence of anterior or posterior capsular tear is considered as a contraindication to the use of CTR as the centrifugal force generated by the ring may cause an extension of the tear with risk of loss of the CTR to the posterior segment. A CTS can be possibly used in such cases with discontinuous rhexis, anterior or posterior capsular tear as it does not create a 360 deg expansile force (Fig. 6.13). The size of the CTR selected depends on the capsular bag dimension which correlates with the axial length and corneal diameter. Thus, horizontal white to white and axial length are used as a guide to select the size [20, 23]. Also, the time of placement has been debatable and depends on the capsular stability, device preferred, and choice of surgeon. Early placement provides capsular stability but may cause increased manipulations and zonular stress compared with placement after cataract removal [24–27].

Capsular phimosis and/or IOL bag displacement are inevitable complication without the use of endocapsular fixation in these patients (Figs. 6.14 and 6.15).

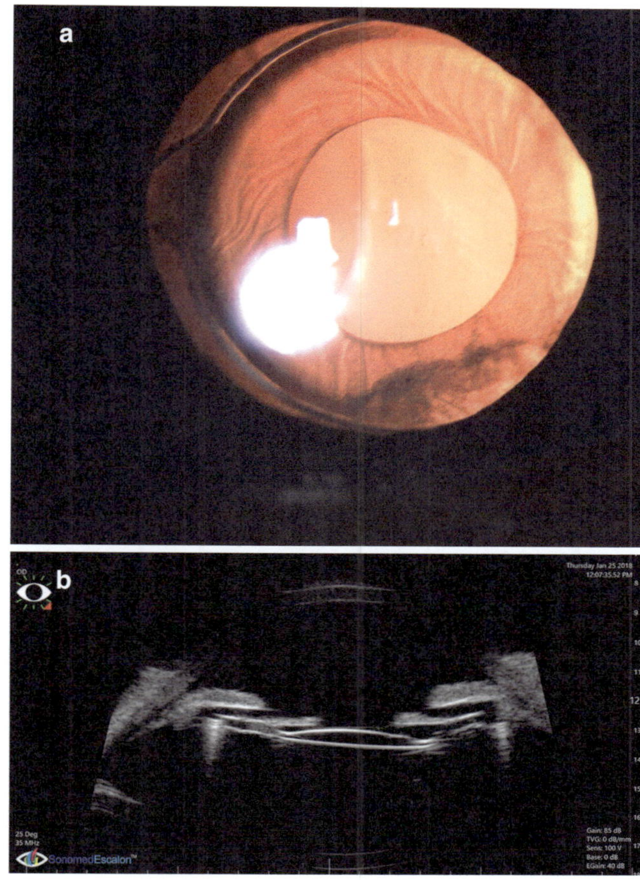

Fig. 6.11 3-year postoperative picture of a 14-year-old girl operated for mild subluxation (2 clock hours) with CTR in situ. (**a**) Clinical picture showing anterior capsular fibrosis with mild contracture. (**b**) Ultrasound biomicroscopy of the same showing IOL in bag, anterior capsular thickening, and minimal tilt, also note the after shadow of CTR

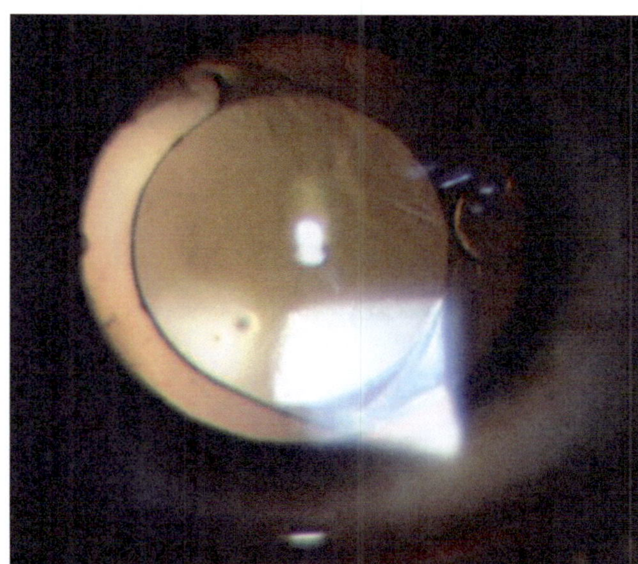

Fig. 6.12 2-year postoperative picture of a 17-year-old boy with IOL and Cionni ring in bag, well-centered IOL

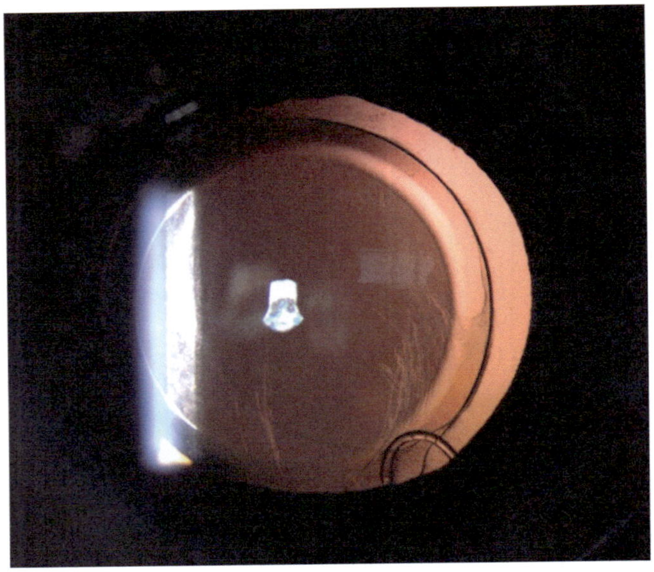

Fig. 6.13 18-month post-operative picture of a 13-year-old girl with IOL in bag and CTS holding IOL in place. Note inferior oval posterior capsular defect, CTS is a better option in these cases than Cionni ring

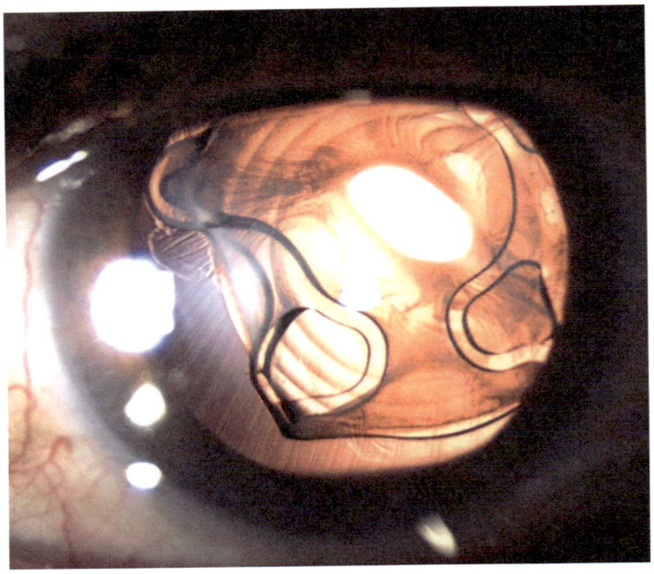

Fig. 6.15 10-year postoperative picture of 15-year-old patient with progressive subluxation. Severe anterior capsular contraction with overriding plate haptic of hydrophilic lens is noted. Note lack of endocapsular fixation and stretched zonules

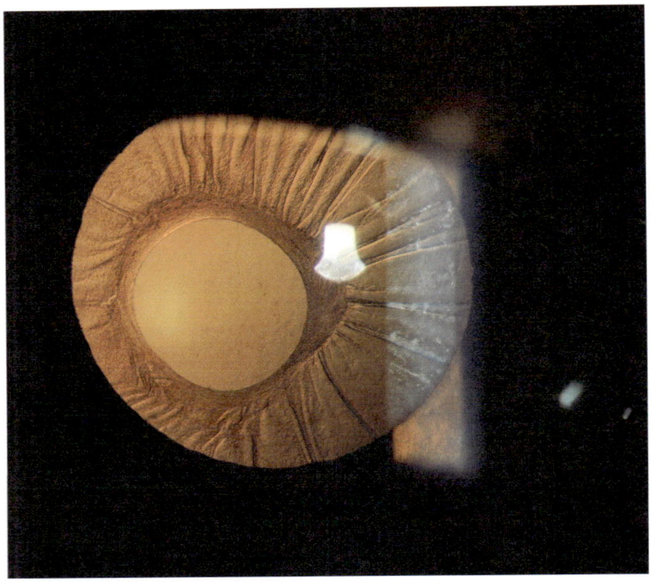

Fig. 6.14 Anterior capsular phimosis with moderate contracture in circular as well as linear pattern

6.5.6 Intraocular Lens (IOL)

In cases with an intact posterior capsule, a single piece IOL is implanted in the bag. However in cases with inadequate capsular support, ACIOL/iris fixated lens or SFIOL can be opt for [28–30] (Fig. 6.16a, b). Scleral suture-fixated IOLs and glued IOLs are being used in cases with subluxated lenses especially in individuals >10 years, those with healthy sclera, absence of any connective tissue disorders, and normal anterior chamber angle [30].

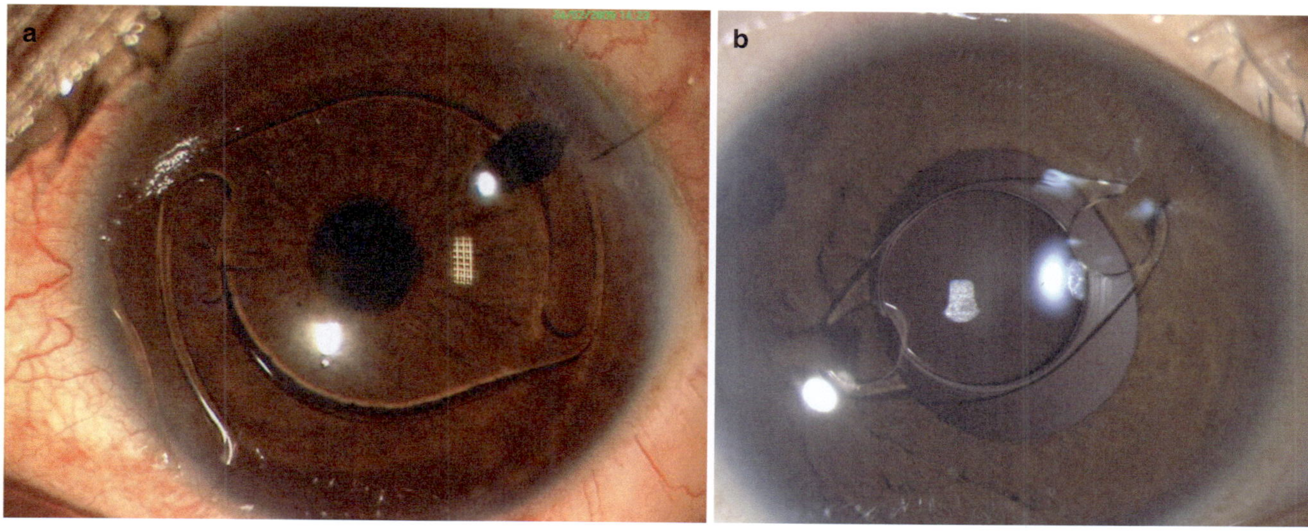

Fig. 6.16 Postoperative picture of cases with severe subluxations. (**a**) ACIOL in place, mid-peripheral iridotomy is patent. (**b**) Iris claw lens in place, peripheral iridotomy is patent

References

1. Nemet AY, Assia EI, Apple DJ, Barequet IS. Current concepts of ocular manifestations in Marfan syndrome. Surv Ophthalmol. 2006;51(6):561–75.
2. Clarke CC. Ectopia lentis: a pathologic and clinical study. Arch Ophthalmol. 1939;21(1):124–53.
3. Faivre L, Dollfus H, Lyonnet S, Alembik Y, Mégarbané A, Samples J, et al. Clinical homogeneity and genetic heterogeneity in Weill-Marchesani syndrome. Am J Med Genet A. 2003;123A(2):204–7.
4. Burke JP, O'Keefe M, Bowell R, Naughten ER. Ocular complications in homocystinuria—early and late treated. Br J Ophthalmol. 1989;73(6):427–31.
5. Tunçbilek E, Alanay Y. Congenital contractural arachnodactyly (Beals syndrome). Orphanet J Rare Dis. 2006;1:20. https://doi.org/10.1186/1750-1172-1-20.
6. Harrison DA, Mullaney PB, Mesfer SA, Awad AH, Dhindsa H. Management of ophthalmic complications of homocystinuria. Ophthalmology. 1998;105(10):1886–90.
7. Cross HE, Jensen AD. Ocular manifestations in the Marfan syndrome and homocystinuria. Am J Ophthalmol. 1973;75(3):405–20.
8. Pavlin CJ, Buys YM, Pathmanathan T. Imaging zonular abnormalities using ultrasound biomicroscopy. Arch Ophthalmol. 1998;116(7):854–7.
9. Waiswol M, Kasahara N. Lens subluxation grading system: predictive value for ectopia lentis surgical outcomes. Einstein. 2009;7:81–7.
10. Hoffman RS, Snyder ME, Devgan U, Allen QB, Yeoh R, Braga-Mele R. Management of the subluxated crystalline lens. J Cataract Refract Surg. 2013;39(12):1904–15.
11. Neely DE, Plager DA. Management of ectopia lentis in children. Ophthalmol Clin N Am. 2001;14(3):493–9.
12. Wu-Chen WY, Letson RD, Summers CG. Functional and structural outcomes following lensectomy for ectopia lentis. J AAPOS. 2005;9(4):353–7.
13. Burk SE, Da Mata AP, Snyder ME, Schneider S, Osher RH, Cionni RJ. Visualizing vitreous using Kenalog suspension. J Cataract Refract Surg. 2003;29(4):645–51.
14. Khokhar S, Aron N, Yadav N, Pillay G, Agarwal E. Modified technique of endocapsular lens aspiration for severely subluxated lenses. Eye. 2017;32:128.
15. Sinha R, Sharma N, Vajpayee RB. Intralenticular bimanual irrigation: aspiration for subluxated lens in Marfan's syndrome. J Cataract Refract Surg. 2005;31(7):1283–6.
16. Praveen MR, Vasavada AR, Singh R. Phacoemulsification in subluxated cataract. Indian J Ophthalmol. 2003;51(2):147.
17. Gimbel HV, Sun R. Clinical applications of capsular tension rings in cataract surgery. Ophthalmic Surg Lasers. 2002;33(1):44–53.
18. Weber CH, Cionni RJ. All about capsular tension rings. Curr Opin Ophthalmol. 2015;26(1):10–5.
19. Menapace R, Findl O, Georgopoulos M, Rainer G, Vass C, Schmetterer K. The capsular tension ring: designs, applications, and techniques. J Cataract Refract Surg. 2000;26(6):898–912.
20. Cionni RJ, Osher RH. Management of profound zonular dialysis or weakness with a new endocapsular ring designed for scleral fixation. J Cataract Refract Surg. 1998;24(10):1299–306.
21. Dong EY, Joo CK. Predictability for proper capsular tension ring size and intraocular lens size. Korean J Ophthalmol. 2001;15(1):22–6.
22. Dietlein TS, Jacobi PC, Konen W, Krieglstein GK. Complications of endocapsular tension ring implantation in a child with Marfan's syndrome. J Cataract Refract Surg. 2000;26(6):937–40.
23. Bayraktar S, Altan T, Küçüksümer Y, Yilmaz OF. Capsular tension ring implantation after capsulorhexis in phacoemulsification of cataracts associated with pseudoexfoliation syndrome. Intraoperative

complications and early postoperative findings. J Cataract Refract Surg. 2001;27(10):1620–8.
24. Blecher MH, Kirk MR. Surgical strategies for the management of zonular compromise. Curr Opin Ophthalmol. 2008;19(1):31–5.
25. Ahmed IIK, Cionni RJ, Kranemann C, Crandall AS. Optimal timing of capsular tension ring implantation: Miyake-Apple video analysis. J Cataract Refract Surg. 2005;31(9):1809–13.
26. Wagoner MD, Cox TA, Ariyasu RG, Jacobs DS, Karp CL, American Academy of Ophthalmology. Intraocular lens implantation in the absence of capsular support: a report by the American Academy of Ophthalmology. Ophthalmology. 2003;110(4):840–59.
27. Hoffman RS, Fine IH, Packer M. Primary anterior chamber intraocular lens for the treatment of severe crystalline lens subluxation. J Cataract Refract Surg. 2009;35(10):1821–5.
28. Luk ASW, Young AL, Cheng LL. Long-term outcome of scleral-fixated intraocular lens implantation. Br J Ophthalmol. 2013;97(10):1308–11.
29. Gabor SGB, Pavlidis MM. Sutureless intrascleral posterior chamber intraocular lens fixation. J Cataract Refract Surg. 2007;33(11):1851–4.
30. Agarwal A, Kumar DA, Jacob S, Baid C, Agarwal A, Srinivasan S. Fibrin glue-assisted sutureless posterior chamber intraocular lens implantation in eyes with deficient posterior capsules. J Cataract Refract Surg. 2008;34(9):1433–8.

Spherophakia: A Rare Condition Affecting Pediatric Eyes

7

Sagnik Sen, Chirakshi Dhull, and Sudarshan Kumar Khokhar

Spherophakia (SP) is a rare disabling developmental disease, which commonly is seen in both eyes associated with high lenticular myopia along with a risk of chronic glaucoma development and often patients present with a systemic syndromic manifestation. Prevalence of spherophakia is unclear because of the rare occurrence of the disease. SP can be seen as an isolated condition or may be familial. Familial cases have been reported in lineage studies and consanguinity has been found to be a characteristic finding in all these reports [1, 2]. Systemic associations have been found with homocysteinemia, Weill–Marchesani syndrome, Marfan's syndrome, Alport's syndrome, hyperlysinemia, congenital rubella syndrome, megalocornea-spherophakia-secondary glaucoma, arrhythmogenic right ventricular dysplasia type 1, spinocerebellar ataxia, etc. [3]. Spherophakia has been seen to commonly occur in patients of Weill–Marchesani syndrome (WMS) and the prevalence of WMS has been estimated at 1:100,000. Data from India has shown that 1.2% of children presenting with lens abnormalities have spherophakia [4].

Pathologically, the lens zonules in spherophakia patients are developmentally hypoplastic and abnormally weak and the crystalline lens becomes spherical because of nonattachment of the weak posterior zonules to the lens equator [5]. The lens does not achieve its normal biconvex shape during childhood and puberty. The spherical lens may undergo subluxation or dislocation from the patellar fossa leading to glaucoma and reduced vision.

7.1 Clinical features

A triad of angle-closure glaucoma, shallow anterior chamber, and high myopia is highly suggestive of SP. Patients usually present with reduced vision or acute eye pain. A lot of patients may have developed amblyopia because of uncorrected lenticular myopia since childhood and amblyopia may be bilateral. Others would be using thick aspheric meniscus lenses for visual rehabilitation.

Clinically, SP is diagnosed when the equator of the entire crystalline lens is visible after full mydriasis (Figs. 7.1 and 7.2). Lens is usually clear and differentiation. Lens may be smaller in size when it is referred to as microspherophakia (Fig. 7.1). Typical golden rings may be seen in distant direct examination, which aids in diagnosis (Fig. 7.3). The intraocular findings are spherical lens, iridodonesis, and axial as well as lenticular myopia.

The physical features reflect the associated syndrome. Marfan syndrome is an autosomal dominant condition causing cardiac, skeletal, and muscular abnormalities along with lens subluxation and SP [3, 6]. Patients have arachnodactyly, tall stature, high arched palate, increased upper segment–lower segment ratio, joint laxity with upward dislocation of the lens. SP is seen in some cases.

Homocystinuria patients present with tall stature and progressive lens subluxation and rarely SP [3]. Homocysteine levels may be raised in the urine and serum. Homocystinuria cases have been seen to be associated with seizures and hemiparesis due to a hypercoagulable state [7]. Patients may also have musculoskeletal or metabolic diseases. However, they usually do not have buphthalmos, abnormal angle anatomy, or increased axial length, which helps differentiate them from primary congenital glaucoma.

WMS is however the commonest association of SP and is an autosomal recessive disorder leading to short stature, brachydactyly, and joint stiffness (Fig. 7.4a–e) [3, 8]. Inferior lens subluxation and SP are commonly seen. Progressive SP may lead to sever progressive myopia.

The lens subluxation can occur superiorly, inferiorly, or anteriorly into the anterior chamber and posteriorly into the vitreous cavity (Fig. 7.5a, b). Most patients have high myopia which can be corrected by spectacles or contact lenses. However, with anterior subluxation of the lens, patients can present with pupillary block glaucoma due to the spontane-

S. Sen
Dr. Rajendra Prasad Centre for Ophthalmic Sciences, All India Institute of Medical Sciences, New Delhi, India

Aravind Eye Hospital, Madurai, India

C. Dhull · S. K. Khokhar (✉)
Dr. Rajendra Prasad Centre for Ophthalmic Sciences, All India Institute of Medical Sciences, New Delhi, India

S. K. Khokhar, C. Dhull (eds.), *Atlas of Pediatric Cataract*, https://doi.org/10.1007/978-981-13-6939-1_7

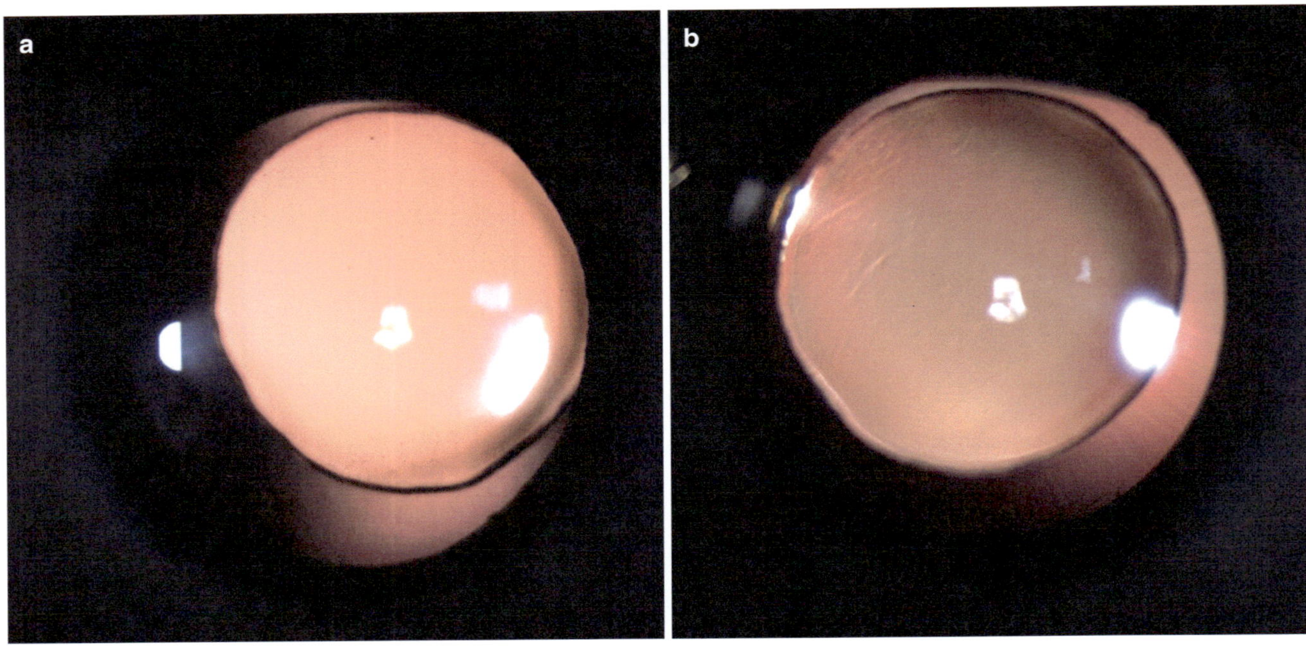

Fig. 7.1 Microspherophakia. (**a** and **b**) Retroillumination picture of right and left eye, respectively, showing small clear lens, with margins of the lens seen 360° along with stretched zonules

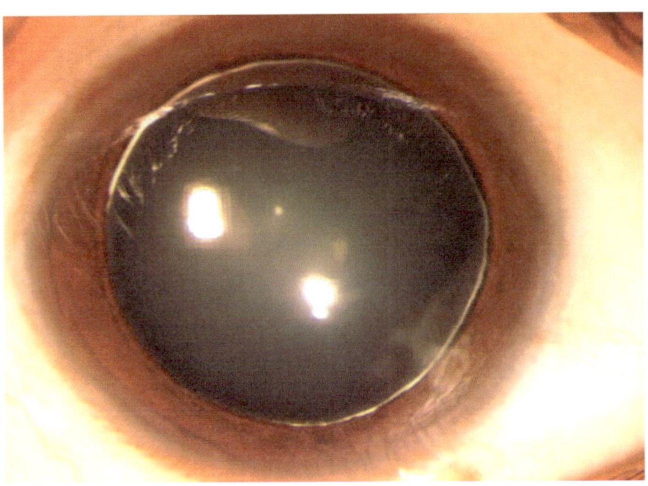

Fig. 7.2 Spherophakia: Slit lamp picture in diffuse illumination showing lens margin in all quadrants except inferonasal, lens appears near normal in size

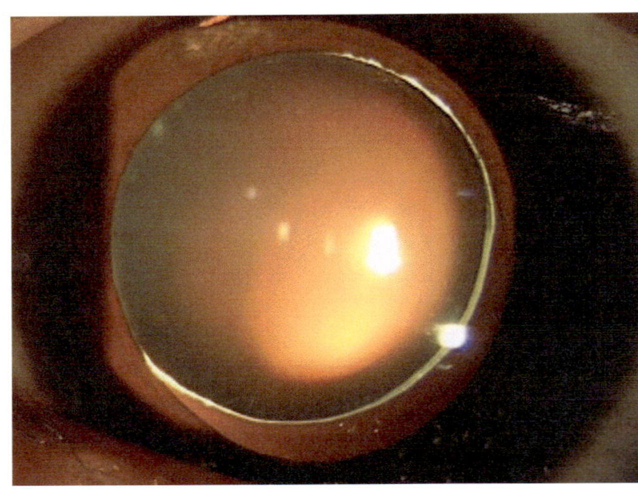

Fig. 7.3 Golden ring sign seen in spherophakia in retroillumination or distant direct examination. Patent peripheral iridotomy is seen supero nasal quadrant of iris

ous shift of iris-lens diaphragm anteriorly [9, 10]. Also, if the lens comes to lie in the anterior chamber, they can present with severe pain due to mechanical angle closure and "inverse glaucoma," since miosis will lead to inability of the subluxated lens to return to the patellar fossa [11] (Fig. 7.6a, b). This condition is deteriorated by miotics and relieved by mydriatic agents [12]. Spontaneous dislocation may be a common cause of lens dislocation [13]. Post-traumatic dislocation may also happen due to the zonules being weak. Movement of the lens into the anterior chamber may be intermittent causing episodic acute glaucoma attacks and may be associated with an eventual retinal detachment due to repeated vitreous traction [10]. Chronic pupillary block may result in trabecular meshwork crowding and if untreated may lead to peripheral anterior synechiae formation with a future risk of raised IOP and secondary glaucoma [14].

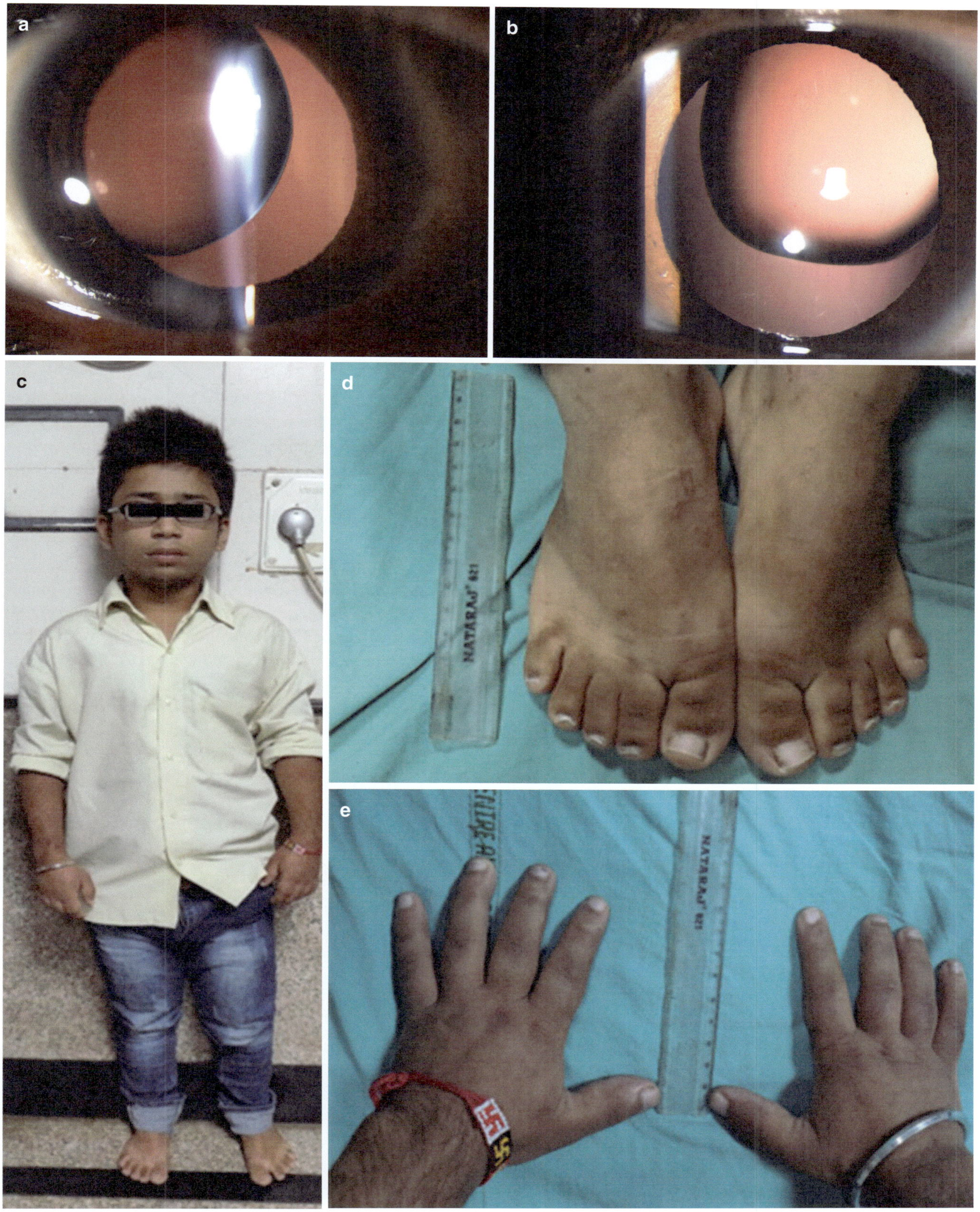

Fig. 7.4 16-year-old boy with Weill–Marchesani syndrome with spherophakia. (**a** and **b**) Retroillumination picture of right and left eye, respectively, showing spherophakia with supero-temporal subluxation and broken zonules. (**c**) Notice short stature of the patient. (**d**) Small feet with short toes. (**e**) Short, stubby fingers are seen

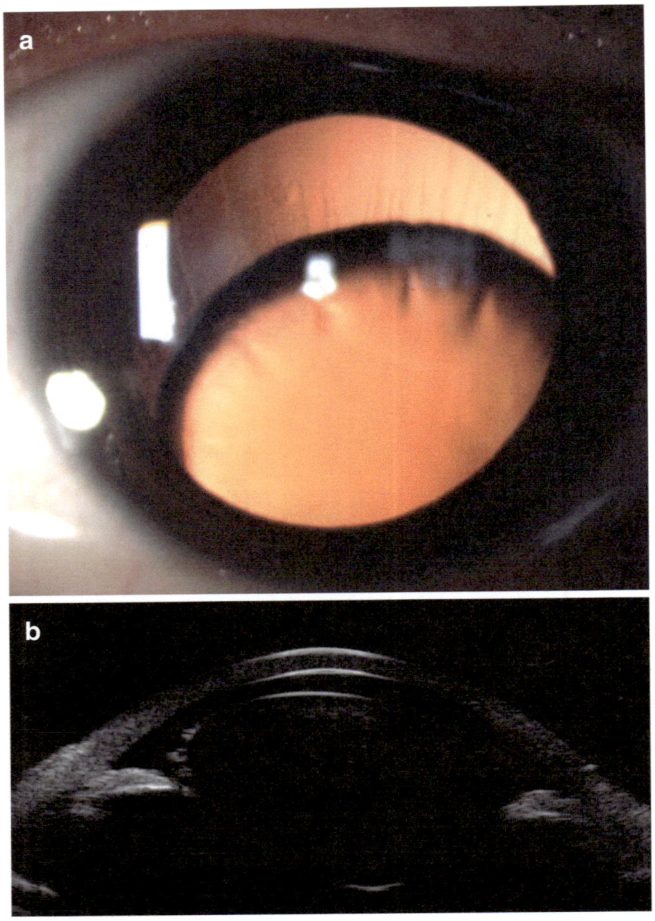

Fig. 7.5 (**a**) Clinical picture of spherophakia with inferiorly subluxated lens with party broken zonules (**b**) UBM of the same showing spontaneous incomplete anterior subluxation in lying down position

7.2 Inheritance

Small round lens presenting as an isolated abnormality without any systemic association is a recessive condition. Non-syndromic SP is rarely found. Familial SP is not associated with systemic diseases and both autosomal recessive and autosomal dominant inheritance have been reported [15–17].

7.3 Genetics

One study found homozygosity in a region of 14q chromosome containing the LTPB2 gene [18]. Another study identified homozygosity for a frameshift mutation in LTBP2 gene [17]. LTBP2 or TGF β-binding protein 2 is a family of proteins having similar structure to fibrillins and these are expressed in the trabecular meshwork, ciliary processes, lens capsule, and lens epithelium. Isolated spherophakia has been said to be caused by a homozygous LTBP2 mutation. A few other studies failed to find such chromosomal homozygosity and said that SP is a heterozygous disease.

Non-syndromic familial lens subluxation cases have been reported to be associated with autosomal recessively inherited ADAMTSL4 gene mutations or with autosomal-dominantly inherited FBN1 mutations [19, 20]. WMS cases have been reported to be associated with ADAMTSL10 gene mutations [20]. Overall, LTBP2, FBN1, and ADAMTS gene mutations are believed to be associated with abnormality of zonules leading to lens subluxation and SP.

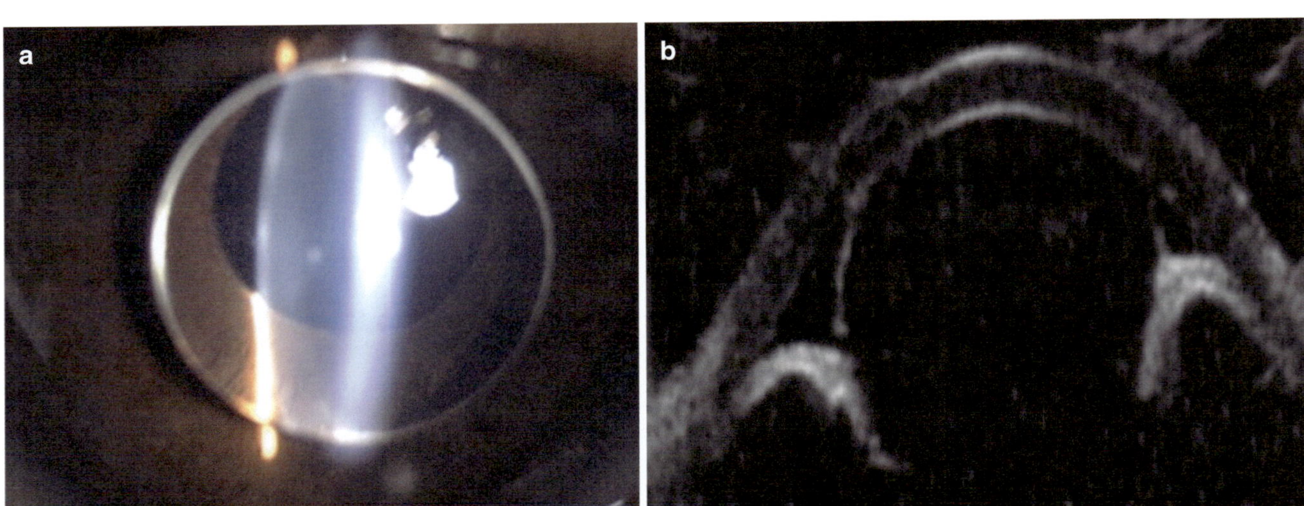

Fig. 7.6 (**a**) Spontaneous anteriorly dislocated lens with small pupil. (**b**) UBM of the same showing pupillary block (source Khokhar et al. [28])

7.4 Investigations

7.4.1 Anterior Segment Optical Coherence Tomography (ASOCT)

High resolution optical coherence tomography of the anterior segment using time-domain or spectral-domain technology may give a cross-sectional image of the cornea, anterior chamber angle and the lenticular anatomy and is useful to determine the shape of the lens and the orientation of the iris-lens diaphragm to identify pupillary block.

7.4.2 Ultrasound Biomicroscopy (UBM)

This technology uses ultrasound waves to produce two-dimensional cross-sectional images of the anterior segment showing morphology of the anterior chamber angle, iris, ciliary body, zonules, and lens. UBM has been used to effectively assess corneal diseases, ciliary body tumors, and congenital cataracts.

7.4.3 B-scan Ultrasonography for Posterior Segment Examination

B-scan ultrasound is useful to assess the status of the retina and vitreous in cases where pupils are poorly dilating or the lens is opacified.

7.4.4 Biometry

Biometry forms an important part of planning during intraocular lens implantation after lens extraction. Immersion ultrasound biometry or IOL Master Optical biometry may be helpful. Since the eyes of SP patients are myopic with longer axial lengths, SRK-T or Holladay I formulae may be useful for intraocular lens power calculation.

7.5 Management Options

7.5.1 Lens Management

Patients of very high lenticular myopia or lens subluxation, anterior or posterior, require lens extraction followed by refractive rehabilitation, which may be in the forms of aphakic spectacles, contact lenses, and intraocular lenses (IOLs) [21]. The type of IOL chosen depends on the surgeon and patient factors. The options include angle-supported anterior chamber IOLs (ACIOL) (Fig. 7.7), iris-enclavated IOLs, posterior chamber IOLs (PCIOL), and scleral-fixated IOL (SFIOL) [22–24]. Angle-supported ACIOLs are associated with corneal endothelial cell loss, peripheral anterior synechiae (PAS) formation, and glaucoma due to chronic anterior chamber irritation, which may be of concern in the younger population [25]. Iris-enclavated lenses avoid the angle-related complications and may be placed anterior [22] or posterior [26] to the iris. Traumatic

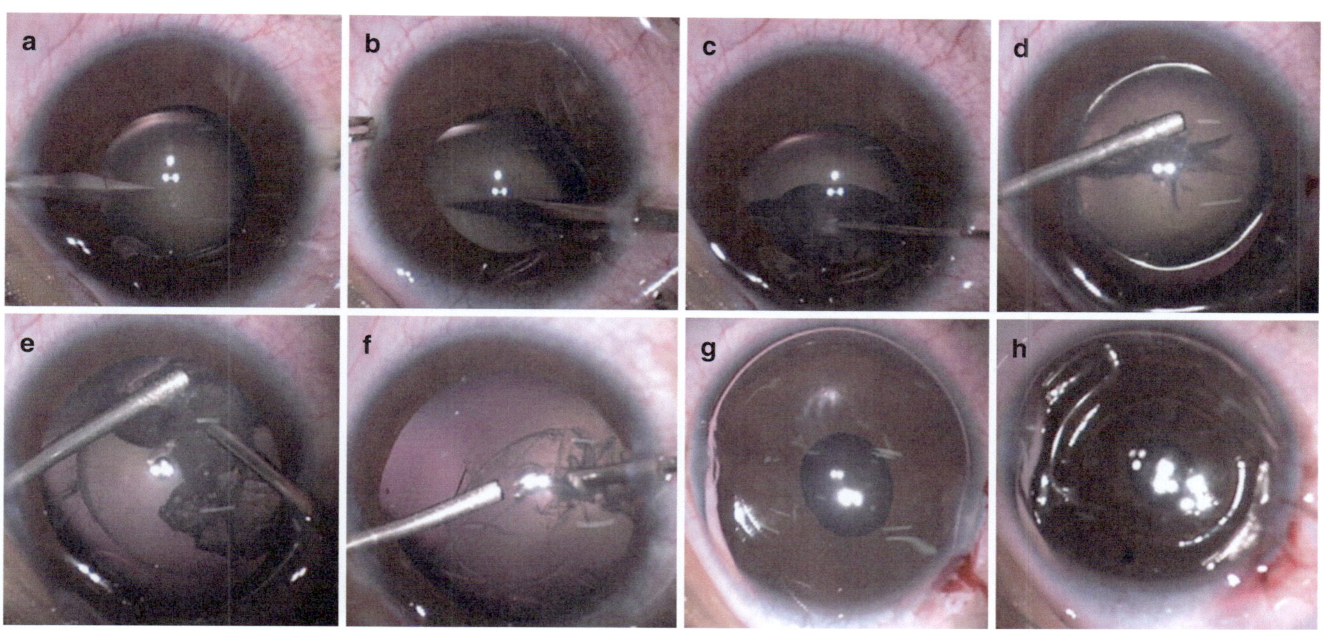

Fig. 7.7 Lensectomy with ACIOL. (**a–c**) Two MVR entry with entry in the lens, (**d**) irrigation port of vitrectomy cutter inside lens, (**e**) lensectomy with cutter, (**f**) capsular bag removed with cutter, (**g**) AC formed with air, (**h**) ACIOL placed under air (source Khokhar et al. [28])

de-enclavations may be a cause for concern with these lenses [27] in pediatric ages. However, on account of iris-enclavated lenses having highly inflated prices, limited availability and affordability as compared to angle-supported lenses, ACIOLs may be of considerable importance in the Indian context [28].

PCIOL placement in the capsular bag is controversial since the zonules are developmentally weak with a possibility of bag-lens complex dropping into the vitreous cavity [29]. We have previously demonstrated a "dual-support technique" of insertion of a capsular tension segment (CTS) with tension ring (CTR) along with PCIOL in a case of spherophakia to help overcome zonular weakness (Fig. 7.8) [30]. We have also seen long-term follow-up of such patients who maintain good centration following dual support (Figs. 7.9 and 7.10).

Scleral-fixated PCIOL (SFIOL) in aphakic children has been performed without angle-related concerns. However, children have more elastic and less rigid sclera as compared to adults. Hence, there is always a chance of scleral dehiscence (Fig. 7.11). Moreover, trans-scleral suture exposure and late onset suture degradation are all possibilities [31]. In patients having corneal white-to-white diameter >13 mm, such as megalocornea, SFIOL, or ACIOL are not preferred, considering IOL instability and decentration, respectively. In such cases, iris-enclavated lenses are the best choice [32]. If IOL is placed in the bag without CTR/CTS, it invariable leads to anterior capsular phimosis, decentration and IOL instability (Fig. 7.12).

After implantation of IOL, the patients have to be followed up for amblyopia treatment. In spite of all efforts, postsurgical cases invariably suffer from some extent of amblyopia because of noncompliance to glasses and amblyopia therapy [33].

7.5.2 Glaucoma Management

Apart from topical and/or systemic medications, pupillary block cases are treated with laser or surgical peripheral iridotomy [27, 34]. Some surgeons have suggested trabeculectomy for control of intraocular pressure [29]. Simple lens extraction may also control IOP to some extent; however, it may be temporary and a trabeculectomy may be required at a later date [29, 31]. Inverse glaucoma cases almost always require lens extraction for immediate control of IOP.

To conclude, spherophakia is a rare ocular disease with multiple systemic associations. Ocular disability may require simple interventions like spectacles or contact lenses or may require lens extraction and intraocular lens implantation. Glaucoma may be associated with the natural history of the disease and may require medical and/or surgical management.

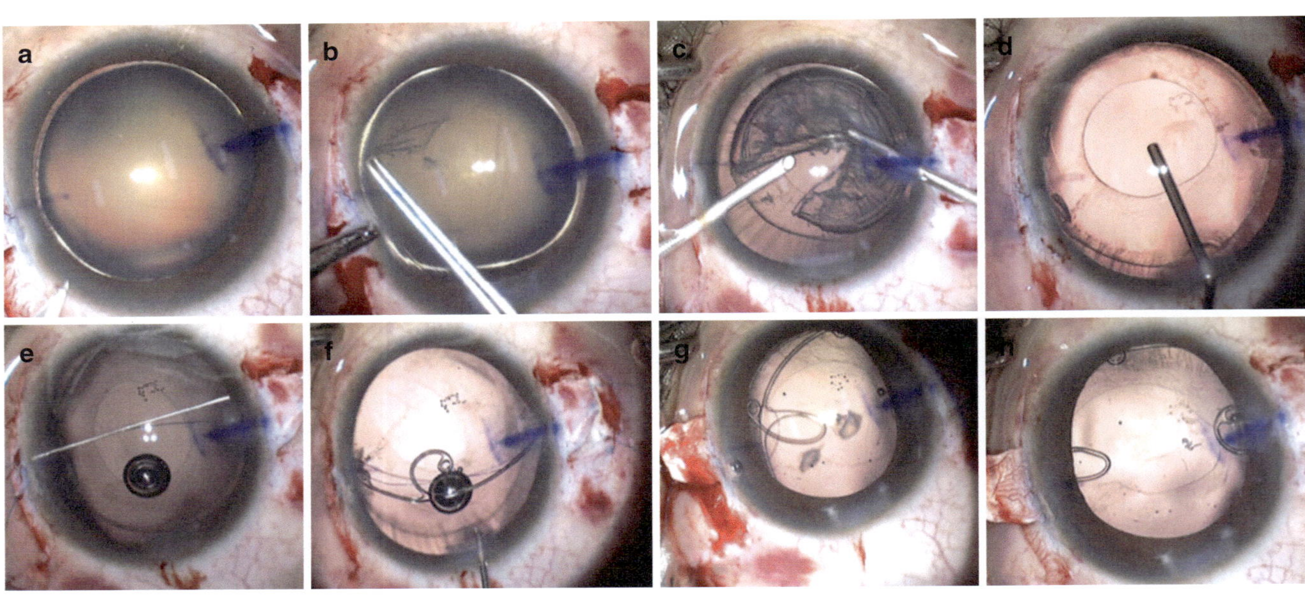

Fig. 7.8 Dual fixation technique. (**a**) Spherophakia with two scleral tunnel 180° across. (**b**) Anterior capsulorhexis completed using Utrata forceps. (**c**) Lensectomy performed inside the bag. (**d**) Intact bag after completion on lensectomy. (**e**) 9-0 prolene being used to fix Cionni ring with sclera. (**f**) Cionni ring in the bag G. CTS in the bag (opposite side). (**h**) Final position after placing IOL with superior and inferior fixation

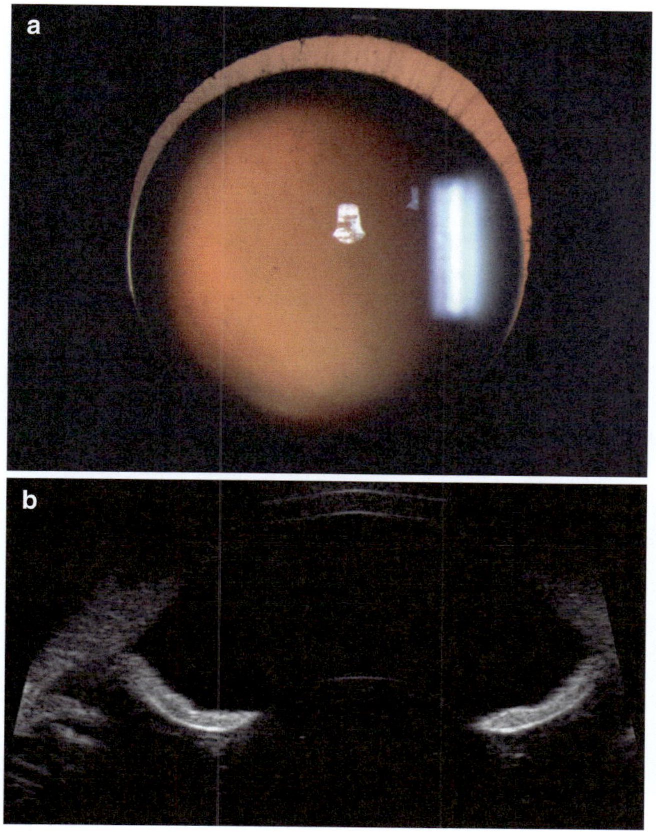

Fig. 7.9 Preoperative picture of a 15-year-old girl with spherophakia. (**a**) Retroillumination picture, (**b**) UBM of the same showing small, globular lens and iris bowing posteriorly

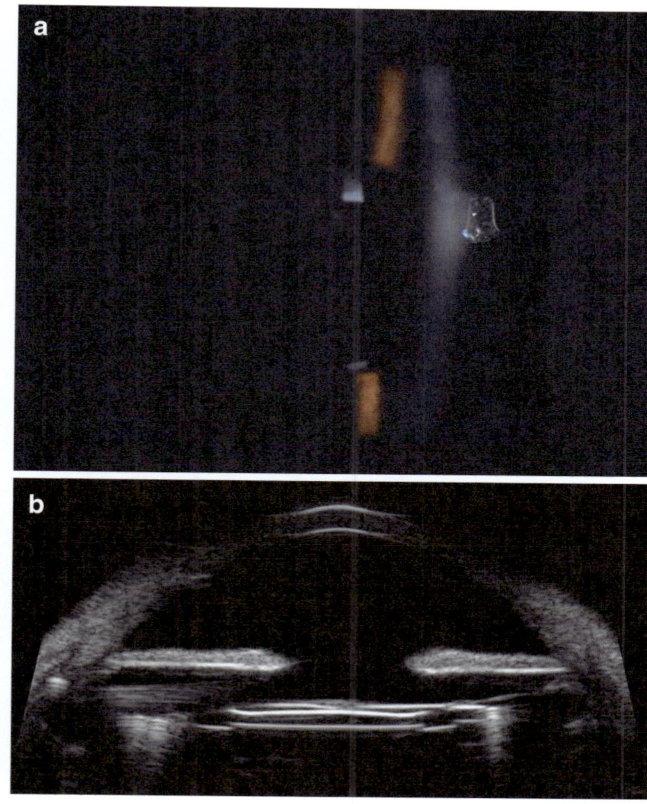

Fig. 7.10 Postoperative picture of the same patient after 3 years. (**a**) Slit examination showing fibrosis of anterior capsule and IOL in bag with no clinical tilt (**b**) UBM of the patient showing IOL in bag with good centration and no tilt. Note the reverberations from both the edges of the IOL-bag complex caused by loop of Cionni ring and CTS

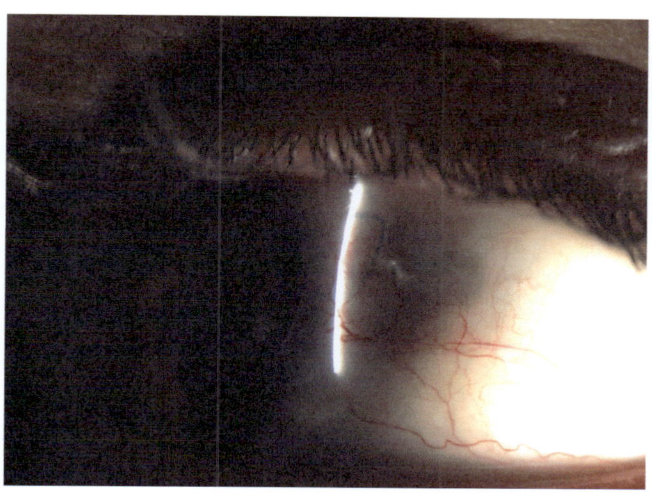

Fig. 7.11 Haptic extrusion in a case of spherophakia 6 months after SFIOL implantation

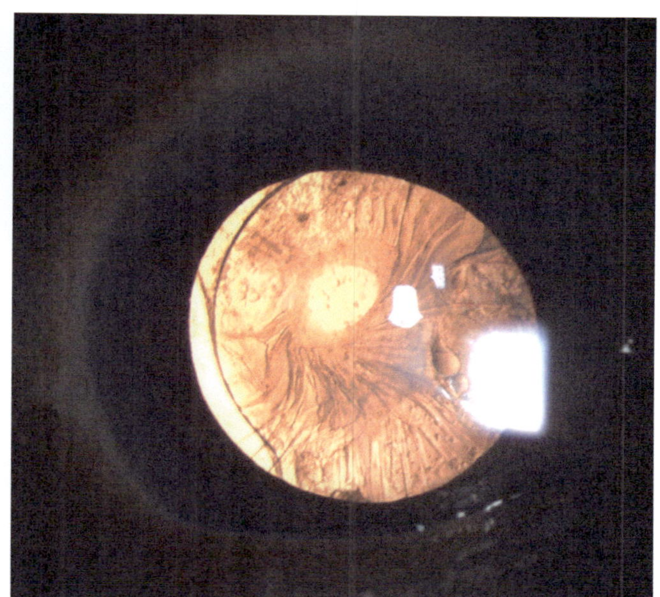

Fig. 7.12 IOL decentration and anterior capsular fibrosis following in the bag IOL placement without CTR in a case of spherophakia

References

1. Ben Yahia S, Ouechtati F, Jelliti B, Nouira S, Chakroun S, Abdelhak S, Khairallah M. Clinical and genetic investigation of isolated spherophakia in a consanguineous Tunisian family. J Hum Genet. 2009;54:550–3.
2. Kumar A, Duvvari MR, et al. A homozygous mutation in LTBP2 causes isolated spherophakia. Hum Genet. 2010;128:365–71.
3. Nelson LB, Maumenee IH. Ectopia lentis. Surv Ophthalmol. 1982;27:143–60.
4. Khokhar S, Agarwal T, Kumar G, Kushmesh R, Tejwani LK. Lenticular abnormalities in children. J Pediatr Ophthalmol Strabismus. 2012;49:32–7.
5. Duke-Elder Sir WS. Normal and abnormal development. Part 2, Congenital deformities. St Louis: CV Mosby Co; 1963. p. 694–6.
6. Easty DL, Sparrow JM. Oxford textbook of ophthalmology, vol. I. Oxford: Oxford University Press; 1999. p. 708.
7. Hossein E, Farah A, et al. Homocystinuria: a rare disorder presenting as cerebral sinovenous thrombosis. Iran J Child Neurol. 2015;9(2):53–7.
8. Verloes Averloes A, Hermia JP, Galand A, Koulischer L, Dodinval P. Glaucoma-lens ectopia-spherophakia-stiffness-shortness (GEMSS) syndrome: a dominant disease with manifestations of Weill-Marchesani syndromes. Am J Med Genet. 1992;44:48–51.
9. Desir J, Sznajer Y, Depasse F, Roulez F, Schrooyen M, Meire F, Abramowicz M. LTBP2 null mutations in an autosomal recessive ocular syndrome with megalocornea, spherophakia, and secondary glaucoma. Eur J Hum Genet. 2010;18:761–7.
10. Khan AO, Aldahmesh MA, Alkuraya FS. Congenital megalocornea with zonular weakness and childhood lens-related secondary glaucoma—a distinct phenotype caused by recessive LTBP2 mutations. Molec. Vis. 2011;17:2570–9.
11. Urbanek J. Glaucoma juvenile inversum. Z Augenheilkd. 1930;71:171–2.
12. Willi M, Kut L, Cotlier E. Pupillary-block glaucoma in the Marchesani syndrome. Arch Ophthalmol. 1973;90:504.
13. Jovanović M, Stefanović I. Spontaneous dislocation of a transparent lens to the anterior chamber--a case report. Srp Arh Celok Lek. 2010;138:486–8.
14. Johnson GJ, Bosanquet RC. Spherophakia in a NewFoundland family: 8-year experience. Can J Ophthalmol. 1983;18:159–64.
15. Johnson VP, Grayson M, Christian JC. Dominant spherophakia. Arch Ophthalmol. 1971;85:534–7.
16. Khan AO, Aldahmesh MA, Al-Ghadeer H, Mohamed JY, Alkuraya FS. Familial spherophakia with short stature caused by a novel homozygous ADAMTS17 mutation. Ophthalmic Genet. 2012;33:235–9.
17. Kumar A, Duvvari MR, Prabhakaran VC, Shetty JS, Murthy GJ, Blanton SH. A homozygous mutation in LTBP2 causes isolated spherophakia. Hum Genet. 2010;128:365–71.
18. Khan AO, Aldahmesh MA, Alkuraya FS. Congenital megalocornea with zonular weakness and childhood lens-related secondary glaucoma—a distinct phenotype caused by recessive LTBP2 mutations. Mol Vis. 2011;17:2570–9.
19. Ahram D, Sato TS, Kohilan A, et al. A homozygous mutation in ADAMTSL4 causes autosomal-recessive isolated ectopia lentis. Am J Hum Genet. 2009;84:274–8.
20. Ades LC, Holman KJ, Brett MS, Edwards MJ, Bennetts B. Ectopia lentis phenotypes and the FBN1 gene. Am J Med Genet A. 2004;126A:284–9.
21. Muralidhar R, Ankush K, Vijayalakshmi P, George VP. Visual outcome and incidence of glaucoma in patients with spherophakia. Eye. 2015;29:350–5.
22. Lifshitz T, Levy J, Klemperer I. Artisan aphakic intraocular lens in children with subluxated crystalline lenses. J Cataract Refract Surg. 2004;30(9):1977–81.
23. Bhattacharjee H, Bhattacharjee K. Clear lens extraction and intraocular lens implantation in a case of spherophakia with secondary angle closure glaucoma. Indian J Ophthalmol. 2010;58(1):67–70.
24. Subbiah S, Thomas PA, Jesudasan CA. Scleral-fixated intraocular lens implantation in spherophakia. Indian J Ophthalmol. 2014;62(5):596–600.
25. McAllister AS, Hirst LW. Visual outcomes and complications of scleral-fixated posterior chamber intraocular lenses. J Cataract Refract Surg. 2011;37:1263–9.
26. Dureau P, De Laage de Meux P, Edelson C, Caputo G. Iris fixation of foldable intraocular lenses for ectopia lentis in children. J Cataract Refract Surg. 2006;32:1109–14.
27. De Silva SR, Arun K, Anandan M, Glover N, Patel CK, Rosen P. Iris-claw intraocular lenses to correct aphakia in the absence of capsule support. J Cataract Refract Surg. 2011;37:1667–72.
28. Khokhar S, Pillay G, Sen S, et al. Clinical spectrum and surgical outcomes in spherophakia: a prospective interventional study. Eye. 2018;32(3):527–36.
29. Khokhar S, Pangtey MS, Sony P, Panda A. Phacoemulsification in a case of spherophakia. J Cataract Refract Surg. 2003;29:845–7.
30. Khokhar S, Gupta S, Kumar G, Rowe N. Capsular tension segment in a case of spherophakia. Cont Lens Anterior Eye. 2012;35:230–2.
31. Lubniewski AJ, Holland EJ, Woodford S. Histologic study of eyes with transsclerally sutured posterior chamber intraocular lenses. Am J Ophthalmol. 1990;110:237–43.
32. Sminia ML, Odenthal MT, Prick LJ, Cobben JM, Mourits MP, Völker-Dieben HJ. Long-term follow-up after bilateral Artisan aphakia intraocular lens implantation in two children with Marfan syndrome. J AAPOS. 2012;16(1):92–4.
33. Romano PE, Kerr NC, Hope GM. Bilateral ametropicfunctional amblyopia in genetic ectopia lentis: its relation to the amount of subluxation, an indicator for early surgical management. Binocul Vis Strabismus Q. 2002;17(3):235–41.
34. Qasem Q, Kirwan C, O'Keefe M. 5-year prospective followup of Artisan phakic intraocular lenses for the correction of myopia, hyperopia and astigmatism. Ophthalmologica. 2010;224:283.

8 Pediatric Traumatic Cataract

Chirakshi Dhull, Sourabh Verma, and Sudarshan Kumar Khokhar

Traumatic cataract is a major cause of visual disability and blindness in children, especially in developing countries [1–3]. Ocular trauma causes 12–46% of all pediatric cataracts [4, 5]. Children are more likely to be affected by it while playing unsupervised. Sharp metallic objects, bow and arrow, wooden sticks, pencils, firecrackers, stones, balls, toys, etc. may cause trauma.

Birmingham Eye Trauma Terminology System is a comprehensive system of eye trauma related terms and has divided eye trauma as [6] Fig. 8.1.

Traumatic cataract is seen more commonly after open globe injury than closed globe injury [7, 8]. Based on the mode, severity, and duration that has passed after the injury a large variety of presentations can be encountered clinically and require a tailored approach for management.

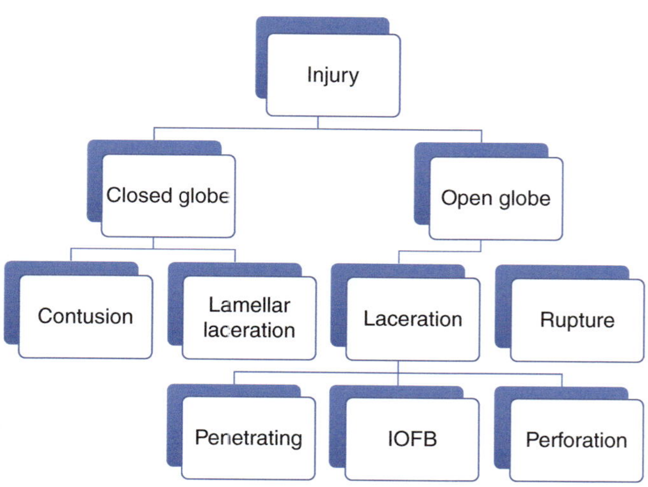

Fig. 8.1 Birmingham Eye Trauma Terminology System for classification of ocular trauma

8.1 Pathogenesis of Traumatic Cataract

In open globe injury, usually breach of anterior and/or posterior capsule is responsible for lens opacification. In closed globe injury, coup-contrecoup injury is generally considered responsible for traumatic cataract [9]. Blunt trauma results in anteroposterior compression and equatorial expansion of globe which can cause damage to lens zonules, capsule, root of iris, angle, and retina. Cataract may also form due to micro-tears of capsule near zonular attachments.

8.2 Clinical Presentation

8.2.1 Open Globe Injuries

Traumatic cataract can present with corneal and/or scleral perforation. Cataract can occur immediately or may progress over time. Presentation may be variable [2, 7, 8, 10, 11].

- Corneal perforation can range from small self-sealed to large perforation with prolapse of iris, lens, and vitreous through the wound (Fig. 8.2a, b). Even after a meticulous repair of such perforations, corneal opacities can decrease final vision because of scattering of light and astigmatism.
- Prolapsed iris tissue in wound sometimes remains stuck to the endothelium because of loss of structural integrity and can present as adherent leukoma after repair (Fig. 8.3).
- Anterior capsule rupture commonly occurs in penetrating trauma. Large ruptures can cause cataract immediately and fluffed up cortical material can be seen in anterior chamber (Fig. 8.4). Small ruptures may be associated with localized cataract (Fig. 8.5). They may progress with time, hence close follow-up is recommended. With time, margins of capsule get fibrosed that provides surgical advantage (Fig. 8.6).

C. Dhull · S. Verma · S. K. Khokhar (✉)
Dr. Rajendra Prasad Centre for Ophthalmic Sciences, All India Institute of Medical Sciences, New Delhi, India

S. K. Khokhar, C. Dhull (eds.), *Atlas of Pediatric Cataract*, https://doi.org/10.1007/978-981-13-6939-1_8

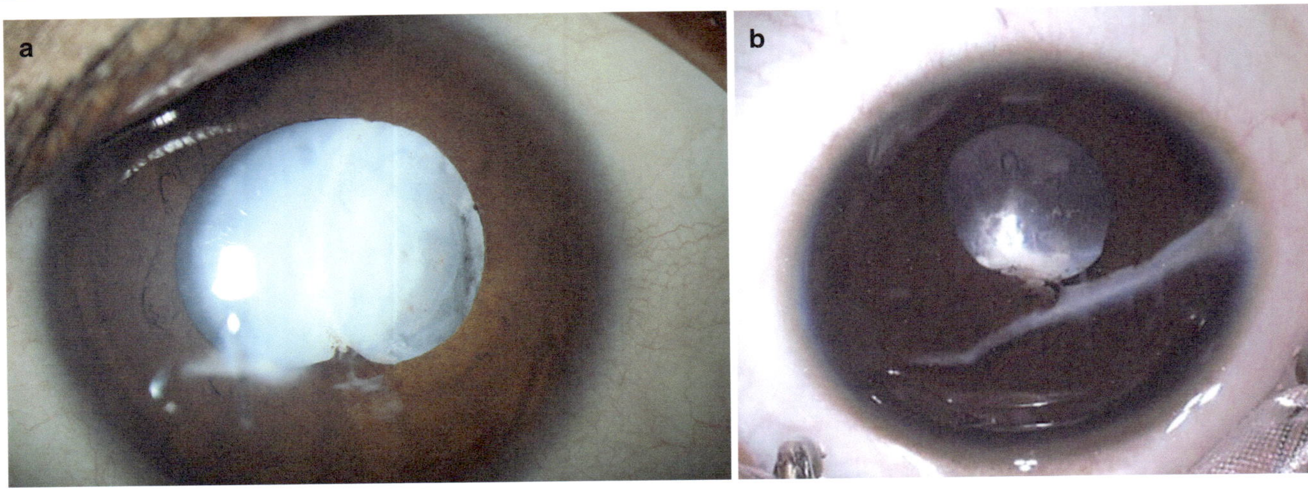

Fig. 8.2 (**a**) Traumatic cataract with small perforation repaired with single suture. (**b**) Large repaired corneal perforation near visual axis with partially absorbed cataract

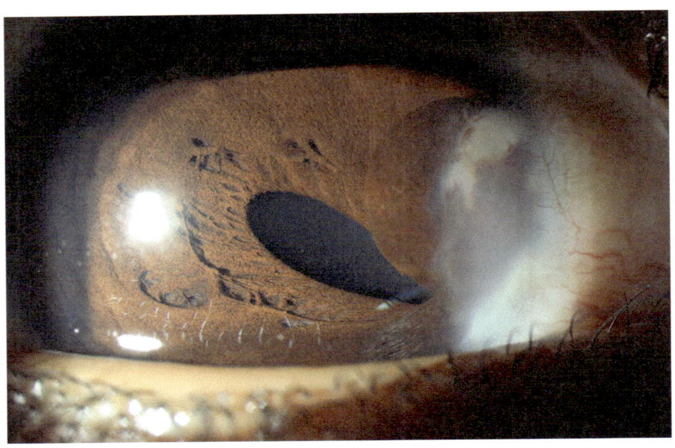

Fig. 8.3 Limbal perforation with iris in wound-forming adherent leukoma with corectopia. Notice bulging of iris nasally due to iris cyst

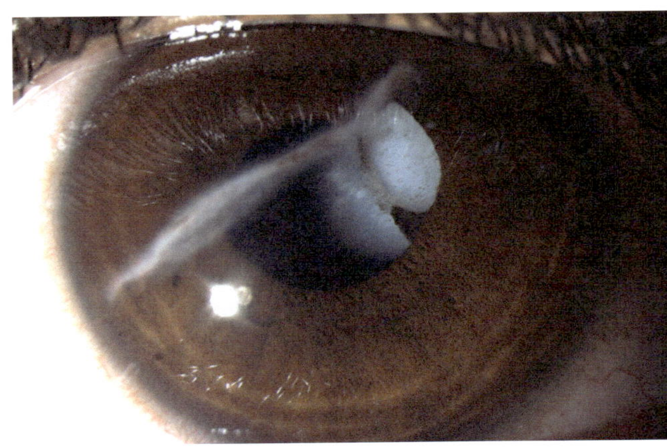

Fig. 8.5 Repaired corneal perforation with ruptured anterior capsule and localized cataract

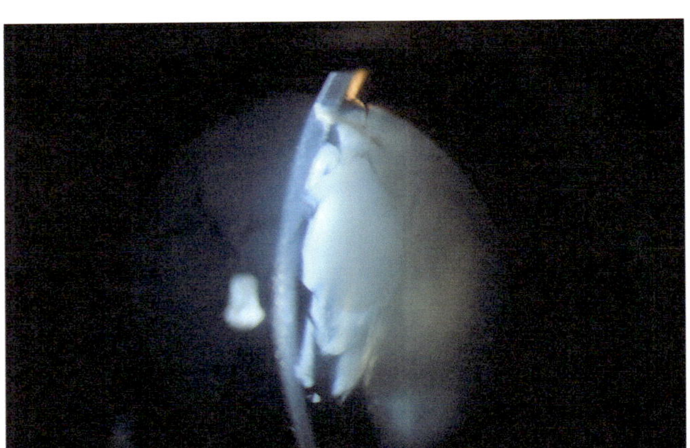

Fig. 8.4 Open globe injury with self-sealed corneal perforation with ruptured anterior capsule and fluffy lens matter in anterior chamber

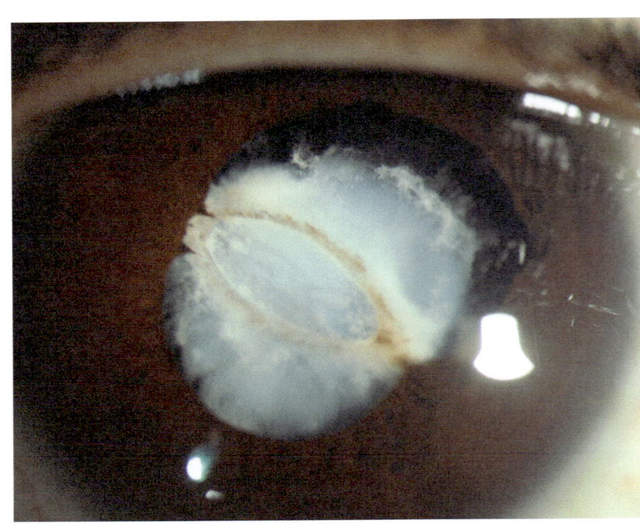

Fig. 8.6 Fibrosed margins of ruptured anterior capsule with membranous cataract

- A sharp object may also penetrate deep enough to rupture both anterior and posterior capsule of lens. Compromised posterior capsular integrity can be picked up on slit lamp examination by the presence of whitish material behind the posterior capsule (Fig. 8.7).
- In long-standing cases cortical matter gets absorbed and a partially absorbed cataractous lens can be encountered (Fig. 8.8).
- Ocular trauma is associated with a retained intraocular foreign body (IOFB). Foreign body might be impacted in cornea (Fig. 8.9a), lying in anterior chamber, impacted in iris (Fig. 8.9b) or lens (Fig. 8.10). Intralenticular foreign bodies may be associated with cataract, which may require cataract surgery along with foreign body removal (Fig. 8.11). In many cases, it penetrates even deeper in posterior segment and iris hole or anterior capsular rupture can be seen along the tract of foreign body.
- Other associations with open globe injury, which have a bearing in management of cataract, include iridodialysis and/or iris defect (Fig. 8.12). Iris cyst may also occur (Fig. 8.13). In rare cases of large scleral or lim-

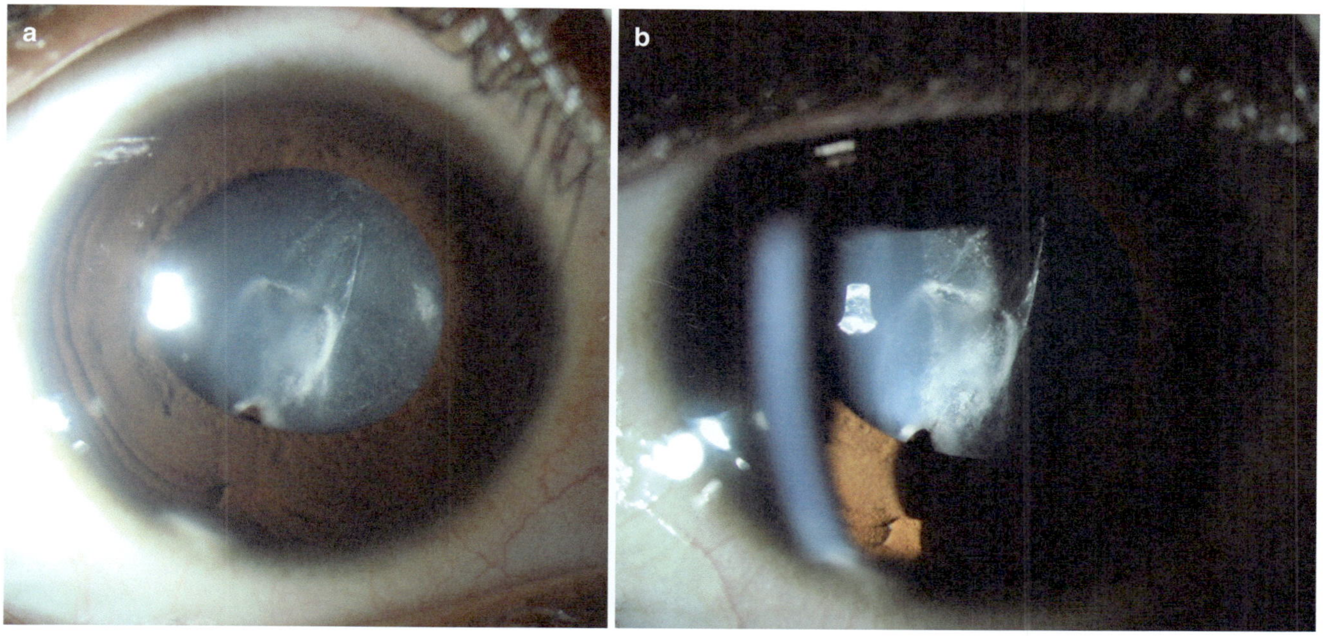

Fig. 8.7 Penetrating injury with posterior capsular defect. (**a**) Diffuse illumination picture showing limbal corneal perforation, iris dimpling, anterior capsular fibrosis posterior capsular defect and (**b**) slit image enhancing posterior capsular defect with white dot sign

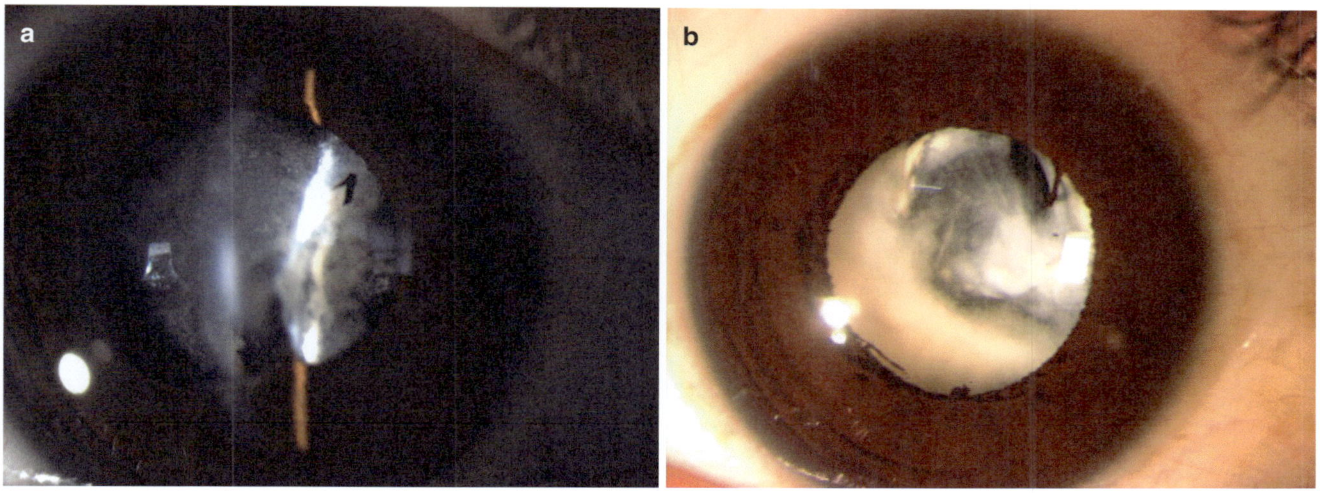

Fig. 8.8 Partially absorbed cataracts. (**a**) 3-year-old child with partially absorbed cataract 2 months post-trauma. Note deep anterior chamber and loss of lens volume. (**b**) 9-year-old child with cataract, 4 years post-trauma with dense fibrosis

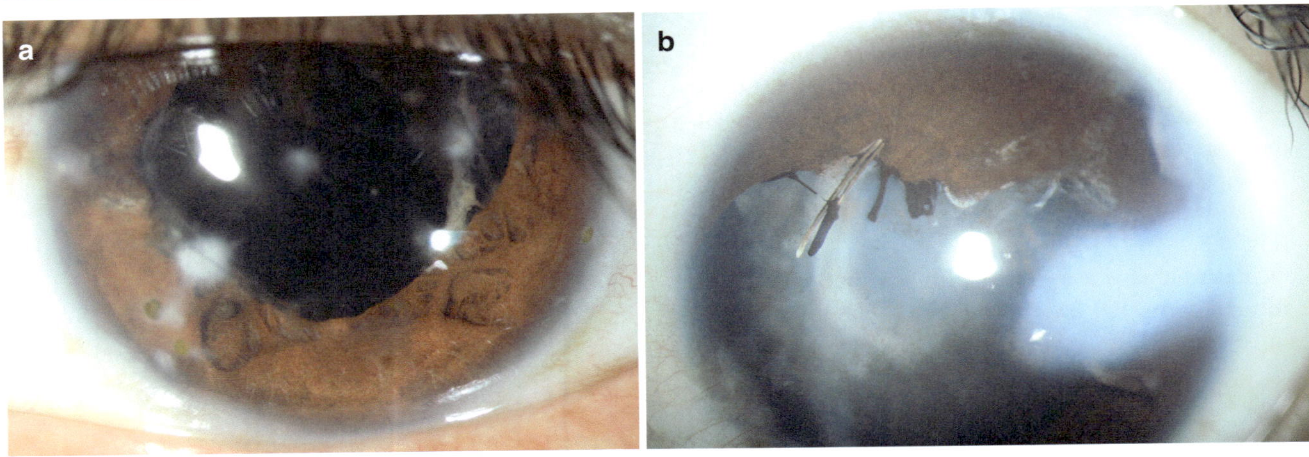

Fig. 8.9 Foreign body (FB). (**a**) Multiple FB: pellet on surface of cornea along with intrastromal FB along with corneal scars and aphakia post pars plana lensectomy and vitrectomy with foreign body removal. (**b**) FB: Two Hair shafts seen in anterior chamber with ends embedded in iris

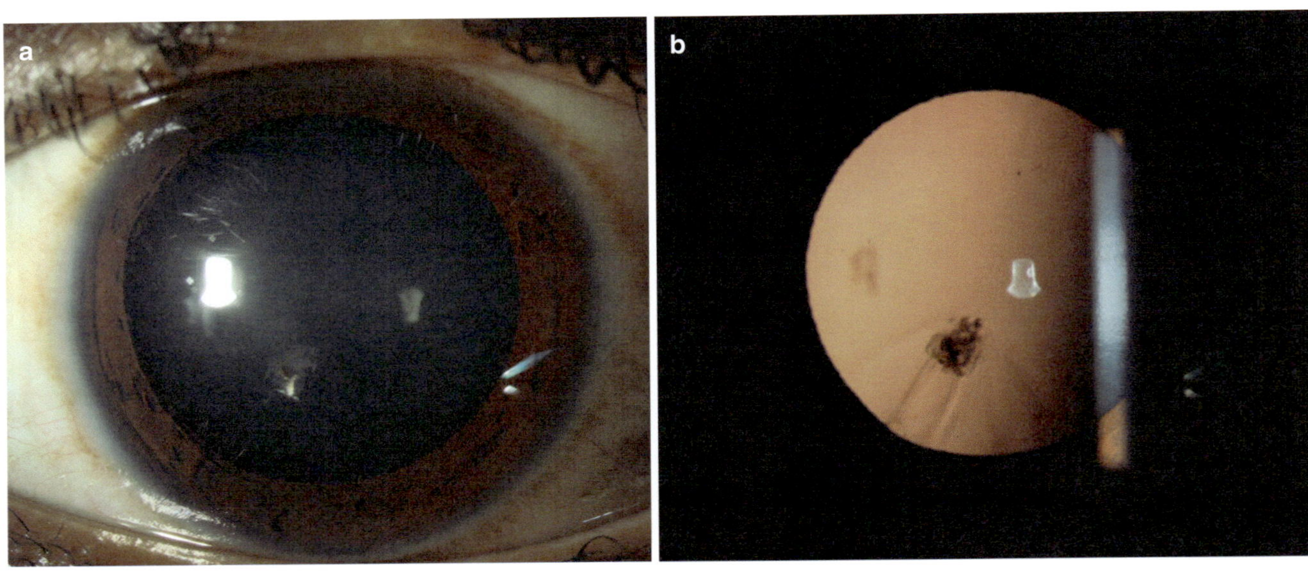

Fig. 8.10 Metallic foreign body on the surface of the lens. This was removed while lens was spared in view of visually insignificant cataract. (**a**) Slit illumination, (**b**) retroillumination

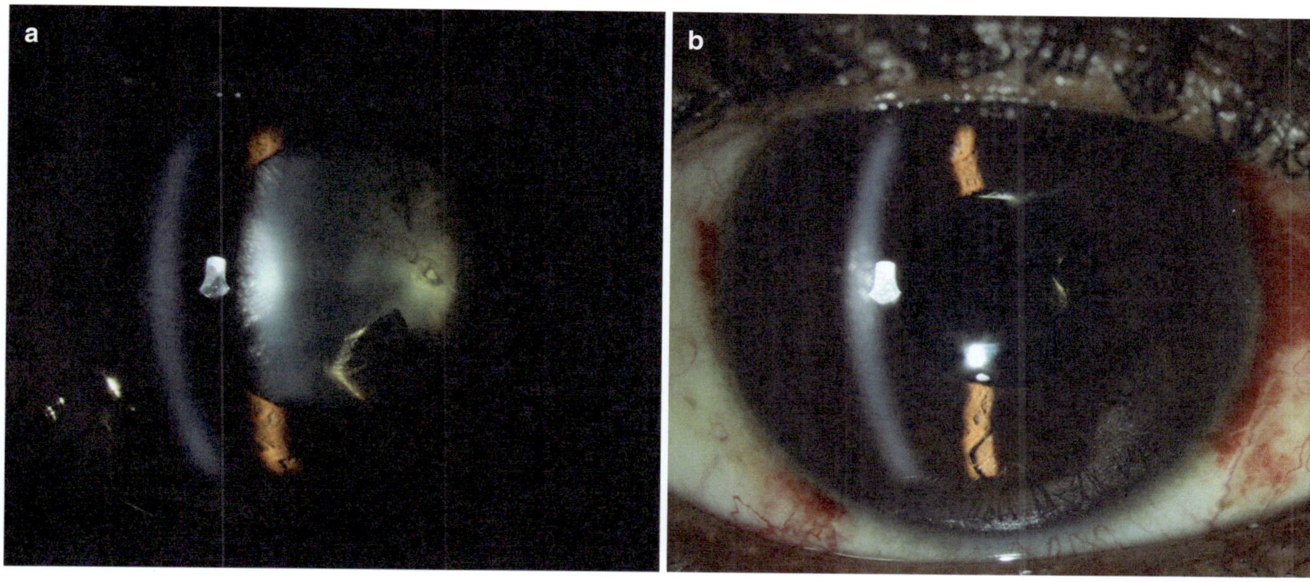

Fig. 8.11 (**a**) Preoperative picture of metallic intralenticular foreign body with posterior subcapsular cataract. (**b**) Postoperative picture of the same with IOL in bag

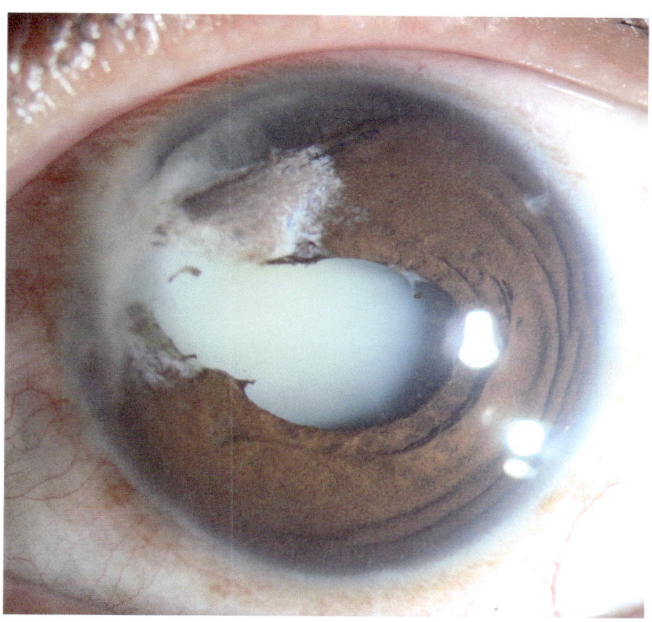

Fig. 8.12 Repaired corneal perforation with iris defect with superior iridodialysis with cataract

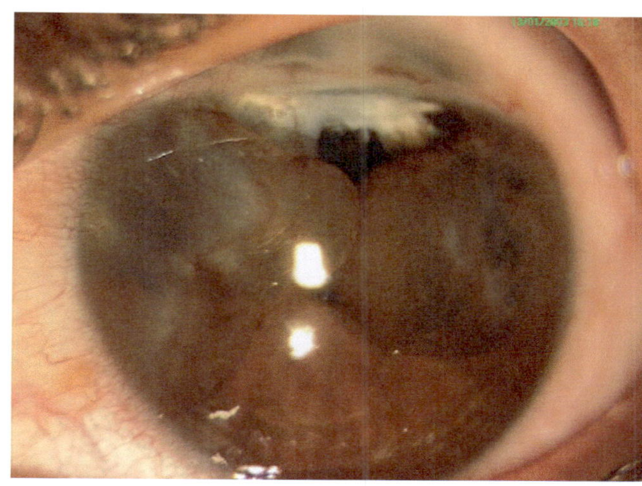

Fig. 8.13 12-year-old girl with large iris cysts seen 9 months after trauma

bal perforation, lens may be seen in subconjunctival space (Fig. 8.14).

- Morphology of cataract may vary from total cataract to partially absorbed or localized cataract. There may be formation of posterior subcapsular cataract without breach of capsule due to inflammation. Sometimes, it has a flower-like pattern resembling rosette cataract (seen in closed globe injury), which can be termed as "pseudorosette cataract" (Fig. 8.15a, b).

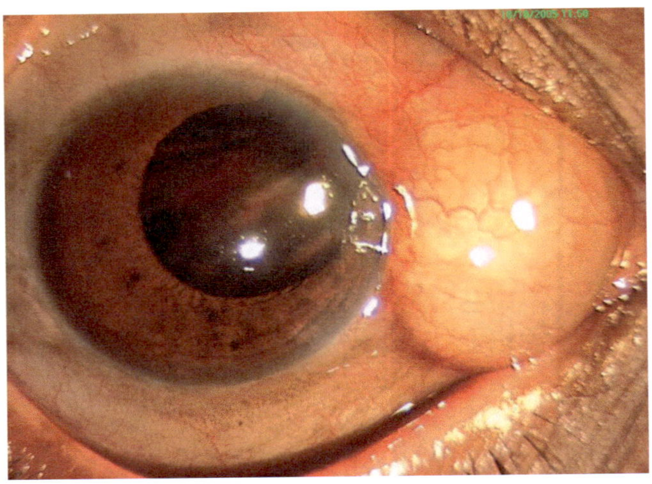

Fig. 8.14 Scleral perforation with aphakia with pseudophacocele (subconjunctival lens)

8.2.2 Closed Globe Injuries

Traumatic cataract may be seen following closed globe injury [2, 7–9]. However, they are generally not seen in immediate period. Hence, close follow-up of eyes with other telltale signs of trauma is recommended.

- A circular ring of brown pigments can be present on anterior lens capsule because of its apposition to a contracted pupillary margin. This is called vossius ring opacity and can be associated with cataract ranging from minor subcapsular opacity to total lenticular opacity (Fig. 8.16a, b).
- Often, initial manifestation is a rosette- or stellate-shaped posterior axial opacities that may be static or progressive in nature and involves posterior lens capsule. Early rosette is characterized by the presence of fine fluid droplets arranged between radiating lens fibers lying just underneath the capsule (Fig. 8.17a, b). Late rosette cataract is found after some months to years and involves deep cortex. Here sutural extensions are shorter and densely packed as compared to early rosette.
- Presence of iridodialysis is one of the hallmarks of blunt trauma. Dialysis may be small or large (Fig. 8.18a, b). Cataract may be localized or diffuse (Fig. 8.19a, b). There may be cyclodialysis as well.
- Zonular damage can result in subluxation of lens with or without cataractous changes [12] (Fig. 8.20a–d). Complete rupture of all the zonules can lead to dislocation of lens into anterior chamber or vitreous cavity (Fig. 8.21).

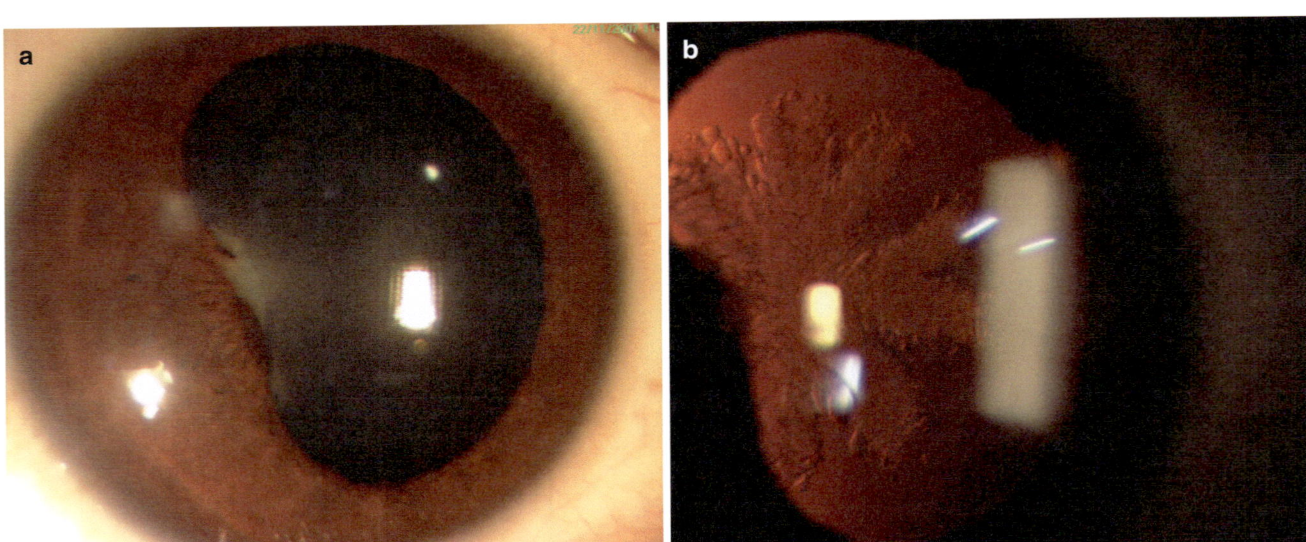

Fig. 8.15 Pseudo-rosette cataract. (**a**) Diffuse illumination picture with self-sealed corneal perforation with posterior synechiae, (**b**) retroillumination picture showing rosette-like cataract

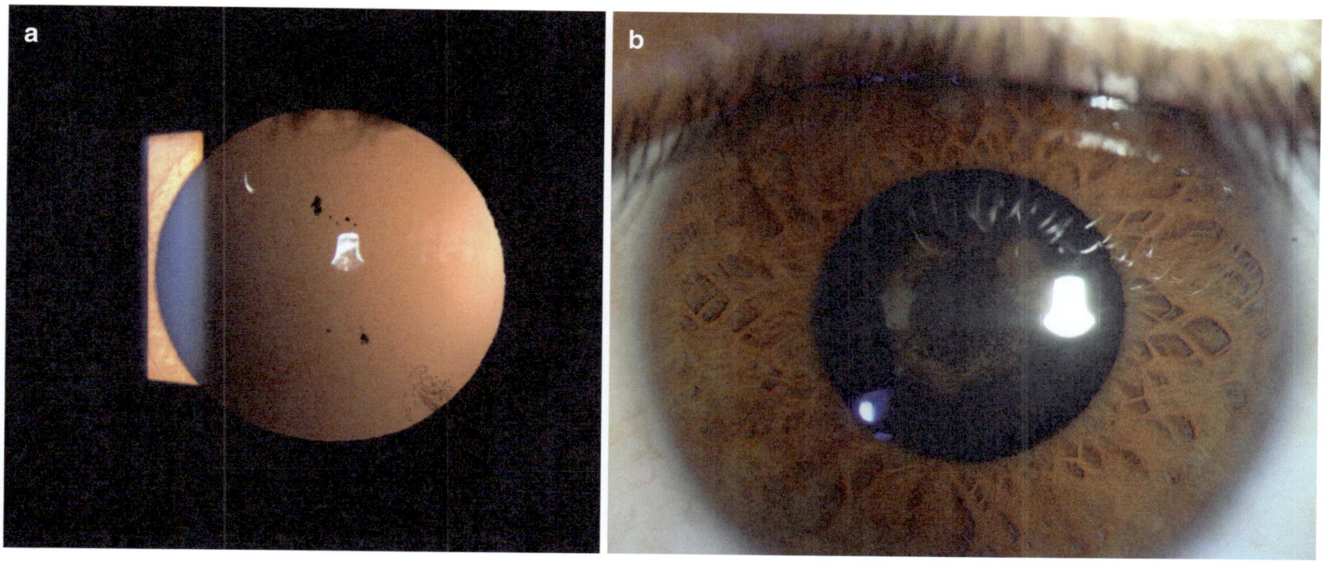

Fig. 8.16 Vossius ring. (**a**) Incomplete ring with few pigment deposits on anterior capsule, (**b**) complete Vossius ring

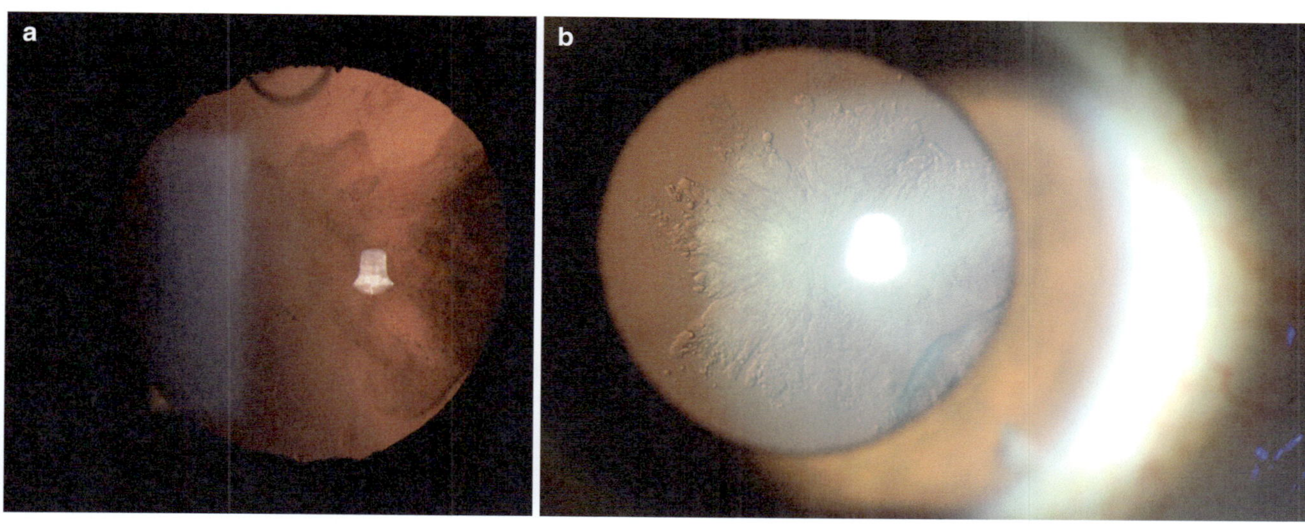

Fig. 8.17 Closed globe injury with rosette cataract. (**a**) Visually insignificant rosette cataract with cortical cataract, (**b**) visually significant rosette cataract

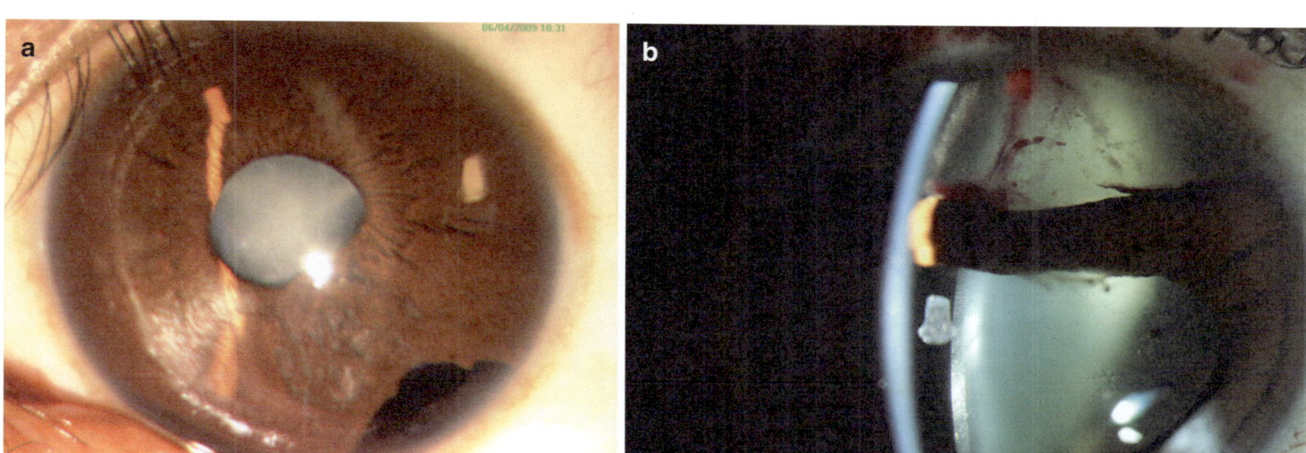

Fig. 8.18 Iridodialysis. (**a**) Small iridodialysis with total cataract, (**b**) large iridodialysis with vitreous in anterior chamber with hyphema

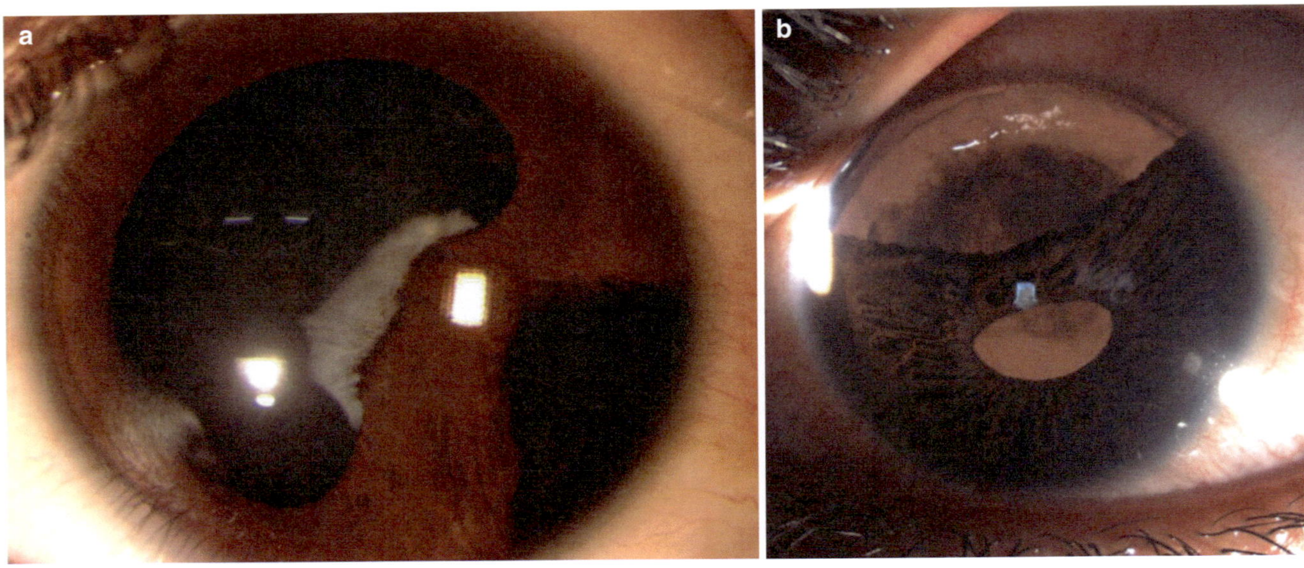

Fig. 8.19 (**a**) Iridodialysis with localized anterior capsular fibrosis, (**b**) iridodialysis with diffuse posterior subcapsular cataract

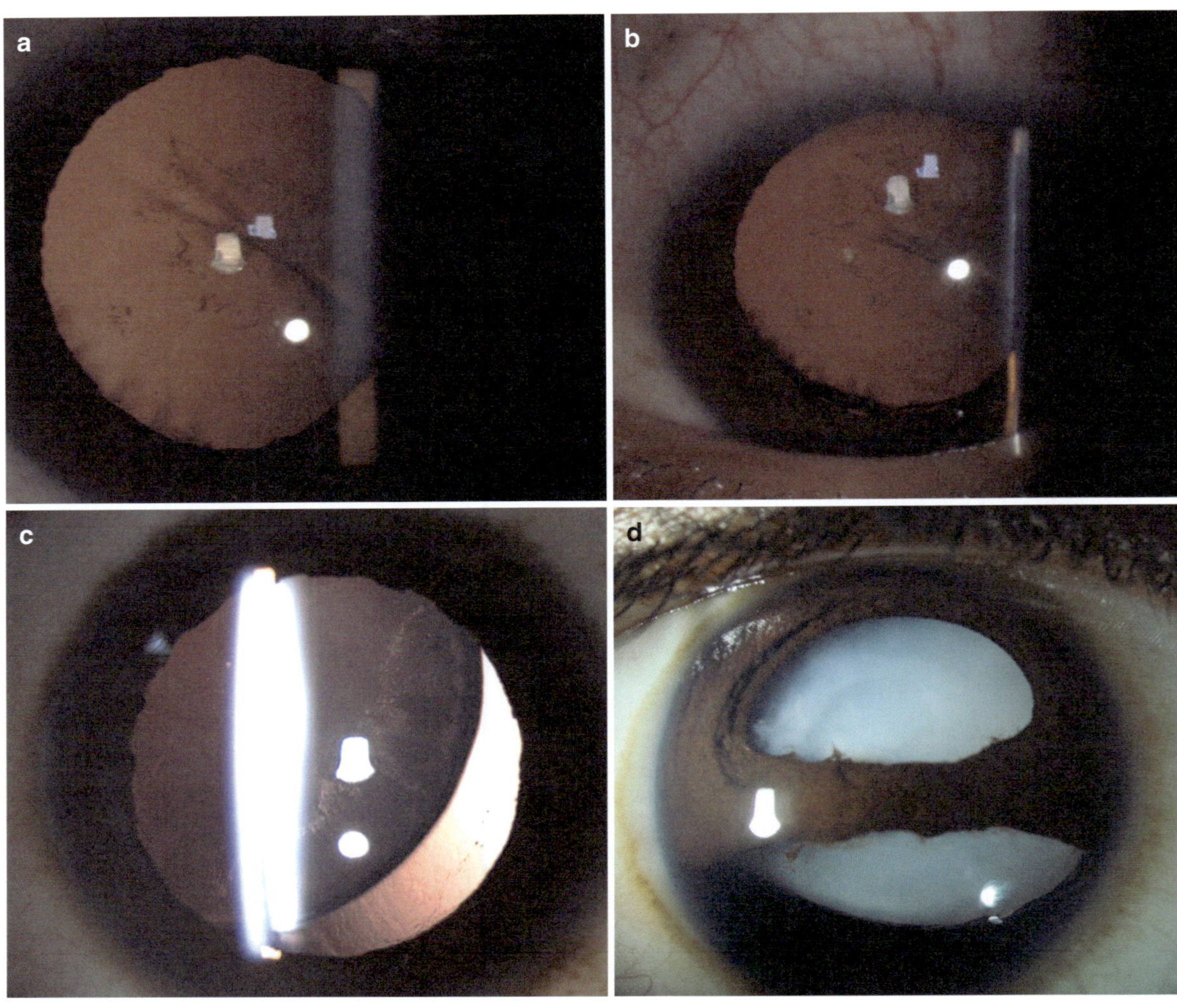

Fig. 8.20 Traumatic anterior subcapsular cataract with sphincter tear with wrinkle in anterior capsule. (**a**) Primary position, (**b**) downgaze position, subluxation missed in primary position is prominent here, (**c**) traumatic subluxation with sphincter tear with pigments behind the posterior capsule without significant cataract, (**d**) traumatic subluxation with total cataract with iridodialysis. Note absence of zonules inferiorly

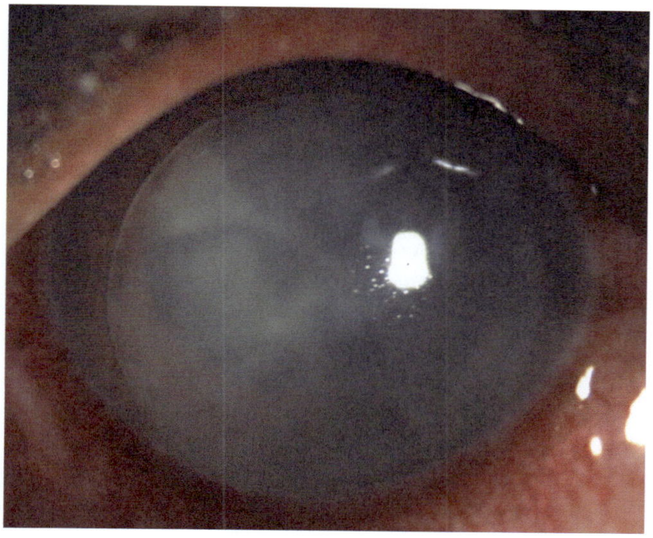

Fig. 8.21 Anteriorly dislocated cataractous lens

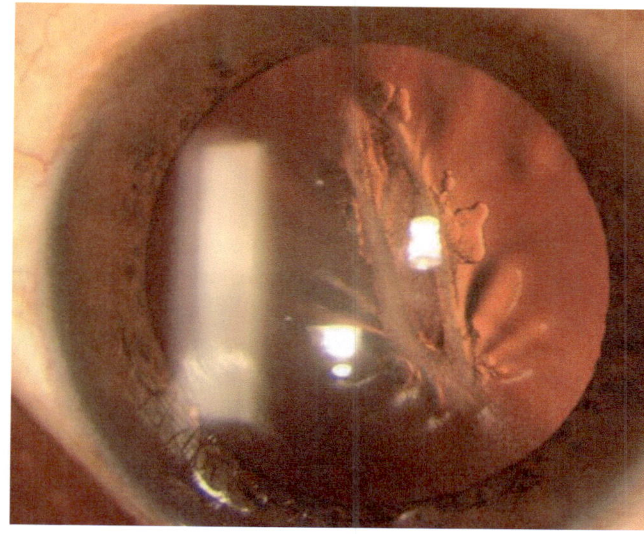

Fig. 8.22 Blunt trauma with tennis ball leading to anterior capsular tear. Tear subsequently became fibrosed with localized cataract

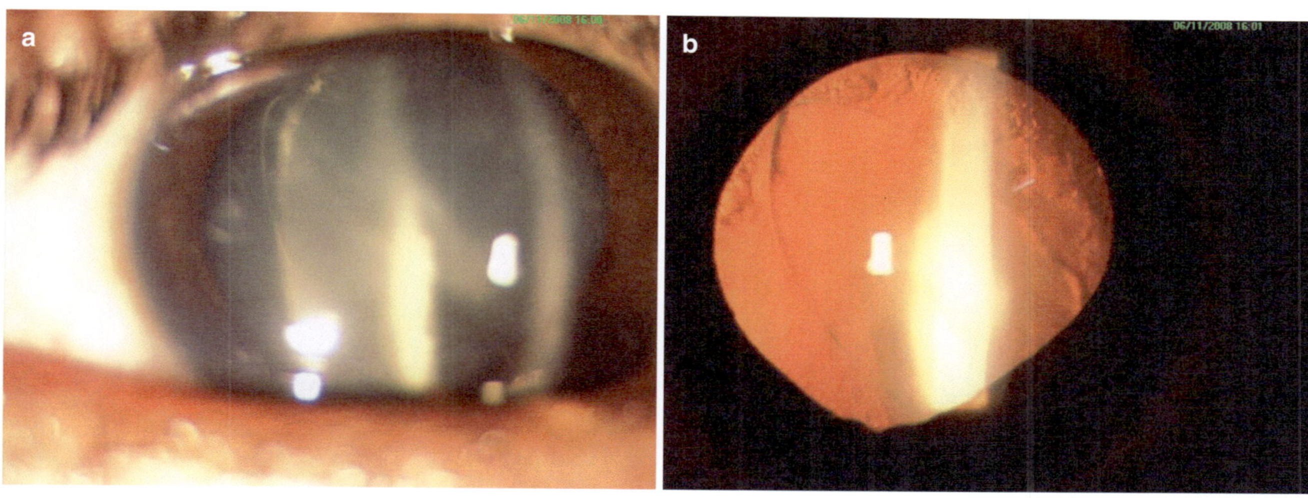

Fig. 8.23 Blunt trauma leading to spindle-shaped posterior capsular defect (PCD), diffuse cataract, and peripheral fluid vacuoles. (**a**) Slit illumination picture showing loss of lens clarity, (**b**) retroillumination showing clearly margins of PCD and fluid vacoules in periphery

- Anterior capsular fibrosis may be seen. Rupture of anterior capsule can occur although it is not as common as open globe injury (Fig. 8.22). Posterior capsular defect may also occur in severe blunt injury (Fig. 8.23).
- All patients should undergo indentation indirect ophthalmoscopy to rule out dialysis or tear and gonioscopy to rule out angle recession [13].

8.3 Investigations

Ultrasonography should be performed in cases where fundus is not visible to rule out retinal detachment or intraocular foreign body. NCCT is a useful tool for localizing the foreign body so that an appropriate approach for management can be decided.

In cases with total lenticular opacity or corneal opacity where lens details are not clear, ultrasound biomicroscopy (UBM) can help us in visualizing lens (Fig. 8.24).

8.4 Surgical Management

In open globe injuries, primary closure of the defect is necessary (Fig. 8.25). Often such injuries are associated with lens capsule rupture with lens material in anterior chamber, which is tolerated well in children. A second surgery can be planned after control of inflammation [14, 15] and removal of sutures, if possible, for accurate IOL power calculation. Some surgeons prefer IOL placement in primary surgery (with perforation repair) [16]. Surgical management of pediatric cataract is discussed in detail in the respective chapter. Pearls helpful in management of traumatic cataract are mentioned below:

- It is useful to stain the capsule with trypan blue to increase its visibility. This step is particularly useful in cases with white cataract and ruptured lens capsule with flocculent lens matter in anterior chamber.
- Cases with anterior capsular plaque or fibrosis might need microincision scissors and forceps to create an opening. Sometimes anterior capsular fibrosis is thick and surgical blade (1 mm) might be needed to give small nicks to assist rhexis.
- A vitrectomy cutter can be used in cases of partially absorbed or fibrosed cataract for anterior and posterior capsulorhexis.
- Hydrodissection should be avoided as structural integrity of posterior capsule is questionable in post-traumatic cases.
- Posterior capsular capsulorrhexis and anterior vitrectomy can reduce the chance of visual axis opacification.
- Capsular tension ring or Cionni ring might be needed in cases with subluxation. This is discussed in detail in respective chapter (Fig. 8.26).
- In case implantation of IOL is not possible, it can be placed in sulcus with or without optic capture (Fig. 8.27a, b).

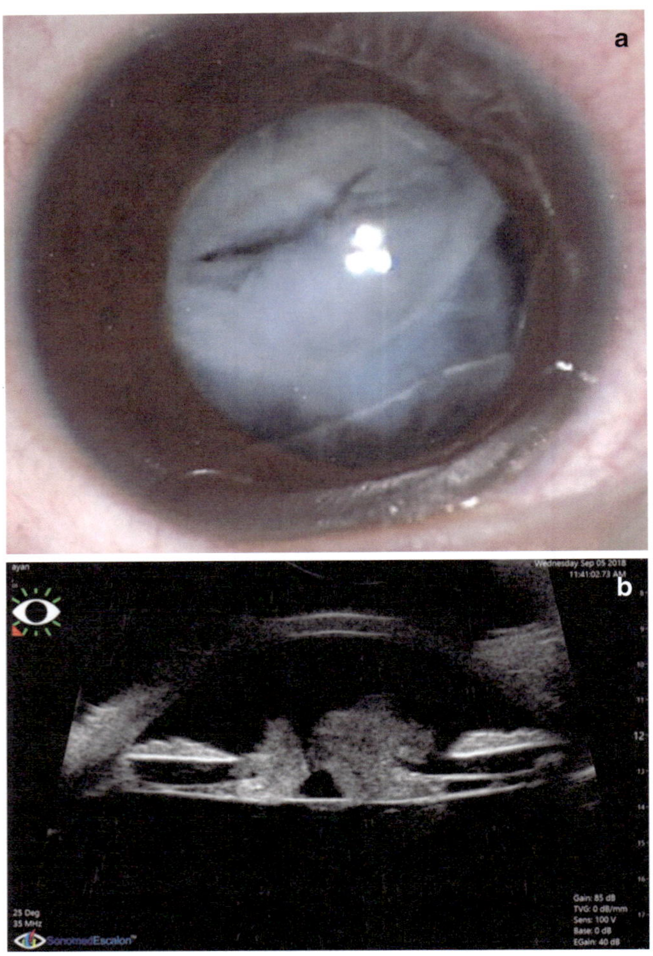

Fig. 8.24 Detection of posterior capsular defect. (**a**) Clinical picture with ruptured anterior capsule and total cataract, (**b**) UBM of the same showing defect in posterior capsule and lens matter in vitreous cavity

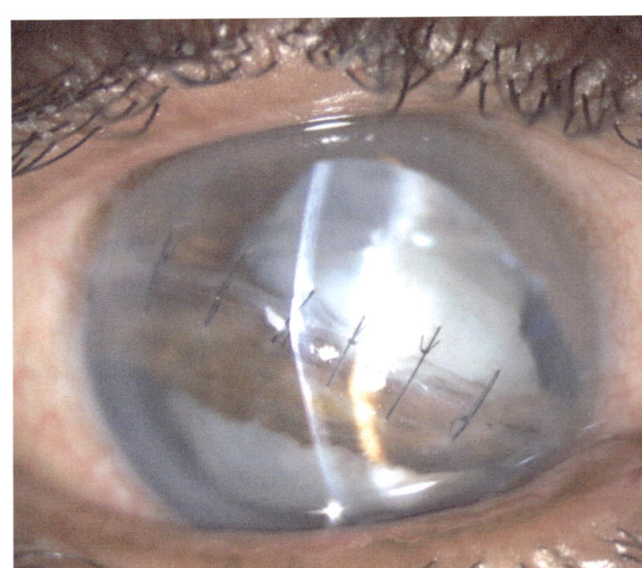

Fig. 8.25 Primary repair of corneal perforation sparing lens despite ruptured anterior capsule and lens matter in anterior chamber

- Iridodialysis and iris tears can be repaired during the surgery by using 9-0 prolene sutures. Similarly associated abnormalities may warrant surgical management.

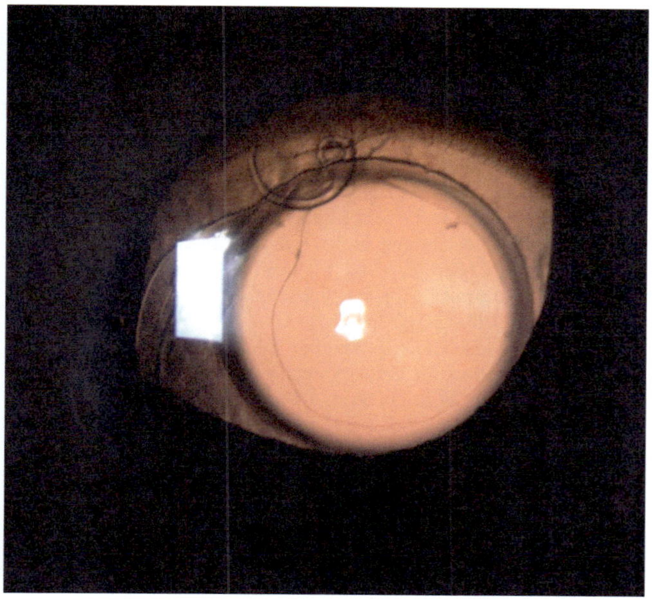

Fig. 8.26 1-year postoperative picture of traumatic subluxation with Cionni fixation

8.5 Postoperative Management and Complications

Higher than usual amount of inflammation is to be expected in such cases and frequent topical and systemic steroids with cycloplegics should be used. Corrective glasses and amblyopia therapy should be started for visual rehabilitation. Final visual outcome is determined by the presence of coexisting corneal scars, glaucoma, and posterior segment pathologies [17, 18]. Postoperative higher rate of visual axis opacification is noted. Other complications include pupillary capture, IOL decentration/posterior dislocation, and iritis. ACIOL and iris fixated IOLs can result in endothelial cell loss and prolonged iritis in long run.

8.6 Conclusion

Prognosis of pediatric eyes suffering from post-traumatic cataract has improved over the years. Meticulous planning before surgery, appropriate surgical technique, and well-tailored postsurgical management are necessary in such cases.

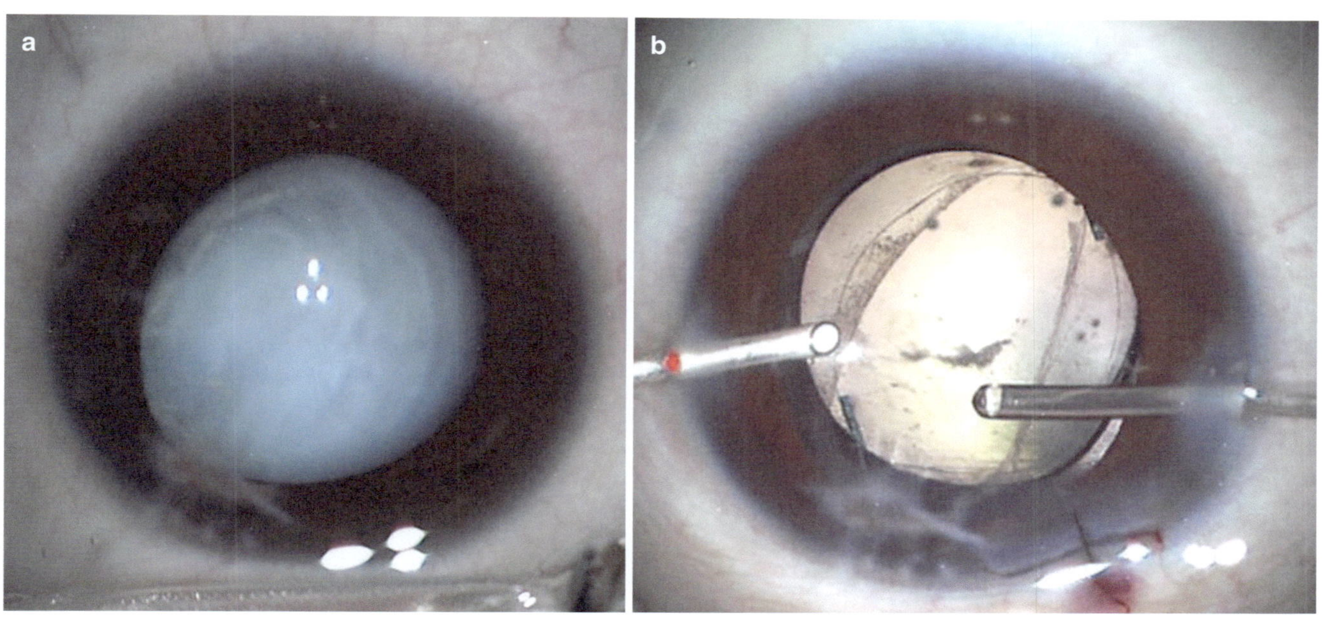

Fig. 8.27 (**a**) Preoperative picture penetrating injury with anterior and posterior capsular defect. (**b**) Intraoperative picture of the same where multipiece IOL has been put with optic capture

References

1. Sharma AK, Aslami AN, Srivastava JP, Iqbal J. Visual outcome of traumatic cataract at a tertiary eye care centre in North India: a prospective study. J Clin Diagn Res. 2016;10:05–8.
2. Adlina AR, Chong YJ, Shatriah I. Clinical profile and visual outcome of traumatic paediatric cataract in suburban Malaysia: a ten-year experience. Singap Med J. 2014;55:253–6.
3. Haavisto AK, Sahraravand A, Holopainen JM, Leivo T. Paediatric eye injuries in Finland—Helsinki eye trauma study. Acta Ophthalmol. 2014;95:392–9.
4. Eckstein M, Vijayalakshmi P, Killedar M, et al. Aetiology of childhood cataract in south India. Br J Ophthalmol. 1996;80:628–32.
5. Shah M, Shah S, Upadhyay P, Agrawal R. Controversies in traumatic cataract classification and management: a review. Can J Ophthalmol. 2013;48:251–8.
6. Kuhn F, Morris R, Witherspoon CD, Mester V. The Birmingham Eye Trauma Terminology system (BETT). J Fr Ophtalmol. 2004 Feb;27(2):206–10.
7. Khokhar S, Agrawal S, Gupta S, Gogia V, Agarwal T. Epidemiology of traumatic lenticular subluxation in India. Int Ophthalmol. 2014;34:197–204.
8. Ram J, Verma N, Gupta N, Chaudhary M. Effect of penetrating and blunt ocular trauma on the outcome of traumatic cataract in children in northern India. J Trauma Acute Care Surg. 2012;73:726–30.
9. Datiles MB, Magno BV. Cataract: clinical types. Duane's ophthalmology. Philadelphia, PA: Lippincott Williams & Wilkins; 2001.
10. Sul S, Gurelik G, Korkmaz S, Ozdek S, Hasanreisoglu B. Pediatric open globe injuries: clinical characteristics and factors associated with poor visual and anatomical success. Graefes Arch Clin Exp Ophthalmol. 2016;254:1405–10.
11. Reddy AK, Ray R, Yen YG. Surgical intervention of traumatic cataracts in children: Epidemiology, complications and outcomes. J AAPOS. 2009;13:170–4.
12. Khokhar S, Gupta S, Yogi R, Gogia V, Agarwal T. Epidemiology and intermediate-term outcomes of open- and closed-globe injuries in traumatic childhood cataract. Eur J Ophthalmol. 2014;24:124–30.
13. Sihota R, Kumar S, Gupta V, Dada T, Kashyap S, Insan R, et al. Early predictors of traumatic glaucoma after closed globe injury: trabecular pigmentation, widened angle recess, and higher baseline intraocular pressure. Arch Ophthalmol. 2008;126(7):921–6.
14. Kamlesh, Dadeya S. Management of paediatric traumatic cataract by epilenticular intraocular lens implantation: long-term visual results and postoperative complications. Eye (Lond). 2004;18:126–30.
15. BenEzra D, Cohen E, Rose L. Traumatic cataract in children: correction of aphakia by contact lens or intraocular lens. Am J Ophthalmol. 1997;123:773–82.
16. Anwar M, Bleik JH, von Noorden GK, et al. Posterior chamber lens implantation for primary repair of corneal lacerations and traumatic cataracts in children. J Pediatr Ophthalmol Strabismus. 1994;31:157–61.
17. Cheema RA, Lukaris AD. Visual recovery in unilateral traumatic pediatric cataracts treated with posterior chamber intraocular lens and anterior vitrectomy in Pakistan. Int Ophthalmol. 1999;23:85–9.
18. Churchill AJ, Noble BA, Etchells DE, et al. Factors affecting visual outcome in children following uniocular traumatic cataract. Eye. 1995;9(Pt3):285–91.

9 Pediatric Uveitic Cataract

Chirakshi Dhull, Barkha Gupta, and Sudarshan Kumar Khokhar

The term "uveitis" refers to a group of conditions in which inflammation affects various components of the uvea, i.e., the iris, ciliary body, and choroid. Uveitis encompasses a myriad of conditions, all of which are characterized by inflammation of the uveal tract either directly or indirectly.

Pediatric uveitis accounts for 5–10% of all uveitis population [1]. Pediatric uveitis is a challenge for an ophthalmologist because of variations in clinical presentation, difficulties in comprehensive eye examination, delayed diagnosis especially in the developing countries, limited management options, and risk of amblyopia. Prolonged duration and increased risks of complications can lead to significant ocular morbidity, and severe vision loss is found in 25–33% of pediatric uveitis cases [2]. In pediatric uveitis, anterior uveitis accounts for 30–40%, posterior uveitis 40–50%, intermediate uveitis 10–20%, and panuveitis 5–10% [3]. As many as 80% of cases of anterior uveitis in the pediatric population are associated with juvenile idiopathic uveitis (JIA) [4]. Complications are frequently already present at the time of diagnosis or referral.

9.1 Cataract in Uveitis

Cataract represents a major complication of uveitis in childhood. It occurs in approximately 35% (range, 20–70%) of the cases of juvenile idiopathic arthritis (JIA)-associated uveitis [5]. It results in reduced visual acuity and can have a detrimental effect on the development and academic achievements of these children.

Apart from JIA (most common cause for pediatric uveitis), other anterior uveitis syndromes can present with complicated cataract leading to ocular morbidity either due to prolonged inflammation or long-term use of corticosteroids (topical or systemic) such as pars planitis, tubercular uveitis, sarcoidosis, VKH, and sympathetic ophthalmia. Masquerade syndrome should be excluded before operating cataract. The most common cause of masquerade syndromes in children include malignancies like retinoblastoma, leukemia, medulloepithelioma, and juvenile xanthogranuloma; inherited retinal degenerations like retinitis pigmentosa; congenital eye disorders like Coat's disease, etc. Leukemia, the most common malignancy of childhood, can often present with the signs of posterior uveitis.

Cataract development and progression can be the result of persistent intraocular inflammation [6], secondary to surgery for uveitis complications (e.g., trabeculectomy and repair of retinal detachments) or as a consequence of uveitis treatment, particularly use of local or systemic corticosteroids [7, 8].

Cataract develops commonly in eyes with panuveitis, chronic anterior uveitis, and intermediate uveitis respectively, whereas it was far less common in those with posterior uveitis, despite extensive use of systemic corticosteroids and local corticosteroids injections, suggesting inflammation as a more significant risk factor [9, 10]. Inflammatory mediators result in structural changes in the eye (i.e., peripheral anterior synechiae, cataract, cystoid macular edema, and formation of vitreous opacities) which is associated with the location of the inflammation, as well as its extent and duration.

9.1.1 Clinical Presentation

Symptoms in small children are generally noted late in the course of disease. In JIA patients, they usually present with systemic features first.

- There may be complaint of red eye with photophobia and pain in older children (Fig. 9.1). Redness may be absent in JIA patients.

C. Dhull · B. Gupta · S. K. Khokhar (✉)
Dr Rajendra Prasad Centre for Ophthalmic Sciences, All India Institute of Medical Sciences, New Delhi, India

S. K. Khokhar, C. Dhull (eds.), *Atlas of Pediatric Cataract*, https://doi.org/10.1007/978-981-13-6939-1_9

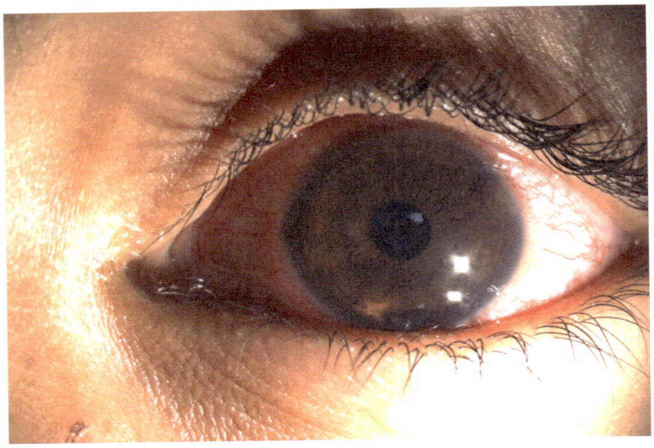

Fig. 9.1 Red eye can be noticed in torch light examination. Flare in the chamber is also noticeable

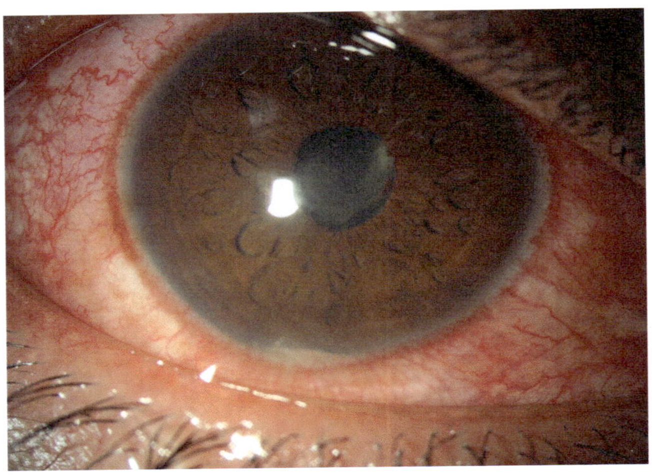

Fig. 9.2 Circumcorneal congestion with fibrinous membrane in anterior chamber with hypopyon

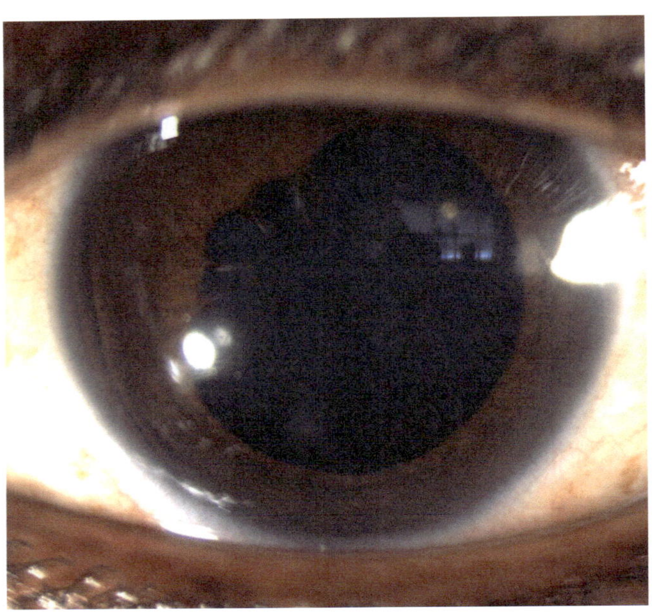

Fig. 9.3 Filiform synechiae seen from 9 to 12 o clock position

- Anterior segment may show presence of cells, flare and keratic precipitates (KPs) in acute stage. There may be presence of hypopyon in the anterior chamber (Fig. 9.2). In such cases, a masquerade syndrome or endophthalmitis must be ruled out.
- As acute phase starts to resolve there may be presence of posterior synechiae. They may be filiform in the early stage (Fig. 9.3) and can be broken by intensive cycloplegics (Fig. 9.4). Multiple synechiae give appearance of festooned pupil (Fig. 9.5).

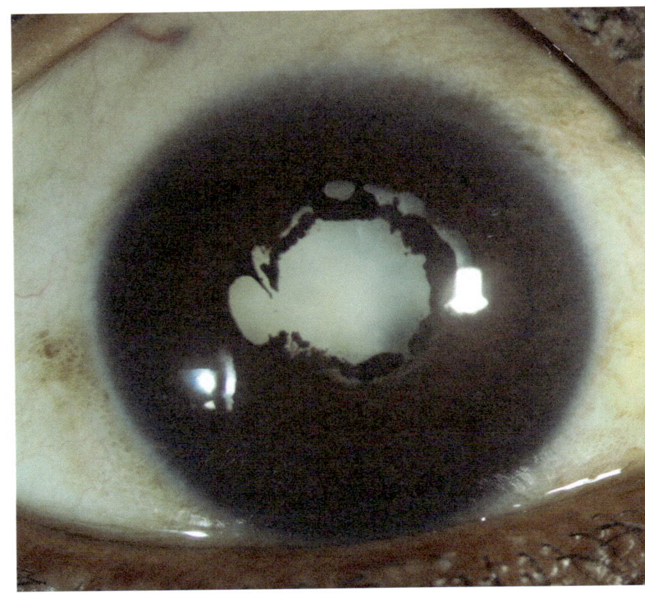

Fig. 9.4 Multiple partially broken synechiae seen leaving pigment impression with total cataract

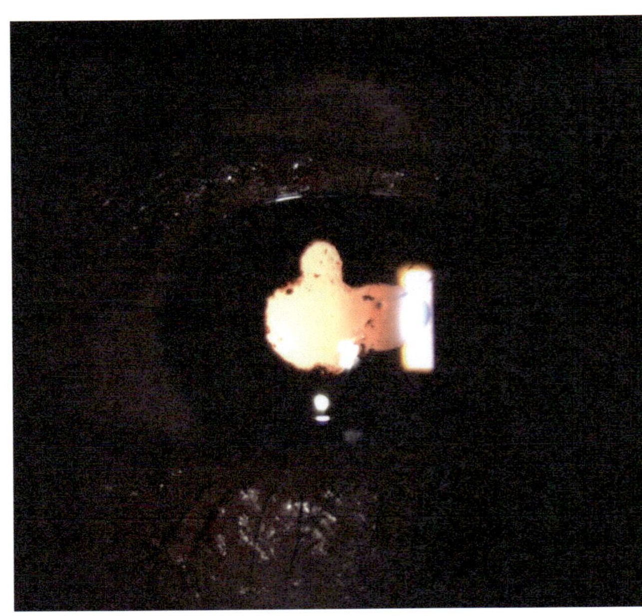

Fig. 9.5 Festooned pupil with clear lens

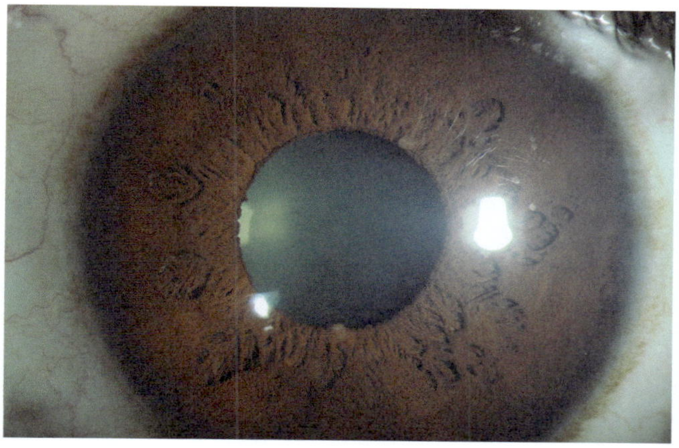

Fig. 9.6 Granulomatous uveitis with koeppe's nodules at 2 and 6 o clock position

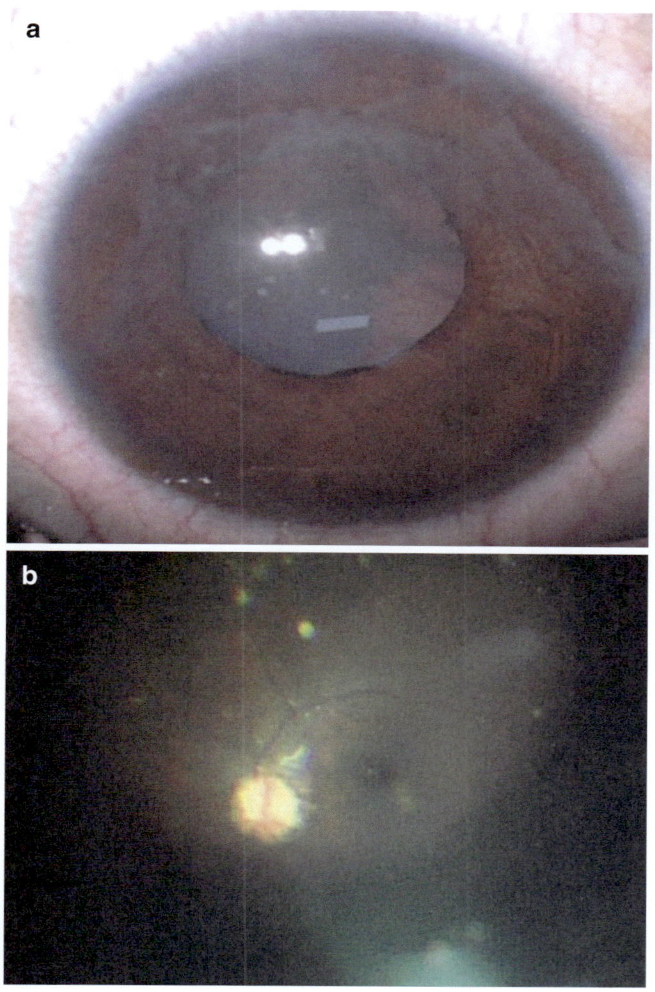

Fig. 9.7 An 8-year-old girl with sarcoidosis. (**a**) Diffuse band-shaped keratopathy with posterior subcapsular cataract, (**b**) intraoperative fundus picture showing media haze, disc granuloma, and sclerosed vessels

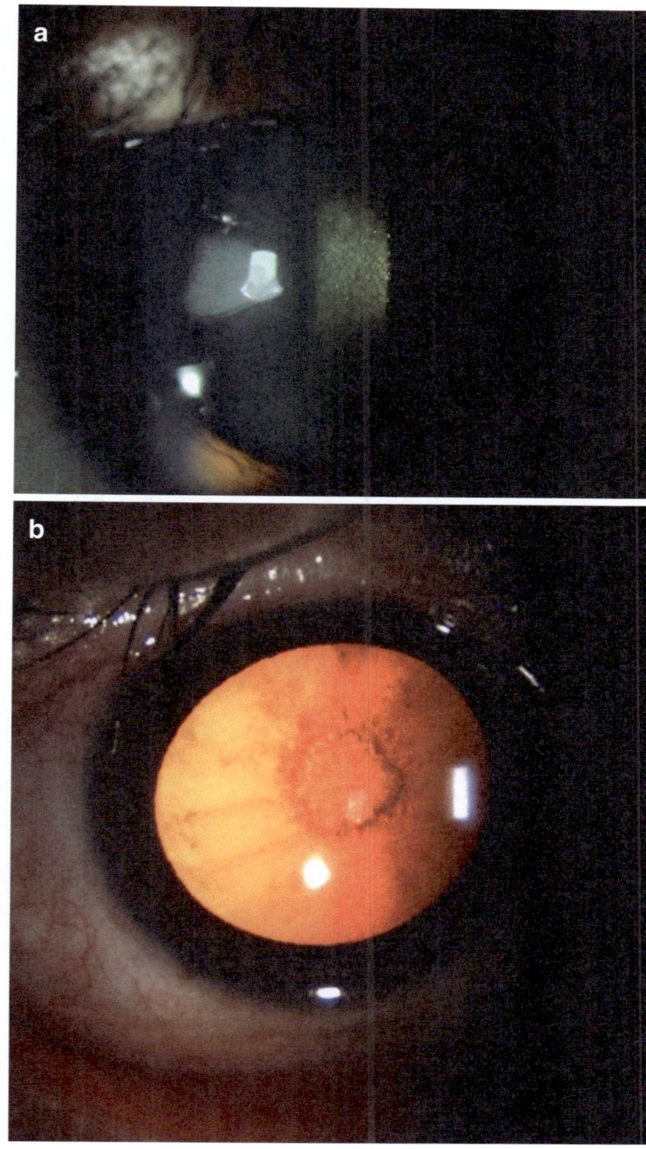

Fig. 9.8 Posterior subcapsular cataract in a patient with pars planitis. (**a**) Slit illumination showing polychromatic luster, (**b**) retroillumination of the same showing central involvement

- In cases of granulomatous uveitis, koeppe's nodules may be seen (Fig. 9.6). Common causes of granulomatous uveitis include tuberculosis and sarcoidosis. These are generally associated with panuveitis (Fig. 9.7).
- Cataract may range from mild posterior subcapsular cataract with polychromatic luster (Fig. 9.8) to total cataract (Fig. 9.9) depending on etiology, chronicity, duration, and associated complications.

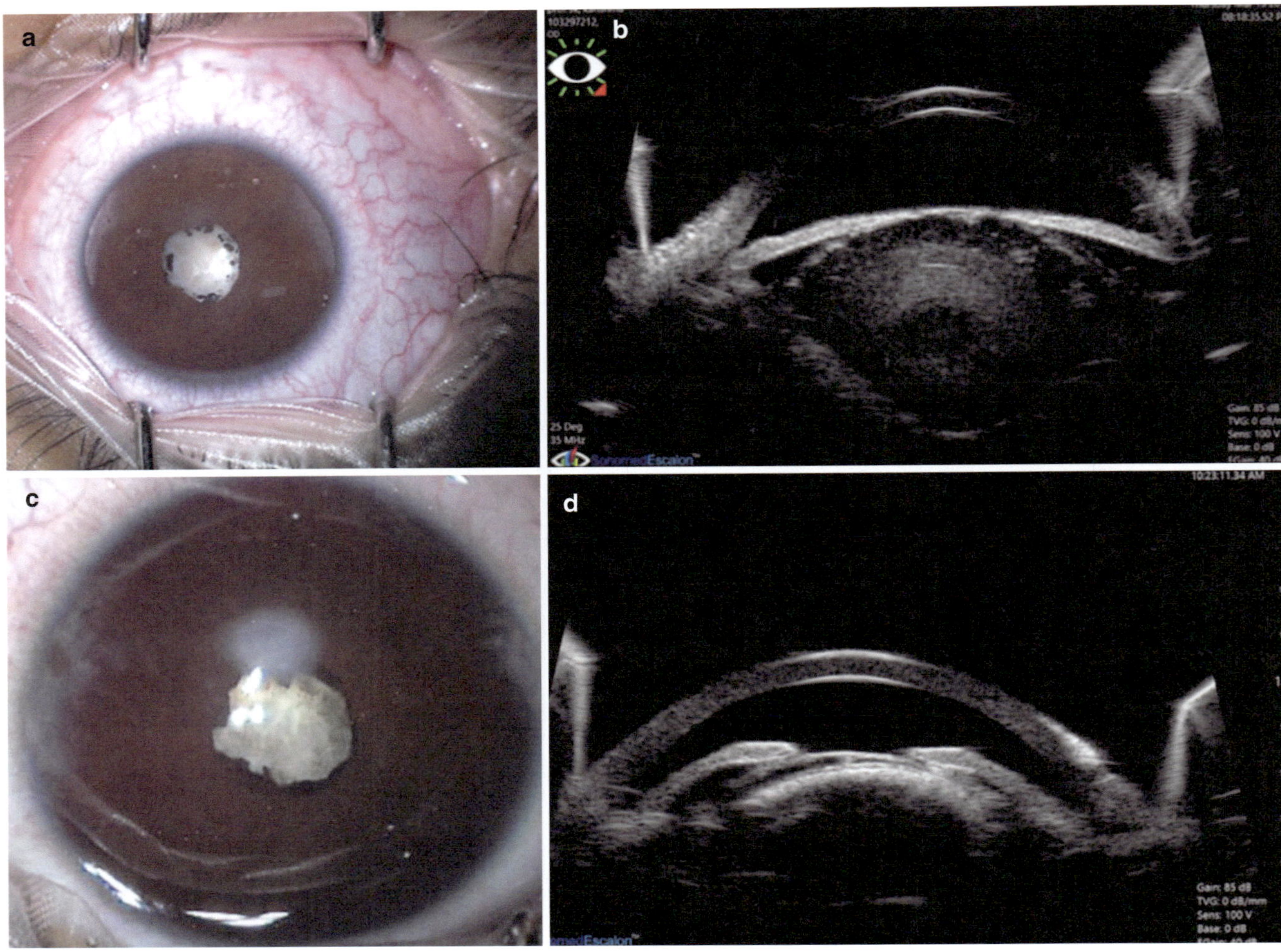

Fig. 9.9 Figure JIA patient OD and OS. (**a** and **c**) Clinical picture showing BSK, total cataract, and posterior synechiae, (**b** and **d**) UBM of the same showing iris position. While OD has seclusion-pupillae, only OS has early iris bombe formation

9.2 Management of Uveitic Cataract

9.2.1 Management of Uveitis

Primary goal of management is early diagnosis and prompt initiation of treatment to achieve complete quiescence of inflammation for prevention of sight-threatening complications.

First-line treatment: topical corticosteroids along with short-acting mydriatics and cycloplegics under observation. Steroids should be administered carefully because of their potential complications like cataract formation, steroid induced ocular-hypertension, and systemic side effects. Prolonged use of mydriatics and cycloplegics can lead to formation of synechiae in dilated position of the pupils. Methotrexate is the most common first-line systemic medication used in JIA [11]. Oral corticosteroids should not be used for long term in children because of their effect on growth and bone metabolism. Methotrexate is usually well tolerated in children; very few develop gastrointestinal side effects, where the drug can be administered intramuscularly or subcutaneously.

9.2.2 Measures to Prevent Cataract Formation [12]

- Uveitis screening: cataract being frequent ophthalmic complication of JIA Uveitis (JIA-U), strategies to prevent and identify cataracts are needed. These preventive strategies involve adherence to early screening and treatment for uveitis.
- Immunosuppressive therapy: methotrexate may reduce the rapidity of cataract formation in JIA-U [13]. Other antimetabolites such as mycophenolate mofetil (MMF) and azathioprine; tumor necrosis factor-α inhibitors such as infliximab and adalimumab; and other biologic agents, including the interleukin-2 receptor inhibitor daclizumab, have also demonstrated efficacy in the treatment of JIA-U and other forms of

pediatric uveitis. Preoperative escalation of immunosuppressive therapy with systemic or locally administered corticosteroids (CS) is advisable prior to surgery if the risk profile is acceptable to the patient. Close collaboration between the ophthalmologist and the treating pediatric rheumatologist is extremely important to ensure a successful surgical outcome.

9.2.3 Cataract Surgery

Cataract surgery in uveitic patients is challenging due to limited surgical exposure from posterior synechiae and fibrinous membranes overlying the anterior lens capsule. There is high risk of postoperative complications such as uncontrolled inflammation leading to early posterior capsular opacification, glaucoma, CME, epiretinal membrane, hypotony, and phthisis bulbi which requires meticulous care [14]. Cataract surgery with IOL implantation still remains controvertial especially in JIA-U. Previously, IOL implant has been associated with increased postoperative inflammation in some cases, e.g., synechiae from fibrin deposition, pupillary membrane formation, hypotony, secondary cataract formation and there may be a possible need for IOL explantation in severe cases. Recent studies have demonstrated favorable overall outcomes with IOL implantation with adequate perioperative corticosteroid management with systemic immunosuppression and postoperative visual rehabilitation with refractive glasses [15, 16].

Counselling of the patient/parents for uveitic cataract surgery: the most important aspect of counselling when planning to perform cataract surgery is explaining the visual prognosis. In addition to general risks involved in surgery, such as infection and other intraoperative complications, it is important to explain that surgery may be complicated and possibly take longer than usual because of ocular complications, such as the presence of synechiae and membranes, and these factors may contribute to postoperative inflammation, delayed visual recovery, the need for strict compliance with medications (systemic immunosuppression may need to be adjusted), and frequent follow-up. Posterior capsule opacification is another frequent complication encountered postoperatively and because of the young age they may require additional surgery.

Perioperative corticosteroid management in addition to systemic immunosuppression: there is a consensus that the uveitis should be inactive for 3 months or longer prior to cataract surgery [9]. Preoperative escalation of immunosuppressive therapy along with systemic or local CS should be done. Oral prednisone is prescribed at a dose of 0.5–1.0 mg/kg 3–7 days prior to surgery [9].

Postoperatively, oral and topical CS should be tapered judiciously based on disease activity [9]. Intravenous or periocular corticosteroids or escalation of CS-sparing immunosuppression may be required in patients developing uveitis flare-up after surgery.

Surgical techniques: the choice of cataract surgery technique depends upon the individual surgeon's skill and experience. Cataract removal by phacoemulsification/lens aspiration is safer for the uveitic cataract as less inflammation is induced than that by a manual extracapsular cataract extraction. During the surgery, the anatomy of the anterior segment should be restored to a state as close to normal as possible.

9.2.4 Intraoperative Challenges

- Band keratopathy obscuring visual axis and field of view: the deposition of calcium in the subepithelial space may warrant ethylenediamine tetra-acetic acid (EDTA) chelation prior to or after cataract surgery (Fig. 9.10a).
- Posterior synechiae: synechiolysis need to be done prior to cataract extraction for which viscoelastic or a blunt spatula (i.e., cycloidal spatula or iris sweep) can be used to dissect the iris adhesions from the lens. However, special care should be taken to avoid manipulating the iris, as perturbation of iris pigment cells contributes to postoperative inflammation.
- Poorly dilating pupil: synechiolysis, viscodilation, and iris hooks can be used. Pupil retainers can also be used, such as Beehler pupil dilator (2 or 3 pronged), to mechanically stretch the pupil in a single injector system; the Malyugin ring which can be injected into the anterior chamber through a 2.2 mm incision and maneuvered to expand and maintain the pupil open at a 6 or 7 mm diameter.
- Peripheral anterior synechiae (PAS) may cause difficulty in creation of wound especially if they are nearly 360° (Fig. 9.10b). In such cases a long 1 mm incision can be made followed by viscoelastic injection in the eye. It can help in breaking PAS in most cases and surgery can be completed.
- Ectropion uvea may increase chances of intraoperative bleeding and postoperative inflammation. These cases are invariably associated with poor visual outcomes (Fig. 9.10c).

9.2.5 IOL Implantation

Alio et al. [16] conducted a multicentre international study evaluating 140 uveitic eyes in 140 patients who underwent phacoemulsification with IOL implantation of hydrophobic acrylic, silicone, polymethyl methacrylate (PMMA), or heparin-coated PMMA lenses. A total of 46% of patients improved to visual acuity (VA) of 20/40 or better [16]. Patients with acrylic lenses showed the least inflammation at postoperative day 1 and at 3-month follow-up, while the

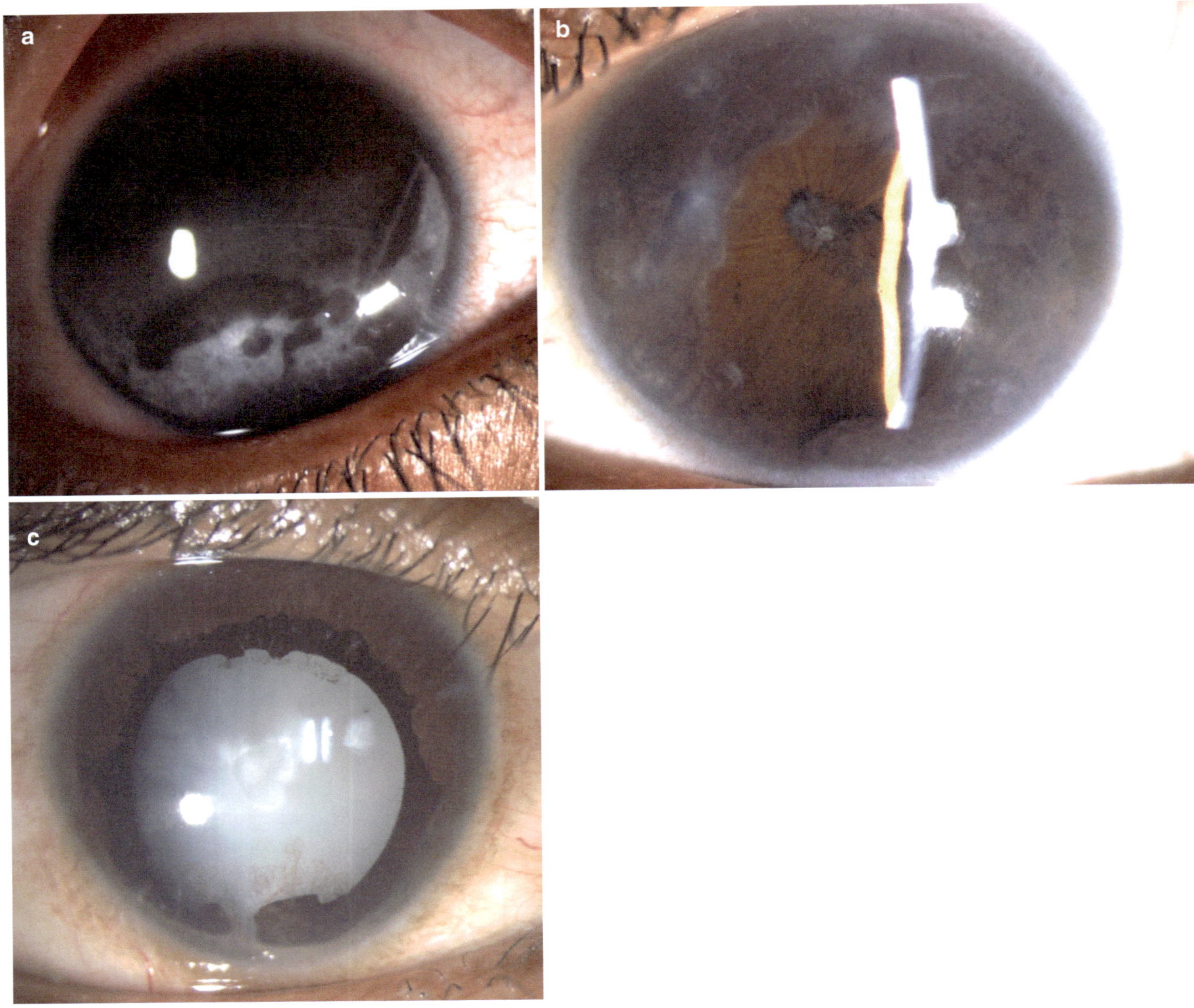

Fig. 9.10 Complications leading to difficult surgery. (**a**) Band-shaped keratopathy, (**b**) extensive peripheral anterior synechiae, Visual axis opacification and its management in uveitic cataract, (**c**) ectropion uvea with vascularization of anterior capsule

acrylic and heparin-coated PMMA lenses showed the lowest incidence of uveitis relapses. The silicone lens group showed the highest rate of posterior capsular opacification, at 34%; for this reason and because of its potential for interfering with vitreoretinal instrumentation, the silicone lens appears less desirable for cataract management in the setting of uveitis. Another study by Papaliodis et al. [17] supported these conclusions and found that acrylic lenses provided better results than heparin-coated PMMA, PMMA, and silicone lens following evaluation of inflammation, posterior capsule opacification, VA, and macular edema.

Limited vitrectomy with or without capsulectomy at time of pediatric cataract surgery: in pediatric patients, posterior capsular opacification and fibrosis may develop (Fig. 9.11), leading to obscuration of the child's visual axis with a reduction in central VA. In older children, Nd:YAG laser capsulotomy may be performed in the clinic and avoids the need for vitrectomy instrumentation at the time of cataract surgery. However, in younger children in whom repeat general anesthesia would be needed for a surgical capsulotomy, limited anterior vitrectomy with posterior capsulotomy should be done following cataract extraction.

9.2.6 Post Op Complications

- Excessive postoperative inflammation: one of the most common postoperative complications. We may need to increase intensity of topical CS and cycloplecis.

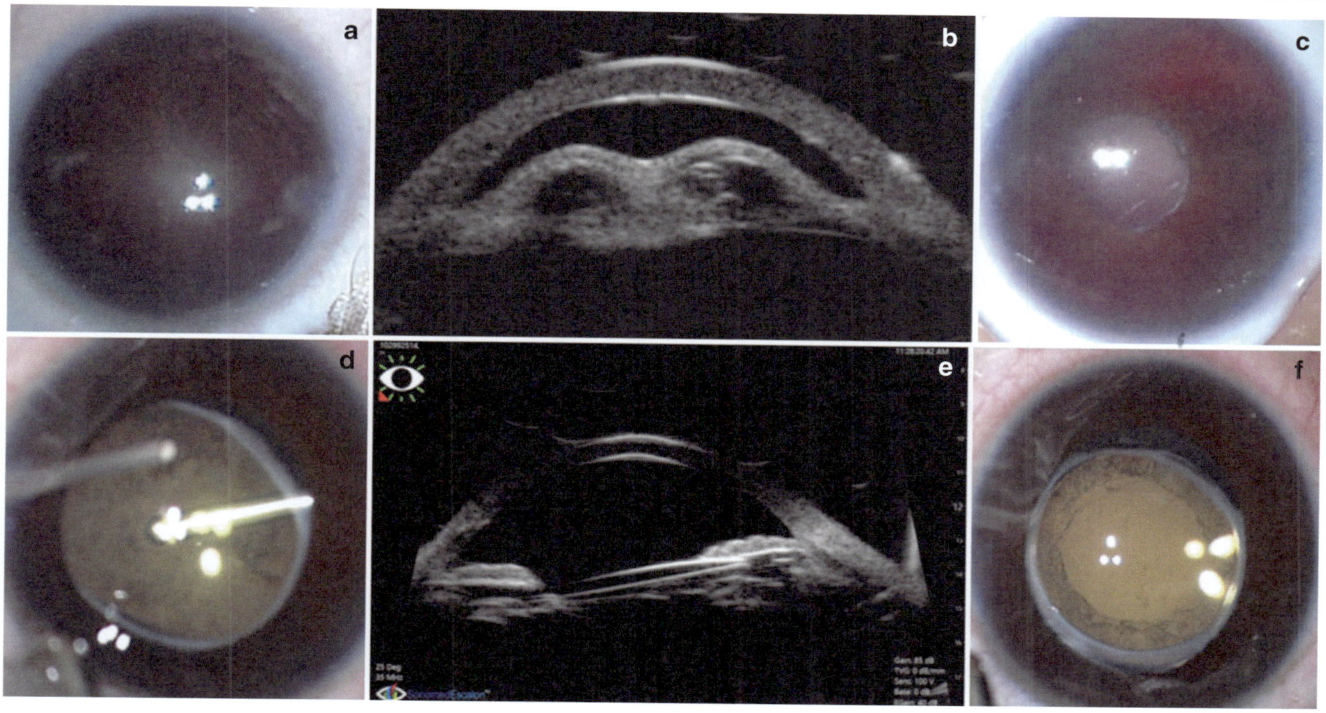

Fig. 9.11 Visual axis opacification (VAO) in pediatric uveitis (**a**). Anterior VAO in JIA patient (**b**). UBM of the same showing iris bombe formation with VAO with aphakia (**c**). Post surgery from anterior route, clear media is seen (**d**). Intraoperative picture showing pars plana membranectomy for posterior VAO (**e**). UBM showing IOL in place and posterior VAO (**f**). Postoperative picture showing clear media and IOL in bag

- Glaucoma: transient rise in IOP can occur during the early postoperative period in eyes with compromised trabecular meshwork or angles. Can be managed with topical and systemic antiglaucoma medications.
- Recurrence of uveitis.
- CME: can be treated with topical CS or topical NSAIDs. However, local periocular or intravitreal CS may be required, particularly in severe cases of CME.
- Posterior capsular opacification: In the late postoperative period, posterior capsular opacification is perhaps the most common complication following any type of cataract surgery. Preventive measures include creating a circular well-centered capsulorhexis which is smaller than the optic size, using an acrylic IOL with a square-edged optic design, meticulous removal of viscoelastic from within the capsular bag and ensuring the optic is stuck on to the posterior capsule at the conclusion of surgery. Judicious control of postoperative inflammation also plays an important role in preventing PCO.
- Amblyopia management: following cataract surgery visual rehabilitation therapy is the integral step for management, patients should be prescribed glasses with occlusion therapy if required (unilateral cataract/anisometropia) and parents should be explained importance of compliance and proper follow-up as advised.

References

1. Edelsten C, Reddy MA, Stanford MR, Graham EM. Visual loss associated with pediatric uveitis in English primary and referral centres. Am J Ophthalmol. 2003;135:676–80.
2. Zierhut M, Michels H, Stübiger N, Besch D, Deuter C, Heiligenhaus A. Uveitis in children. Int Ophthalmol Clin. 2005;45:135–56.
3. Ben Ezra D, Cohen E, Maftzir G. Patterns of intraocular inflammation in children. Bull Soc Belg Ophthalmol. 2001;(279):25–38.
4. O'Brien JM, Albert DM, Foster CS. Juvenile rheumatoid arthritis. In: Albert DM, Jakobiec FA, editors. Principles and practice of ophthalmology: clinical practice, vol. 5. Philadelphia: WB Saunders; 1994. p. 2873–86.
5. Edelsten C, Lee V, Bentley CR, et al. An evaluation of baseline risk factors predicting severity in juvenile idiopathic arthritis associated uveitis and another chronic anterior uveitis in early childhood. Br J Ophthalmol. 2002;86:51–6.
6. Thorne JE, Woreta FA, Dunn JP, Jabs DA. Risk of cataract development among children with juvenile idiopathic arthritis-related uveitis treated with topical corticosteroids. Ophthalmology. 2010;117(7):1436–41.
7. Sallam A, Taylor SR, Habot-Wilner Z, et al. Repeat intravitreal triamcinolone acetonide injections in uveitic macular oedema. Acta Ophthalmol. 2011.
8. Tomkins-Netzer O, Taylor SRJ, Bar A, et al. Treatment with repeat dexamethasone implants results in long-term disease control in eyes with noninfectious uveitis. Ophthalmology. 2014;121(8):1649–54.

9. Blum-Hareuveni T, Seguin-Greenstein S, Kramer M, Hareuveni G, Sharon Y, Friling R, Sharief L, Lightman S, Tomkins-Netzer O. Risk factors for the development of cataract in children with uveitis. Am J Ophthalmol. 2017;177:139–43.
10. Holland GN. A reconsideration of anterior chamber flare and its clinical relevance for children with chronic anterior uveitis (an American ophthalmological society thesis). Trans Am Ophthalmol Soc. 2007;105:344–64.
11. Shah SS, Lewder CY, Schmitt MA, Wilke WS, Kaminsky GS, Geisler DM. xLow-dose methotrexate therapy for ocular inflammatory disease. Ophthalmology. 1992;99:1419–23.
12. Angeles-Han S, Yeh S. Prevention and management of cataracts in children with juvenile idiopathic arthritis–associated uveitis. Curr Rheumatol Rep. 2012;14(2):142–9.
13. Sarsens KM, Roth ova A, Van De Viewer DA, Stigma JS, De Boer JH. Risk factors for the development of cataract requiring surgery in uveitis associated with juvenile idiopathic arthritis. Am J Ophthalmol. 2007;144(4):574–9.
14. Acevedo S, Quinones K, Rao V, et al. Cataract surgery in children with juvenile idiopathic arthritis associated uveitis. Int Ophthalmol Clin. 2008;48:1–7.
15. Sijssens KM, Los LI, Rothova A, et al. Long-term ocular complications in aphakic versus pseudophakic eyes of children with juvenile idiopathic arthritis-associated uveitis. Br J Ophthalmol. 2010;94:1145–9.
16. Alio JL, Chipont E, BenEzra D, Fakhry MA. Comparative performance of intraocular lenses in eyes with cataract and uveitis. J Cataract Refract Surg. 2002;28:2096–108.
17. Papaliodis GN, Nguyen QD, Samson CM, Foster CS. Intraocular lens tolerance in surgery for cataracta complicata: assessment of four implant materials. Semin Ophthalmol. 2002;17:120–3.

Cataract with Infective Etiology

10

Chirakshi Dhull and Sudarshan Kumar Khokhar

Infectious etiology may play a role in cataract formation during embryogenesis [1, 2]. Toxoplasma, Rubella, Cytomegalovirus (CMV), Herpes Simplex virus (HSV), and others including syphilis commonly referred to as TORCH infections have been associated with congenital cataract formation especially in developing countries [3–5]. In addition to childhood cataract, ocular manifestations of TORCH infections include chorioretinitis, microphthalmos, keratitis, iridocyclitis, iris atrophy, glaucoma, optic neuritis, and retinitis [6].

Immunoglobulin (Ig) M and Ig G titers have been used in detection of TORCH infections [3–5, 7–9]. Mahalakshmi and coworkers reported the presence of IgM antibodies in association with congenital cataract [3]. They detected CMV Ig M in 17.8% followed by rubella virus in 8.4% cases among 593 infants with congenital cataract. Ig M for HSV and Toxoplasma has been associated with congenital cataract in various reports [4, 5, 7–9].

There may be an overlap in presentation of these infections. While cataracts are commonly associated with congenital rubella, chorioretinitis is more commonly seen with **congenital toxoplasmosis** (Fig. 10.1). The other common ocular manifestations of congenital toxoplasmosis include

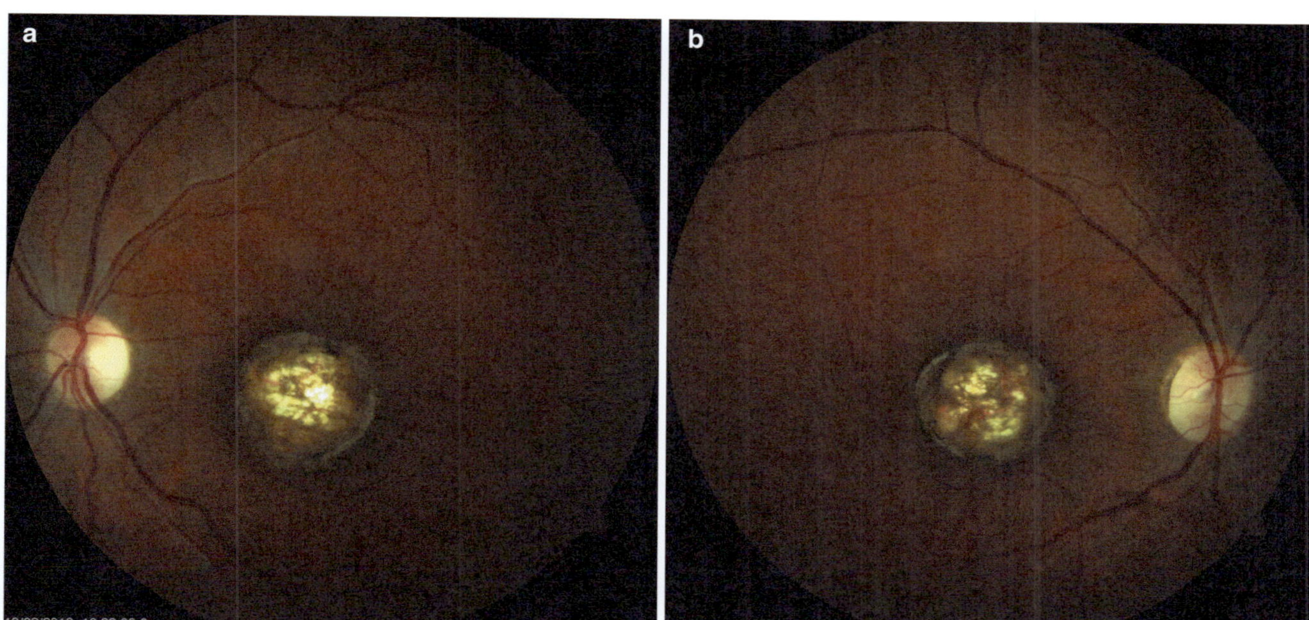

Fig. 10.1 (**a** and **b**) Right and left eye fundus picture of inactive congenital toxoplasma with typical punched out macular scar (Courtesy Dr. Shreyas Themkar, Karnataka, India)

C. Dhull · S. K. Khokhar (✉)
Dr Rajendra Prasad Centre for Ophthalmic Sciences, All India Institute of Medical Sciences, New Delhi, India

S. K. Khokhar, C. Dhull (eds.), *Atlas of Pediatric Cataract*, https://doi.org/10.1007/978-981-13-6939-1_10

microphthalmos, squint, iridocyclitis, cataract, and glaucoma [10–13]. **CMV infection** has also been implicated in congenital cataract. Other ocular manifestations include retinitis, optic atrophy, disc anomaly, microphthalmos, keratitis, and glaucoma [6, 14–16]. H Raghu et al. found **HSV** 1 in 4 cases of congenital cataract [4]. Both HSV 1 and 2 have been implicated in neonatal infections and more commonly associated with conjunctivitis and keratitis along with other features common to TORCH infections [6]. In this chapter, we will discuss cataract associated with congenital rubella syndrome in detail which remains a major challenge in developing countries.

10.1 Congenital Rubella Syndrome

Rubella infection as a cause of congenital cataract was first conclusively put forward by Gregg in 1941 during epidemic of rubella in Australia [17]. His idea of maternally transmitted infections causing ocular and systemic disease remains a milestone in ophthalmology and epidemiology. Despite being eradicated in most developed nation, it still remains an important cause of congenital cataract in developing countries and immigrant population from developing countries [3, 18, 19].

10.1.1 Clinical Presentation

Congenital rubella syndrome (CRS) is described as a multisystem disorder with a classical triad of congenital heart disease, deafness, and cataract [14]. World health organization (WHO) has given clinical criteria for CRS [20]. The criteria include the presence of >2 clinical features from group A, or one feature from group A and >1 from group B in the following list (Table 10.1).

Table 10.1 WHO criteria for diagnosis of CRS [20]

Group A	Group B
Sensorineural hearing impairment	Purpura
Congenital heart disease	Splenomegaly
Pigmentary retinopathy	Microcephaly
Cataract(s)	Developmental delay
Congenital glaucoma	Meningoencephalitis
	Radiolucent bone disease
	Jaundice with onset within 24 h of birth

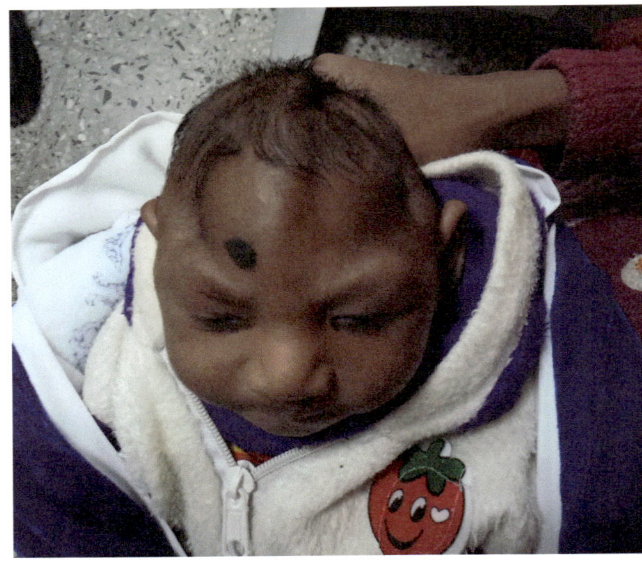

Fig. 10.2 A 6-week-old infant with CRS with microcephaly

Cardiovascular abnormality includes patent ductus arteriosus (PDA) (most common) along with atrial septal defect, pulmonary stenosis, and ventricular septal defect [21]. Neurological abnormalities include microcephaly, hearing disorder, developmental delay, mental retardation, seizure disorder, and speech abnormality [21, 22] (Fig. 10.2).

Ocular features include the following, and the presence of these features should raise a suspicion of CRS [22–24]:

- Microphthalmos (Fig. 10.3).
- Presence of cloudy cornea or corneal opacity (Fig. 10.4).
- Iris atrophy, iritis, iridocyclitis, or iris hypoplasia. Non-dilating pupil may also be seen (Fig. 10.5).
- Congenital cataract may be total, nuclear, or membraneous in nature. Central cataract with peripheral clear area may be seen (Fig. 10.6).
- Angle abnormalities and glaucoma may be seen.
- Pigmentary retinopathy typically salt and pepper retinopathy is seen (Fig. 10.7). Associated maculopathy may be seen. Rubella virus infection of RPE has been associated defective phagocytosis of the RPE in vitro [25]. In rare cases, subretinal neovascularization is seen [13].
- Presence of squint or nystagmus may be seen.
- Other abnormalities include optic atrophy, optic neuritis, lens absorption, keratoconus, corneal hydrops, or even phthisis bulbi may be rarely associated [13].

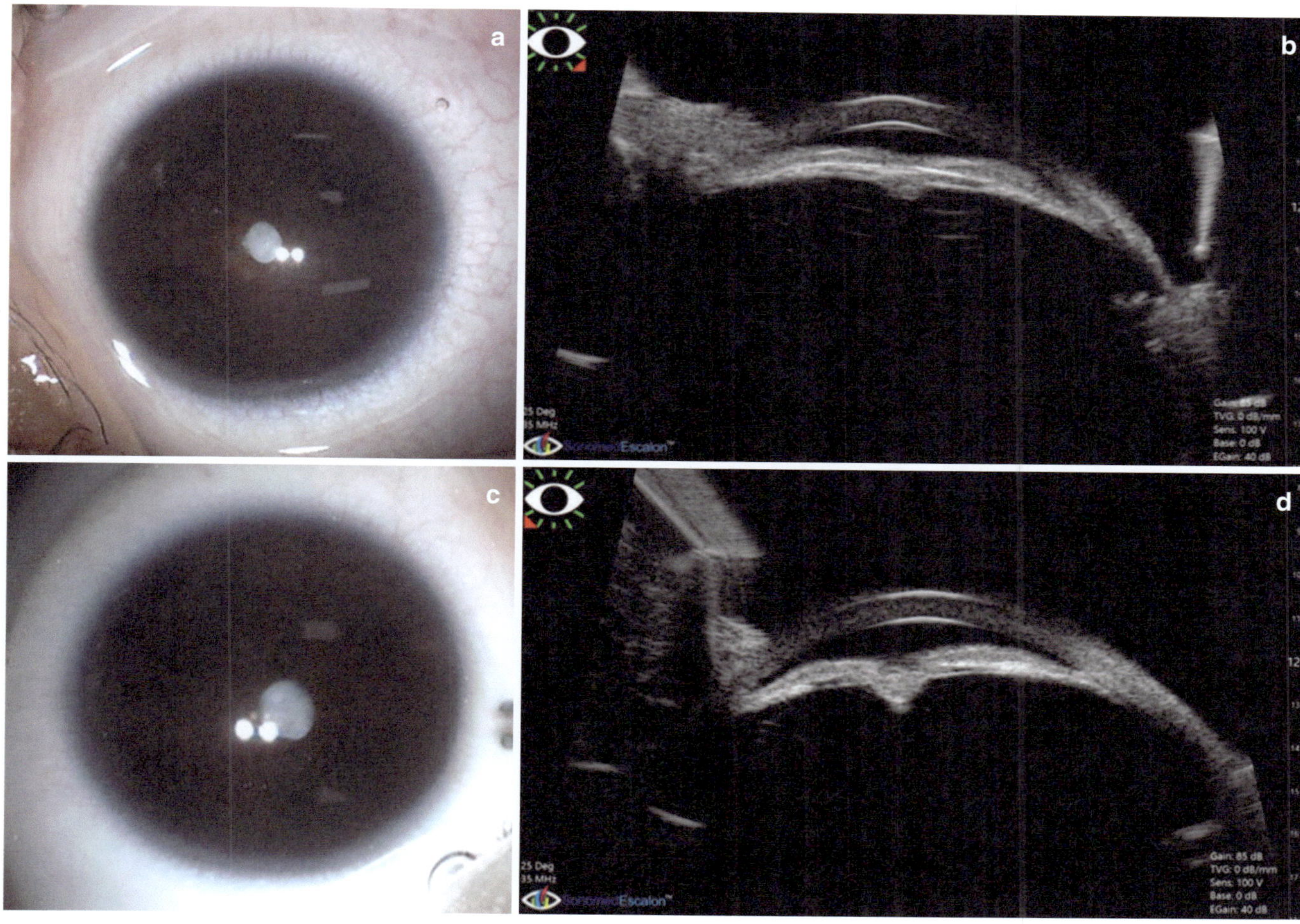

Fig. 10.3 Microphthalmos in a 2-month-old infant with congenital cataract. (**a** and **c**) Clinical picture showing small pupil, atrophy iris, and cataract of right and left eye, respectively, (**b** and **d**) ultrasound biomicroscopy of the same showing microphthalmos, microcornea, shallow anterior chamber, and membranous cataract

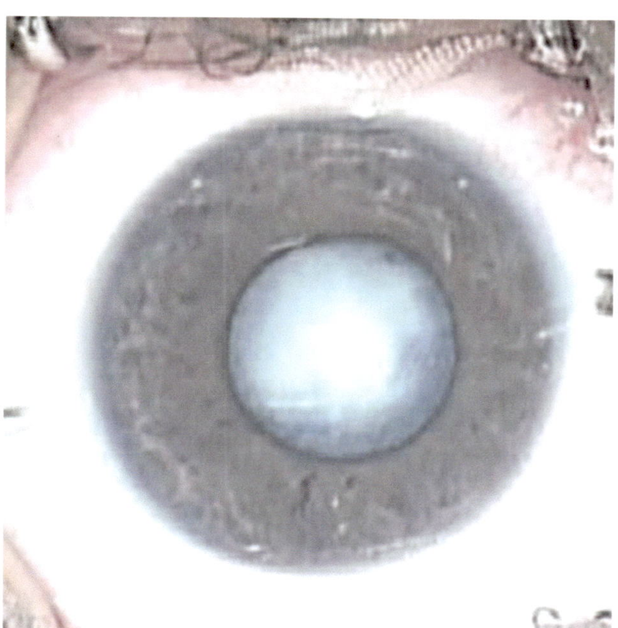

Fig. 10.4 Infant with CRS with hazy cornea, atrophic iris, and cataract

10.1.2 Management

Investigation for diagnosis include Ig M and Ig G antibody, direct detection of virus, or reverse transcription PCR [20]. General principles of management of pediatric cataract remain the same and are discussed in detail in respective chapters.

Special considerations include the following:

- Small size of the globe may cause difficulty in surgery and increase chances of tissue manipulation. Insertion of IOL in these cases is less likely.
- Corneal haze may cause difficulty in surgery and there is greater postoperative risk of corneal edema [26] (Fig. 10.8).
- Non-dilating pupil may require pupilloplasty to reduce risk of VAO formation.
- Nature and morphology of cataract may have a bearing on surgical management. In case of membraneous cataract, if the size of eye is adequate IOL may be placed in sulcus after removal of cataract (Fig. 10.9).

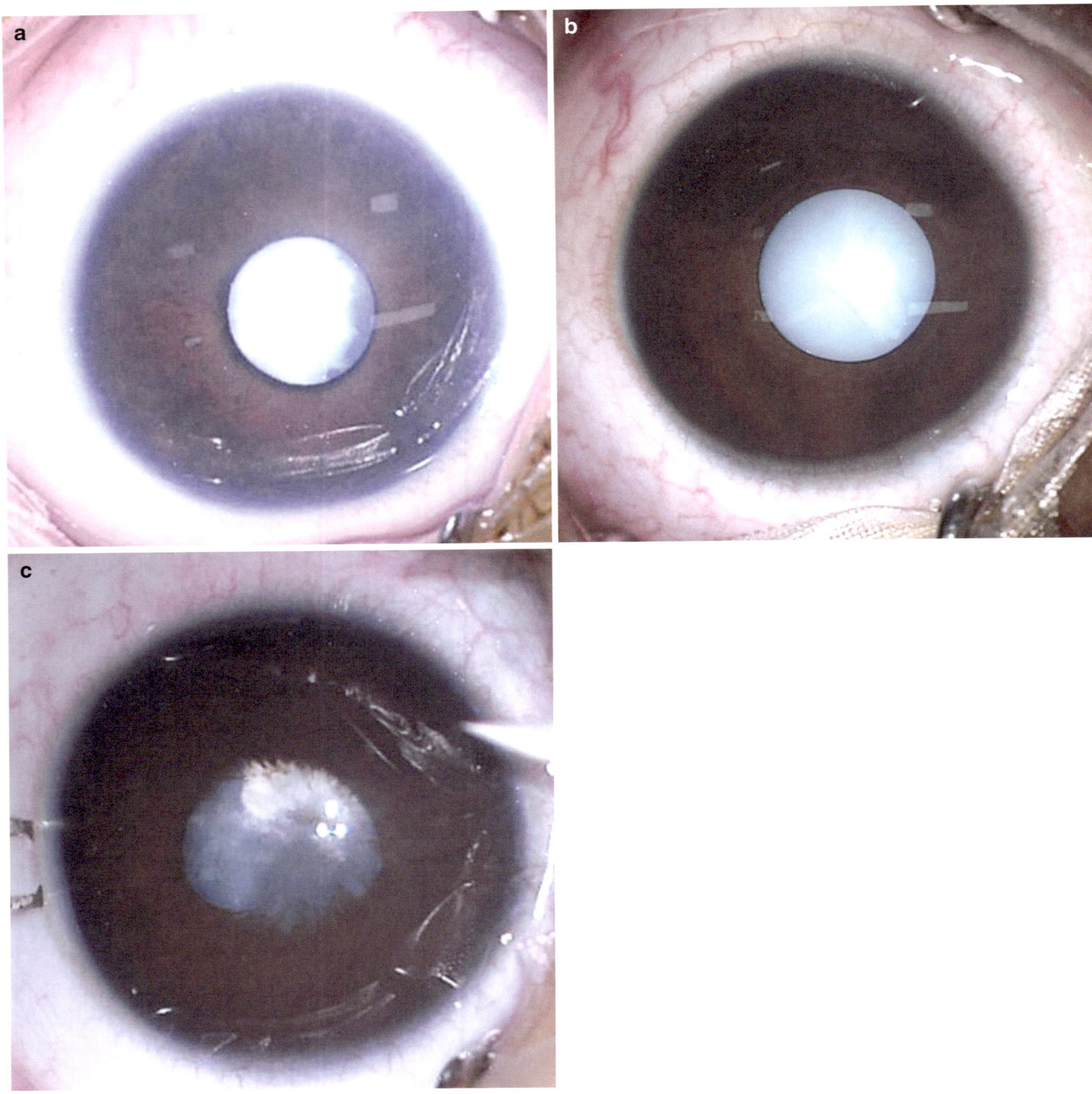

Fig. 10.5 Iris abnormality in CRS. (**a**) Non-dilating pupil with patch iris atrophy with membraneous cataract. (**b**) Diffuse iris atrophy with absence of normal iris pattern along with total cataract with anterior capsular plaque. (**c**) Posterior synechiae along with iris atrophy and membranous calcified cataract

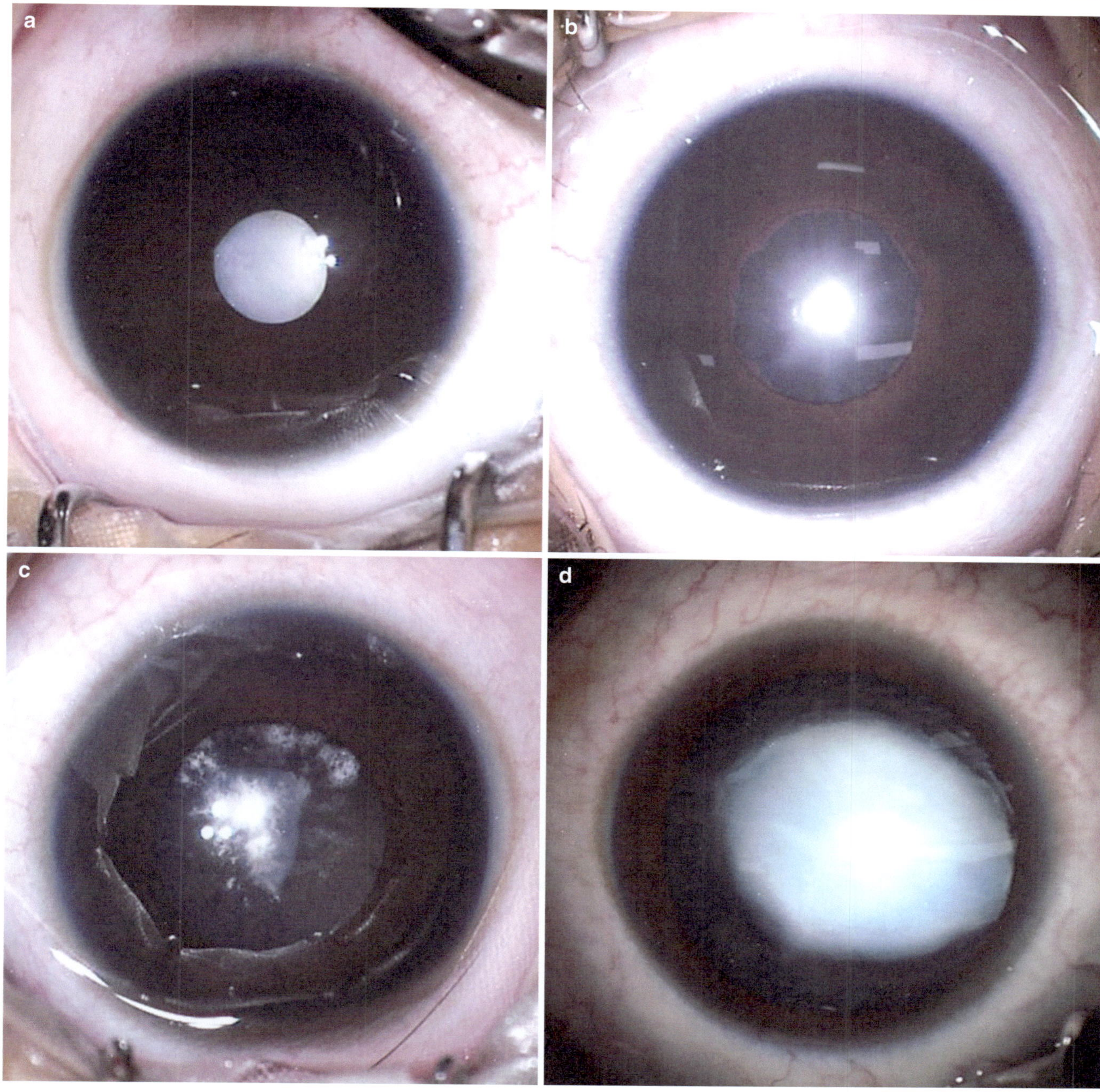

Fig. 10.6 Various morphology of cataract in CRS. (**a**) Total cataract, (**b**) nuclear cataract, (**c**) absorbed cataract, (**d**) membranous cataract

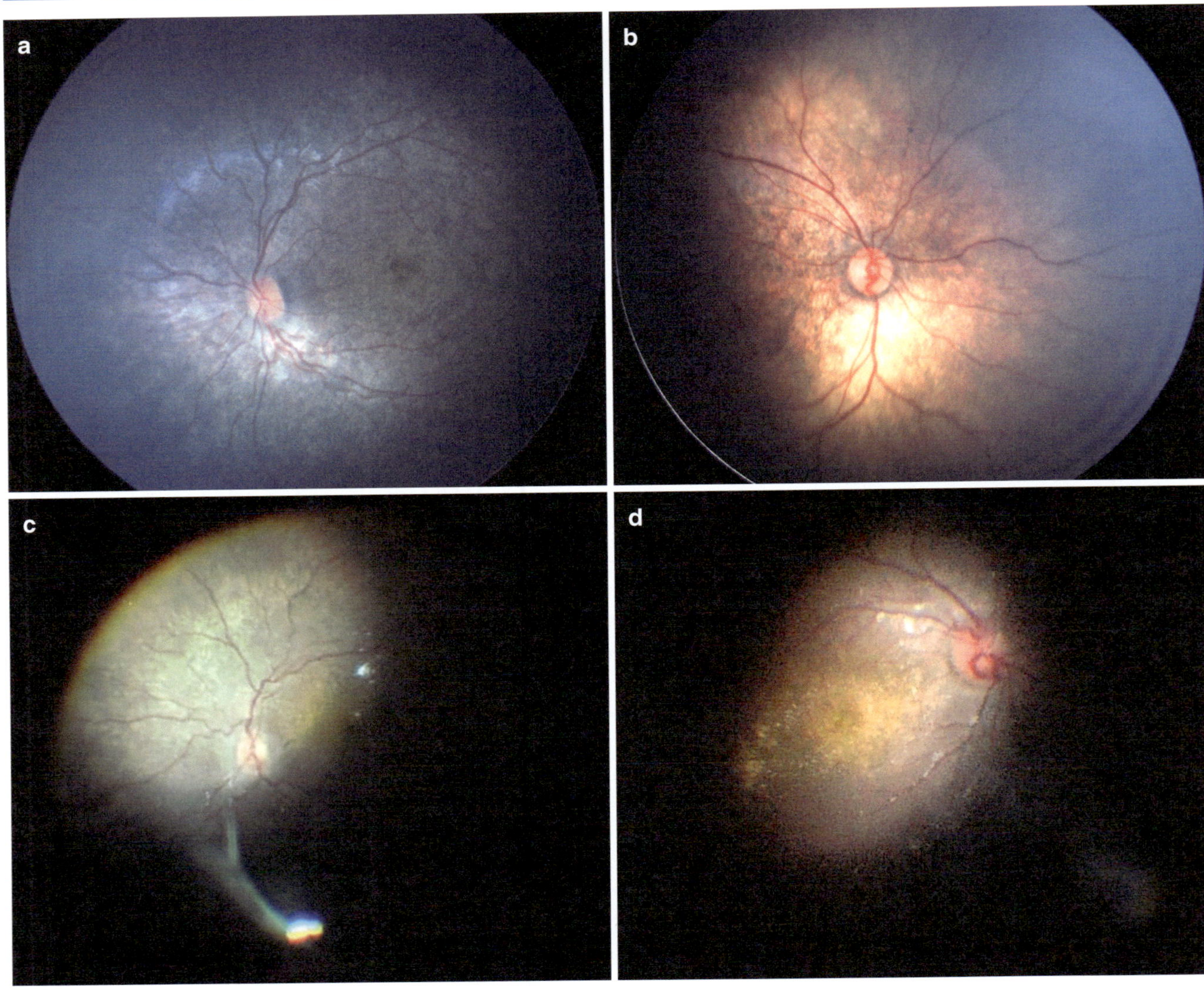

Fig. 10.7 Pigmentary retinopathy in CRS. (**a**) Retcam picture of mild salt and pepper retinopathy at posterior pole. (**b**) Salt and pepper retinopathy with associated chorioretinal atrophy. (**c**) Intraoperative fundus view with wide angle viewing system showing diffuse pigmentary retinopathy. (**d**) Intraoperative fundus view with wide angle viewing system showing Rubella maculopathy

- Risk of postoperative glaucoma is higher in these patients [26].
- Visual outcome may be affected due to associated complications. Pigmentary retinopathy usually does not affect visual outcome [26, 27].

TORCH infections remain an important cause of childhood cataracts especially in developing country. Identifying the etiology helps in planning and prognostication since higher rate of complications is acceptable in these patients [27]. Early surgery and visual rehabilitation with glasses and contact lens is generally possible in most cases.

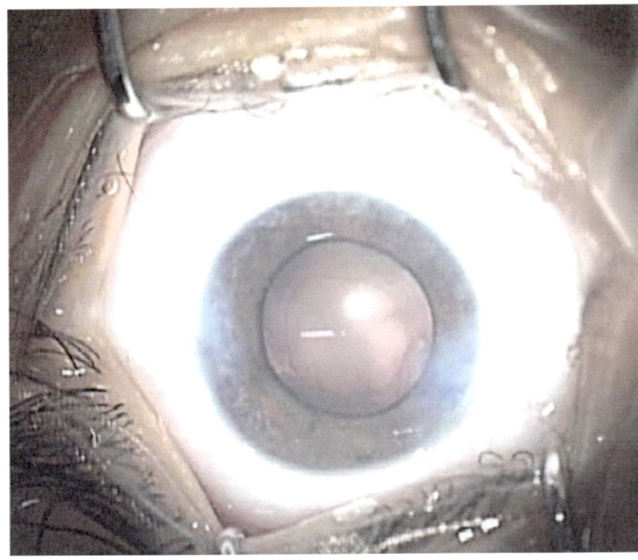

Fig. 10.8 Postoperative picture of a 3-month-old patient with CRS with corneal edema

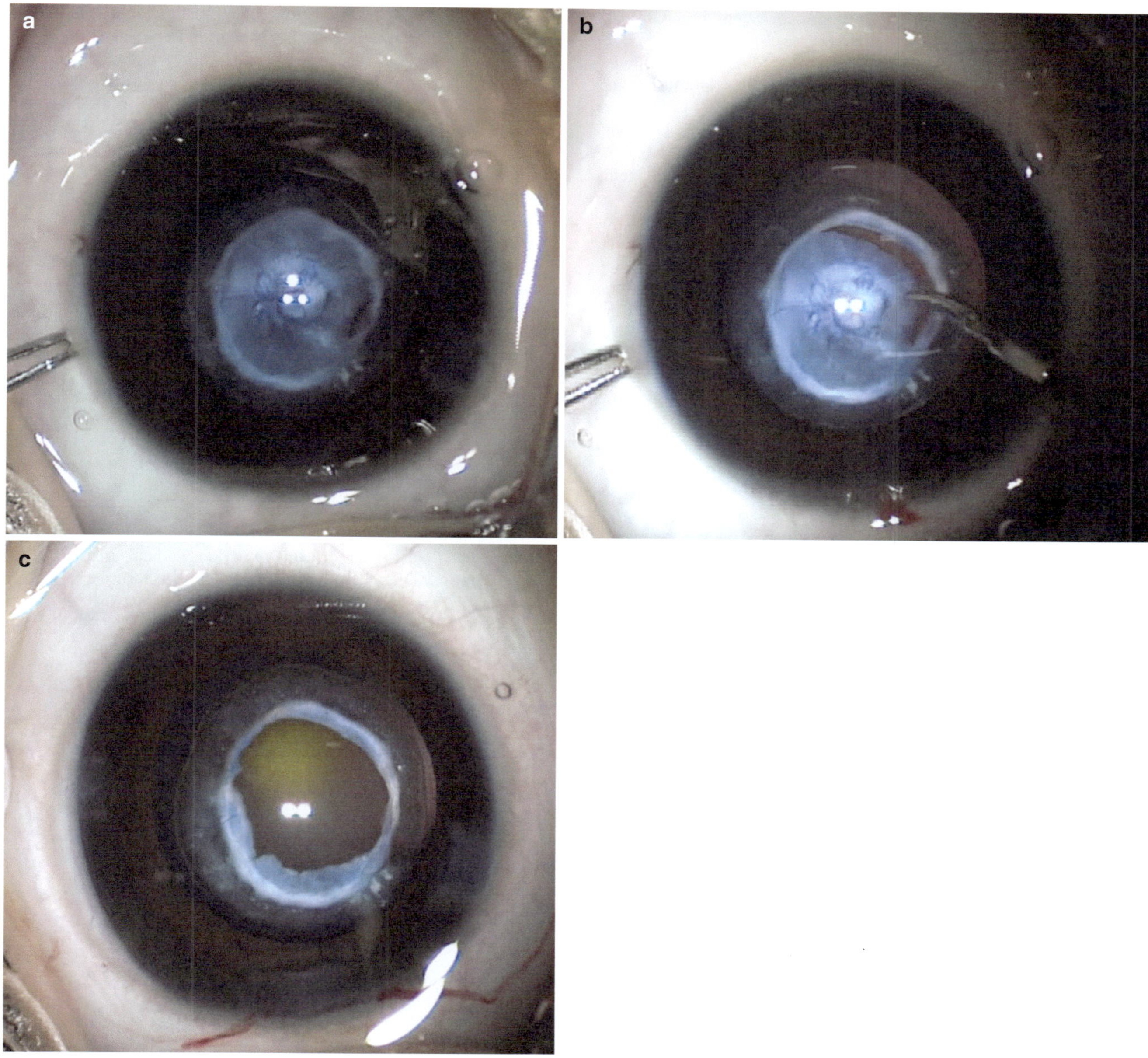

Fig. 10.9 Intraoperative picture of a 6-month-old patient with CRS with membranous cataract (**a**) Nick is given in the fused anterior and posterior capsule. (**b**) Microincision forceps is used for making central 4 mm opening. (**c**) After making opening and performing anterior vitrectomy 360 support is present for IOL insertion in sulcus. Notice small size of lens along with peripheral visible zonules, hence 4 mm opening is made, leaving adequate rim for support. Also notice altered glow because of the presence of pigmentary retinopathy

References

1. Matoba A. Ocular viral infections. Pediatr Infect Dis. 1984;3:358–68.
2. Cotlier E. Congenital varicella cataract. Am J Ophthalmol. 1978;86:627–9.
3. Mahalakshmi B, Therese KL, Devipriya U, Pushpalatha V, Margarita S, Madhavan HN. Infectious aetiology of congenital cataract based on TORCHES screening in a tertiary eye hospital in Chennai, Tamil Nadu, India. Indian J Med Res. 2010;131:559–64.
4. Raghu H, Subhan S, Jose RJ, Gangopadhyay N, Bhende J, Sharma S. Herpes simplex virus-1-associated congenital cataract. Am J Ophthalmol. 2004;138:313–4.
5. Madhavan HN. Laboratory investigations on viral and chlamydia trachomatis infections of the eye: Sankara Nethralaya experiences. Indian J Ophthalmol. 1999;47:241–6.
6. Mets MB. Eye manifestations of intrauterine infections. Ophthalmol Clin N Am. 2001;14:521–31.
7. Mahalakshmi B, Therese KL, Shyamala G, Devipriya U, Madhavan HN. Toxoplasma gondii detection by nested polymerase chain reaction in lens aspirate and peripheral blood leukocyte in congenital cataract patients - the first report from a tertiary eye hospital in India. Curr Rye Res. 2007;32:653–7.
8. Shyamala G, Sowmya P, Madhavan HN, Malathi J. Relative efficiency of polymerase chain reaction and enzyme-linked immunosorbant assay in determination of viral etiology in congenital cataract in infants. J Postgrad Med. 2008;54:17–20.

9. Lu B, Yang Y. Detection of TORCH pathogens in children with congenital cataracts. Exp Ther Med. 2016;12(2):1159–64.
10. Vutova K, Peicheva Z, Popova A, Markova V, Mincheva N, Todorov T. Congenital toxoplasmosis: eye manifestations in infants and children. Ann Trop Paediatr. 2002;22:213–8.
11. Datta S, Banerjee DP. Chorioretinitis in congenital toxoplasmosis. Indian Pediatr. 2003;40:790–1.
12. Mittal V, Bhatia R, Singh VK, Sengal S. Low incidence of congenital toxoplasmosis in Indian children. J Trop Pediatr. 1995;41:62–3.
13. O'Neill JF. The ocular manifestations of congenital infection: a study of the early effect and long-term outcome of maternally transmitted rubella and toxoplasmosis. Trans Am Ophthalmol Soc. 1998;96:813–79.
14. Boniuk I. The cytomegalovirus and the eye. Int Ophthalmol Clin. 1972;12:169–90.
15. Tarkkanen A, Merenmies L, Holmstrom T. Ocular involvement in congenital cytomegalic inclusion disease. J Pediatr Ophthalmol. 1972;9:82–6.
16. Hittner HM, Desmond MM, Montgomery JR. Optic nerve manifestations of human congenital cytomegalovirus infection. Am J Ophthalmol. 1976;81:661–5.
17. Gregg NM. Congenital cataract following German measles in the mother. Trans Ophthalmol Soc Aust. 1941;3:35–46.
18. Papania MJ, Wallace GS, Rota PA, Icenogle JP, Fiebelkorn AP, Armstrong GL, Reef SE, Redd SB, Abernathy ES, Barskey AE, Hao L, McLean HQ, Rota JS, Bellini WJ, Seward JF. Elimination of endemic measles, rubella, and congenital rubella syndrome from the Western hemisphere; the US experience. JAMA Pediatr. 2014;168:148–55.
19. Sheridan E, Aitken C, Jeffries D, Hird M, Thayalasekaran P. Congenital rubella syndrome: a risk in immigrant populations. Lancet. 2002;359:674–5.
20. World Health Organization. Surveillance guidelines for measles, rubella and congenital rubella syndrome in the WHO European Region. http://www.euro.who.int/__data/assets/pdf_file/0018/79020/e93035-2013.pdf?ua=1.
21. Cooper LZ, Ziring PR, Ockerse AB, Fedun BA, Kiely B, Krugman S. Rubella clinical manifestations and management. Am J Dis Child. 1969;118:18–9.
22. Vijayalakshmi P, Kakkar G, Samprathi A, et al. Ocular manifestations of congenital rubella syndrome in a developing country. Indian J Ophthalmol. 2002;50:307–11.
23. Vijayalakshmi P, Rajasundari TA, Prasad NM, et al. Prevalence of eye signs in congenital rubella syndrome in South India: a role for population screening. Br J Ophthalmol. 2007;91:1467–70.
24. Boger WP III, Petersen RA, Robb RM. Spontaneous absorption of the lens in the congenital rubella syndrome. Arch Ophthalmol. 1981;99:433–4.
25. Williams LL, Lew HM, Davidorf FH, et al. Altered membrane fatty acids of cultured human retinal pigment epithelium persistently infected with rubella virus may affect secondary cellular function. Arch Virol. 1994;134:379–92.
26. Vijayalakshmi P, Srivastava KK, Poornima B, et al. Visual outcome of cataract surgery in children with congenital rubella syndrome. J AAPOS. 2003;7:91–5.
27. Shah SK, Praveen MR, Vasavada AR, Vasavada VA, Carelli R, Trivedi RH, Rasoebala V. Long-term longitudinal assessment of postoperative outcomes after congenital cataract surgery in children with congenital rubella syndrome. J Cataract Refract Surg. 2014;40:2091–8.

Cataract in Childhood Glaucoma and Anterior Segment Dysgenesis

11

Sudarshan Kumar Khokhar, Yogita Gupta, Abhidnya Surve, and Chirakshi Dhull

Cataracts can occur in association with ocular or systemic comorbidities. Presence of these comorbidities may alter the presentation and management of lens conditions. In this chapter we will be discussing two such comorbidities: childhood glaucomas and anterior segment dysgenesis. Although childhood glaucoma and anterior segment dysgenesis are separate entities, they have been clubbed together since anterior segment dysgenesis is associated with glaucoma in significant number of cases and few cases of presumed primary congenital glaucoma may actually be glauocomas secondary to anterior segment dysgenesis.

11.1 Childhood Glaucoma

Primary congenital glaucoma (PCG) is an anomaly affecting anterior chamber angle which leads to obstruction of aqueous outflow, increased intraocular pressure (IOP) and optic nerve damage [1]. Buphthalmos is used to describe visible enlargement of the eyeball at birth or early childhood due to an uncontrolled glaucoma [2]. High intraocular pressure (IOP) causes increase in axial length and corneal dimensions of the eye, leading to axial myopia, stretched limbus, corneal thinning, and visibly enlarged eyeballs. The common causes of buphthalmos include primary congenital glaucoma (PCG), Sturge–Weber syndrome, neurofibromatosis and aniridia [2].

The incidence of PCG is one in every 10,000–15,000 live births which accounts for 0.01–0.04% of total blindness [3]. It is bilateral in up to 80% of cases and two-thirds of the cases are males. Most cases are sporadic (90%) [4]. However, in the remaining 10% there appears to be a strong familial pattern.

11.1.1 Clinical Presentation

Vision loss in glaucoma eyes in children may occur secondary to an uncorrected refractive error, corneal opacity, optic nerve damage, amblyopia or per se cataracts. Examination findings may be variable. However, following points should be noted:

- Progressive myopia and high astigmatism may be seen.
- Cornea may be hazy and presence of Haab striae is a common finding (Fig. 11.1), which may obscure vision.
- Cataract may be anterior or posterior subcapsular cataract, total or less commonly cortical or zonular cataract (Fig. 11.2). Cataract may be primary or more commonly secondary to trabeculectomy in 6–58% cases [5–7].
- Bleb in post trabeculectomy eyes with buphthalmos may be thin cystic and rarely associated with other complications (Fig. 11.3).
- Fundus examination may reveal advanced cupping which may be reversible (to some extent) in small children. Features associated with pathological myopia (e.g. tesselated fundus) may be seen.

11.1.2 Investigations

In addition to usual investigations, ultrasound biomicroscopy can aid in measurement of angle to angle and bag diameter to plan for surgery (Fig. 11.4). UBM also helps to assess anterior segment structures, anterior chamber depth (ACD), angle anomalies, abnormal iris insertion, sulcus-to-sulcus measurement and identifies lax zonules and/or pre-exisiting posterior capsular defect preoperatively [8].

S. K. Khokhar · Y. Gupta · A. Surve · C. Dhull (✉)
Dr. Rajendra Prasad Centre for Ophthalmic Sciences, All India Institute of Medical Sciences, New Delhi, India

S. K. Khokhar, C. Dhull (eds.), *Atlas of Pediatric Cataract*, https://doi.org/10.1007/978-981-13-6939-1_11

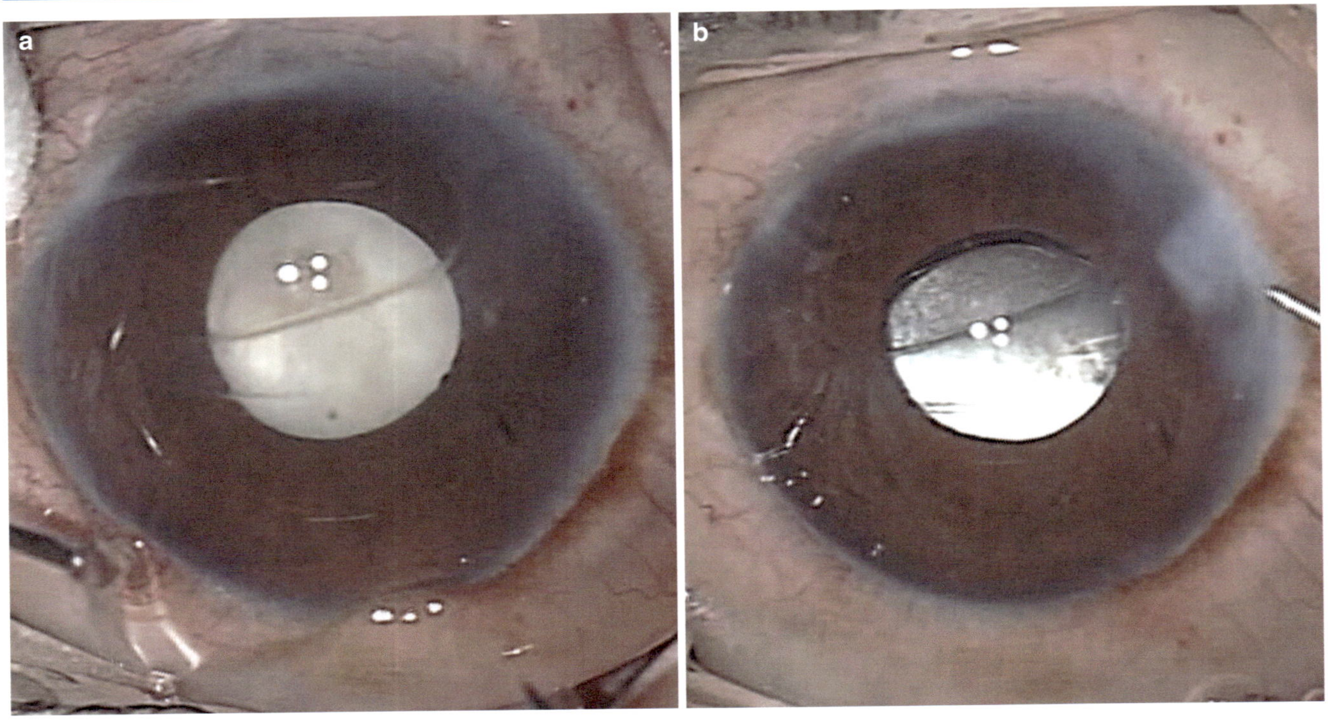

Fig. 11.1 Congenital glaucoma with Haab striae and total cataract. (**a**) Preoperative picture with large superior and multiple peripheral Haab striae seen in cornea, (**b**) postoperative picture of same case with IOL in situ and more pronounced Haab striae

11.1.3 Management of Cataract in Buphthalmic Eyes

The surgical challenges faced by pediatric surgeons while operating for cataract in buphthalmic eyes include the following:

- Corneal haze may cause difficulty in visualization during surgery (Fig. 11.5).
- Very deep anterior chamber (AC) result in difficult instrumentation. Intraoperatively, anterior chamber depth may show frequent fluctuations due to low scleral rigidity in these stretched eyes.
- Phacodonesis, lax lens zonules, liquefied vitreous, and, thus, a weak posterior capsular support can lead to inadvertent complications. There is increased risk of vitreous loss in these patients.
- Highly elastic anterior and posterior capsule may cause continuous curvilinear capsulorhexis (CCC) to be a challenging step.
- Wound closure in eyes with raised pressure may be difficult. All wounds must be well-sutured at the end of surgery in these eyes as postoperatively shallow AC is often noted.
- Intraocular lens (IOL) power calculation remains difficult. Post trabeculectomy buphthalmic eyes have a shift towards with-the-rule astigmatism [9, 10]. As most of these eyes are high myopic, IOL power calculation should be done using appropriate IOL formulae, e.g., SRK-T for axial lengths >24.5 mm. Many a times, no single IOL power formulae might be able to predict the correct emmetropic power of implant for buphthalmic eyes.
- Large eye size and bag dimensions that may lead to postoperative intraocular lens (IOL) decentration [11, 12]. But if bag size appears to be large on UBM, surgeon should plan multipiece IOL in sulcus with optic capture in bag (i.e., optic in bag and haptic in sulcus) (Fig. 11.6). Iris fixated and customized IOLs have also been described for such eyes [12].
- Postoperatively, there are high chances of visual axis opacification (VAO) formation owing to an inflammatory response and formation of dense capsular fibrosis.

11.1.4 Surgical Outcomes

Temporary cessation of ocular growth is reported after adequate IOP control in eyes with AL > 22 mm and in children aged 3 months or older [13].

Our experience with 31 eyes of primary congenital glaucoma (post trabeculectomy) with visually significant cataract undergoing lens aspiration surgery showed a mean best corrected visual acuity of 6/60 (Snellen's) at one year postoperatively. Reasonably predictable refractive results were obtained in these eyes, provided intraocular pressure was well controlled [14].

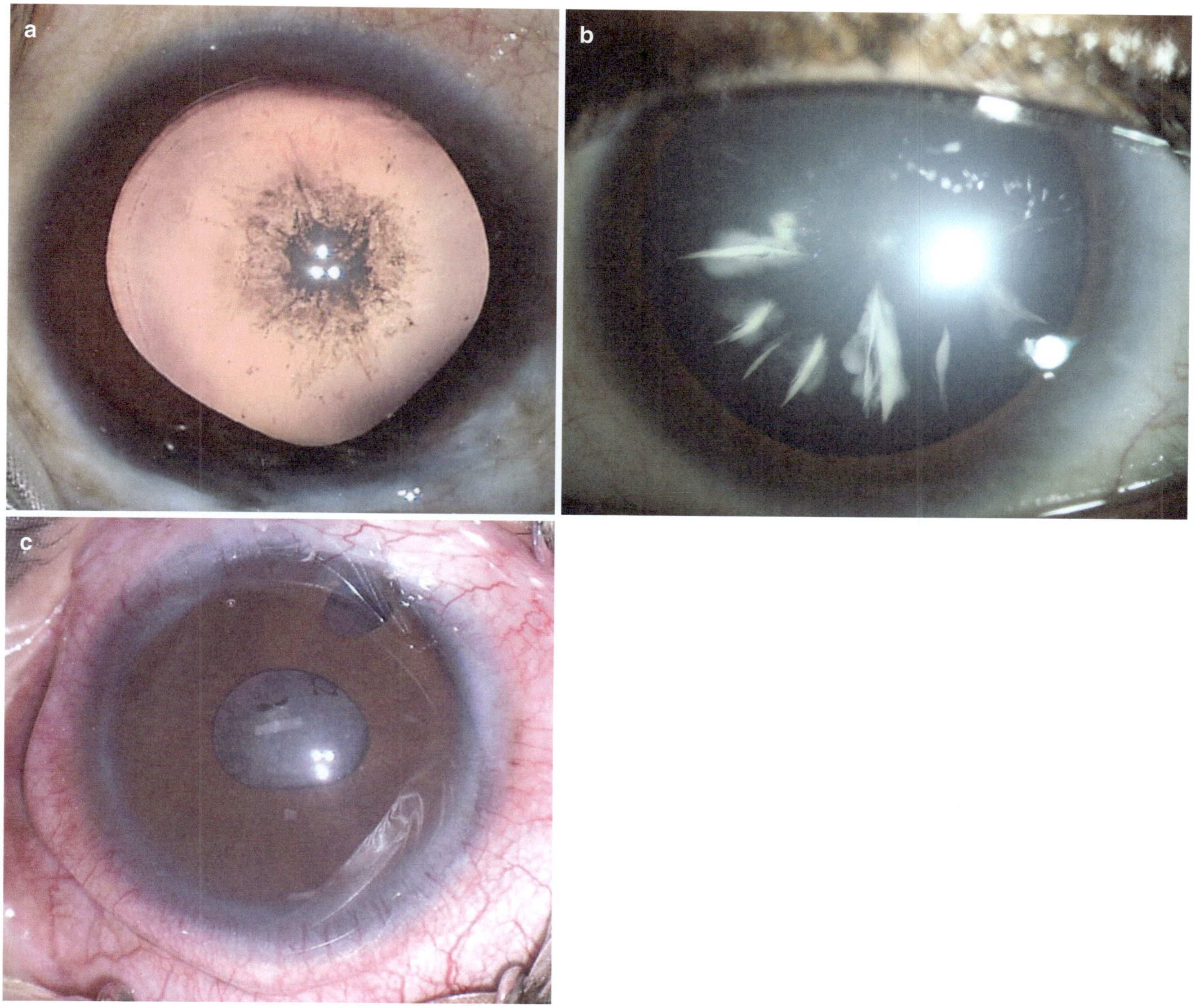

Fig. 11.2 Morphology in cataract with childhood glaucoma post trabeculectomy. (**a**) Posterior subcapsular cataract, (**b**) cortical cataract, (**c**) diffuse cataract with large superonasal peripheral iridotomy

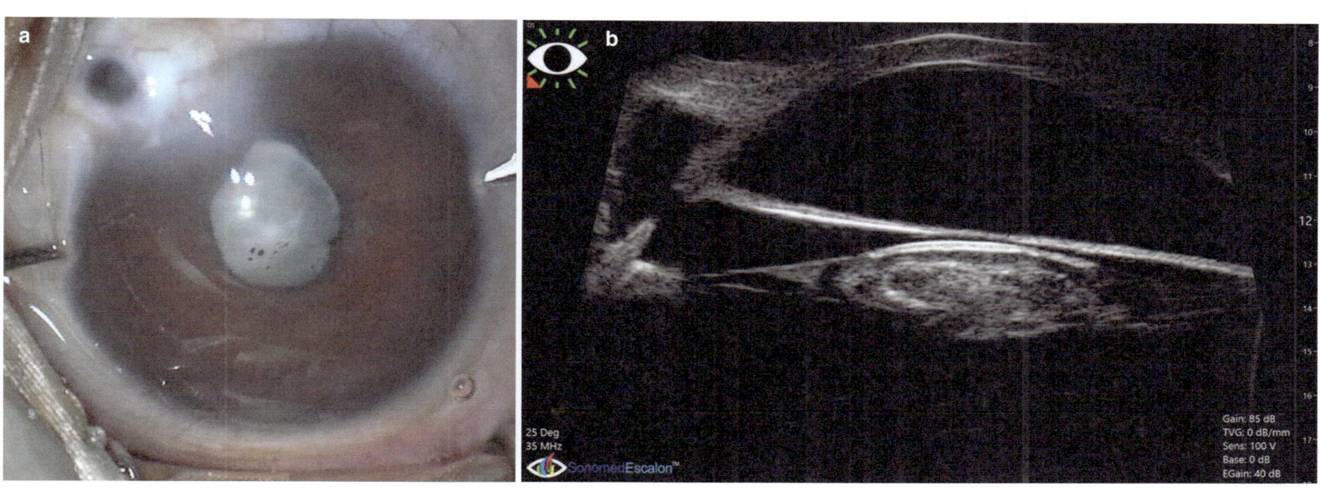

Fig. 11.3 Post trabeculectomy thin cystic bleb with iris prolapse from the ostium and total cataract. (**a**) Clinical picture, (**b**) ultrasound biomicroscopy of the same case showing patent ostium and elevated bleb

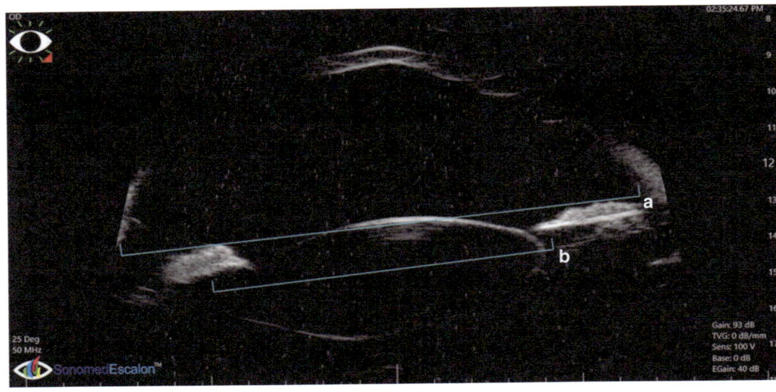

Fig. 11.4 Ultrasound biomicroscopy showing dimensions of a buphthalmic eye. Complete white-to-white examination is not possible in single view. (**a**) angle to angle distance, (**b**) bag diameter

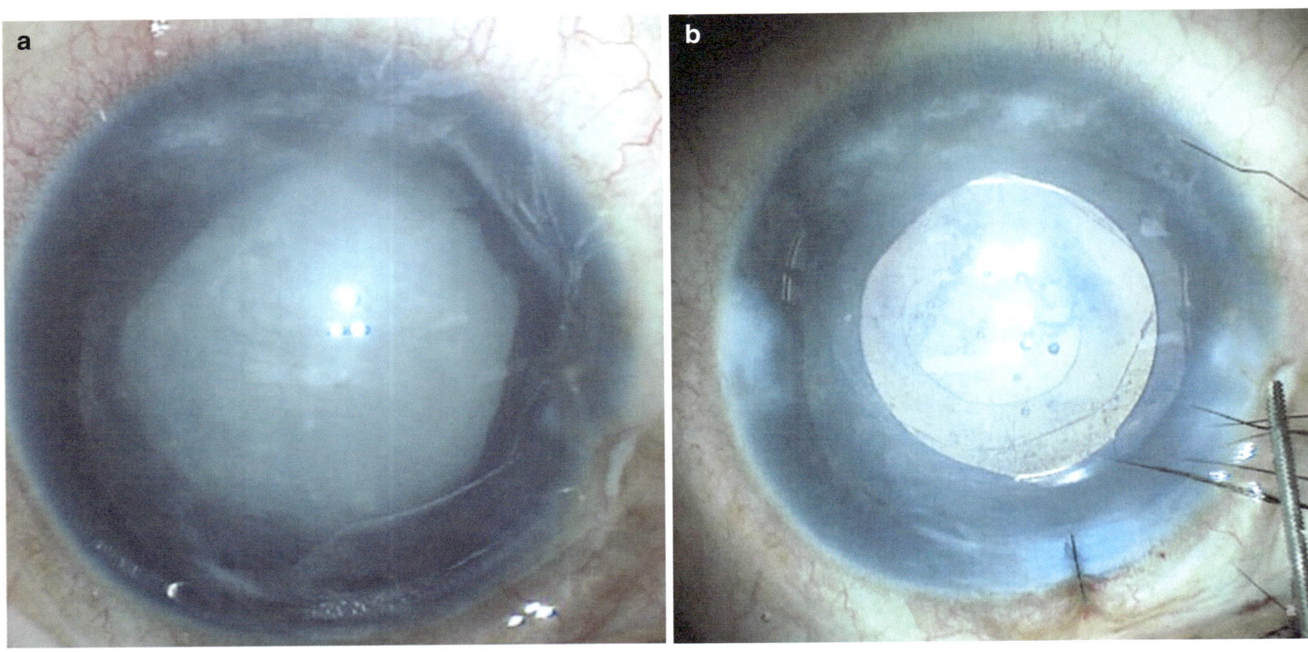

Fig. 11.5 A 6-year-old child with congenital glaucoma with corneal haze with atrophic iris. (**a**) Preoperative picture with total cataract, (**b**) postoperative picture with circular anterior and posterior capsulorhexis and IOL in bag

Thus, besides control of IOP, visual rehabilitation of buphthalmic eyes involves appropriate management for amblyopia, keratoplasty for corneal opacity, and timely cataract surgery for visually significant cataract. Buphthalmic eyes undergoing cataract surgery can achieve successful refractive and visual outcomes if careful preoperative planning is carried out regarding the choice of IOL type and IOL power, taking into consideration the adequacy of intraocular pressure control, accurate biometry, assessment of bag size, and use of appropriate IOL power formulae.

11.2 Anterior Segment Dysgenesis

Anterior segment dysgenesis (ASD) is a group of disorders arising from abnormal development in cornea, iris, lens, and angle structures. This spectrum includes Axenfeld's anomaly, Rieger's anomaly, Axenfeld–Rieger syndrome (ARS), Peters anomaly, sclerocornea, aniridia, posterior keratoconus, and iridogoniodysgenesis. They occur often due to abnormalities in neural crest differentiation and migration. Various classification systems are used for describing ASD depending either on their clinical features or area of involve-

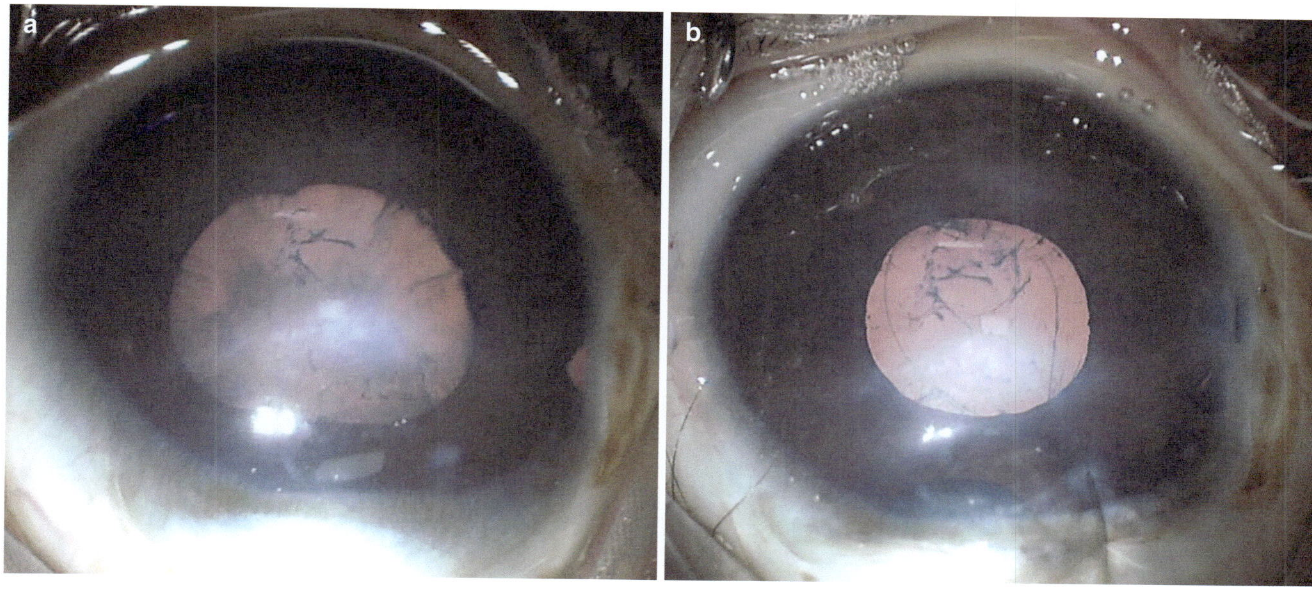

Fig. 11.6 A 15-month-old child with congenital glaucoma with corneal haze with Haab striae and large cornea (buphthalmos). (**a**) Preoperative picture with anterior and posterior subcapsular cataract, (**b**) postoperative picture with IOL in sulcus with optic capture with anterior and posterior capsulorhexis (bag complex) for better centration

ment [15–17]. Lens abnormalities are not uncommon in cases with ASD. Townsend, Font and Zimmerman have classified ASD based on involvement as Descemet layer defect alone or associated with lens abnormalities or with iris stromal abnormalities. This involvement of lens suggested the effects of primary mesenchymal defect on the development of lens [17].

11.2.1 Embryology

The surface ectoderm of developing human embryo invaginates and forms lens vesicle in the embryonic cup at sixth week of gestation. Then, neural-crest derived tissue migrates in three waves beneath this surface ectoderm. The surface ectoderm forms the corneal epithelium. The three waves forms endothelium, corneal stroma, and iris stroma. Any arrest in the development of these layers may affect further development of anterior chamber leading to different presentations of ASD [18].

11.2.2 Genetics

Many genes are involved in the ASD with variable degrees of penetrance. Forty percent cases occur due to involvement of PITX2 (4q25) and FOXC1 (6p25). Typically, PITX2 disruption is associated with ARS with ocular and dental abnormalities, and FOXC1 is associated with ARS with hearing or cardiac abnormalities. Others associated with ARS include PAX6 (11p13) and FOXO1A (13q14) [19, 20]. ARS has autosomal dominant inheritance pattern in 70% cases. In Peter's anomaly, rare cases have been attributed to PITX2, FOXC1, and PAX6 mutations, but the majority of cases are sporadic [21–23].

11.2.3 Clinical Features

- Axenfeld–Rieger syndrome.

Axenfeld anomaly presents as posterior embryotoxon (Fig. 11.7) (anteriorly displaced Schwalbe's line) and iris strands adhered to the anteriorly displaced Schwalbe's line. Rieger anomaly includes posterior embryotoxon, pseudopolycoria, and iris atrophy (Fig. 11.8) while Rieger syndrome is Rieger anomaly along with systemic findings including facial bone defects, hypertelorism, telecanthus, maxillary hypoplasia, dental abnormalities (microdontia and hypodontia), umbilical abnormalities, or pituitary involvement. Thus, they are now considered as a spectrum of disorder termed as Axenfeld–Rieger syndrome (Fig. 11.9). It may vary from subtle changes in the angle to severe ocular changes. Systemic involvement may also include cardiac and endocrine system. Fifty percent cases with ARS are associated with glaucoma [24, 25].

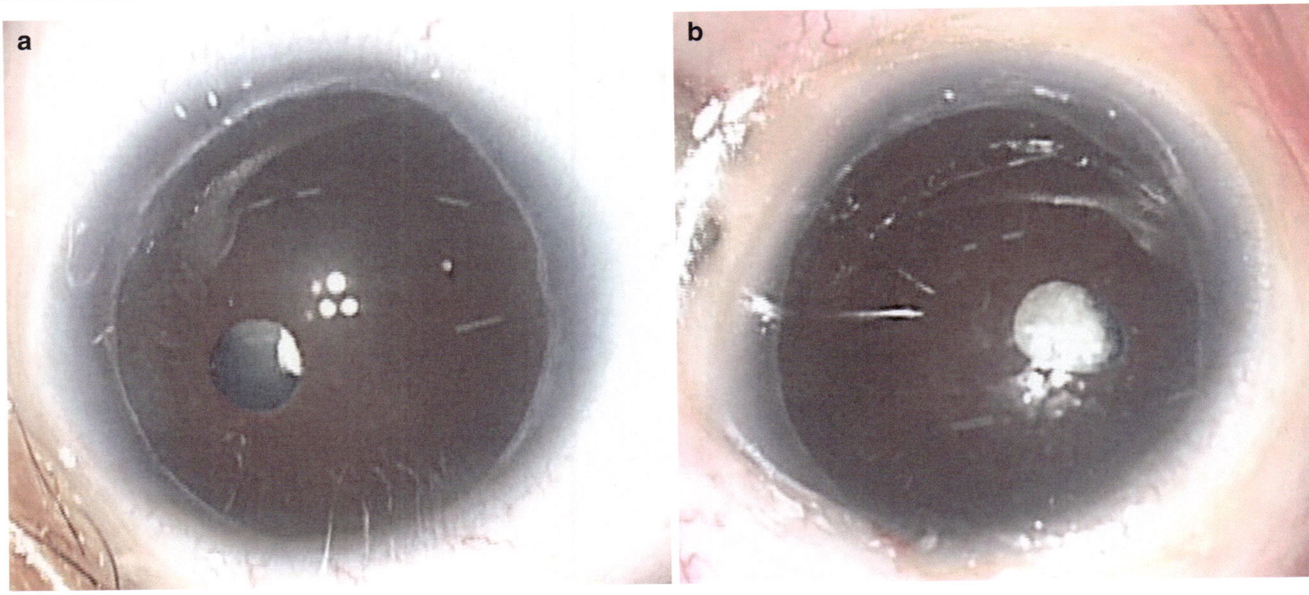

Fig. 11.7 Mild variant of Axenfeld–Rieger syndrome. (**a**, **b**) Posterior embryotoxon in a 9-month-old child with cataract in right and left eye, respectively. Also notice presence of corectopia in both eyes

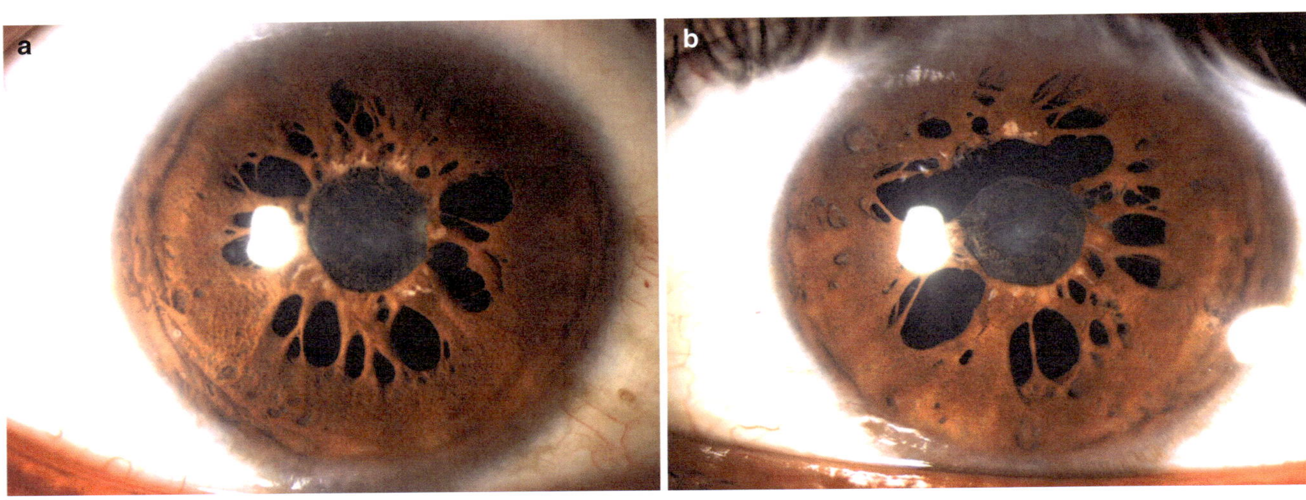

Fig. 11.8 (**a**, **b**) Rieger anomaly—polycoria and iris atrophy in a 7-year-old girl in right and left eye, respectively

- Peters Anomaly.

Peter syndrome is characterized by a shallow anterior chamber, synechiae between iris and cornea, and central corneal opacity. It occurs due to defect in endothelium, Descemet membrane and posterior stroma due to the defect in the migration of the neural crest cells. This syndrome can vary in severity with ocular findings ranging from unilateral mild central corneal opacity to severe bilateral microphthalmia, corneal opacification, cataract, and glaucoma. Eighty percent cases have bilateral presentation. The Peters anomaly has been further divided into type I and type II. Type I Peters anomaly is categorized by central corneal opacity and iridocorneal adhesions (Fig. 11.10). Type II Peters anomaly has a more severe phenotype with corneal opacity and lens involvement with iridocorneal touch with or without cataract (Fig. 11.11). The Peters plus syndrome includes the anterior segment findings with systemic developmental anomalies. These include craniofacial dysmorphism, cleft lip/palate, short stature, brachydactyly, ear abnormalities, and mental retardation [26, 27].

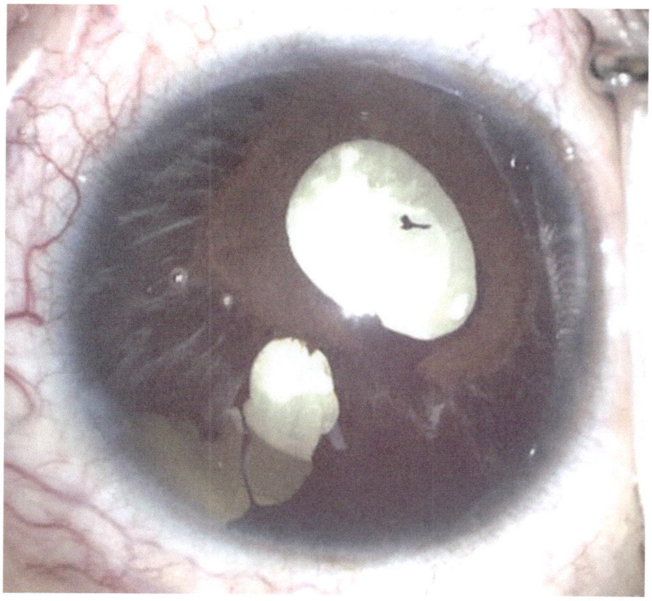

Fig. 11.9 Severe variant of Axenfeld–Rieger syndrome—posterior embryotoxon with corectopia, iris atrophy and polycoria along with total cataract

- Aniridia.

Aniridia is a rare congenital disorder characterized by iris hypoplasia along with other abnormalities of the eye [28] . Ocular abnormalities include dry eye, aniridia associated keratopathy (AAK) (Fig. 11.12), angle abnormalities, glaucoma, cataract, foveal hypoplasia, optic nerve hypoplasia, nystagmus, or strabismus [29–31]. Cataract morphology may be anterior or posterior subcapsular, lamellar, cortical, total or a combination of the above [28] (Fig. 11.13). Zonular weakness may be seen and ectopia lentis may be associated in some patients [28]. This can be managed with placement of capsular tension ring in mild cases (Fig. 11.14). Anterior polar or pyramidal cataract may be associated with aniridia along with remnants of persistent fetal vasculature [32] (Fig. 11.15).

11.2.4 Differential Diagnosis

The differential diagnosis of ASD includes obstetric trauma, congenital glaucoma, intrauterine infections like rubella, herpes simplex virus, and bacterial infections, iridocorneo-

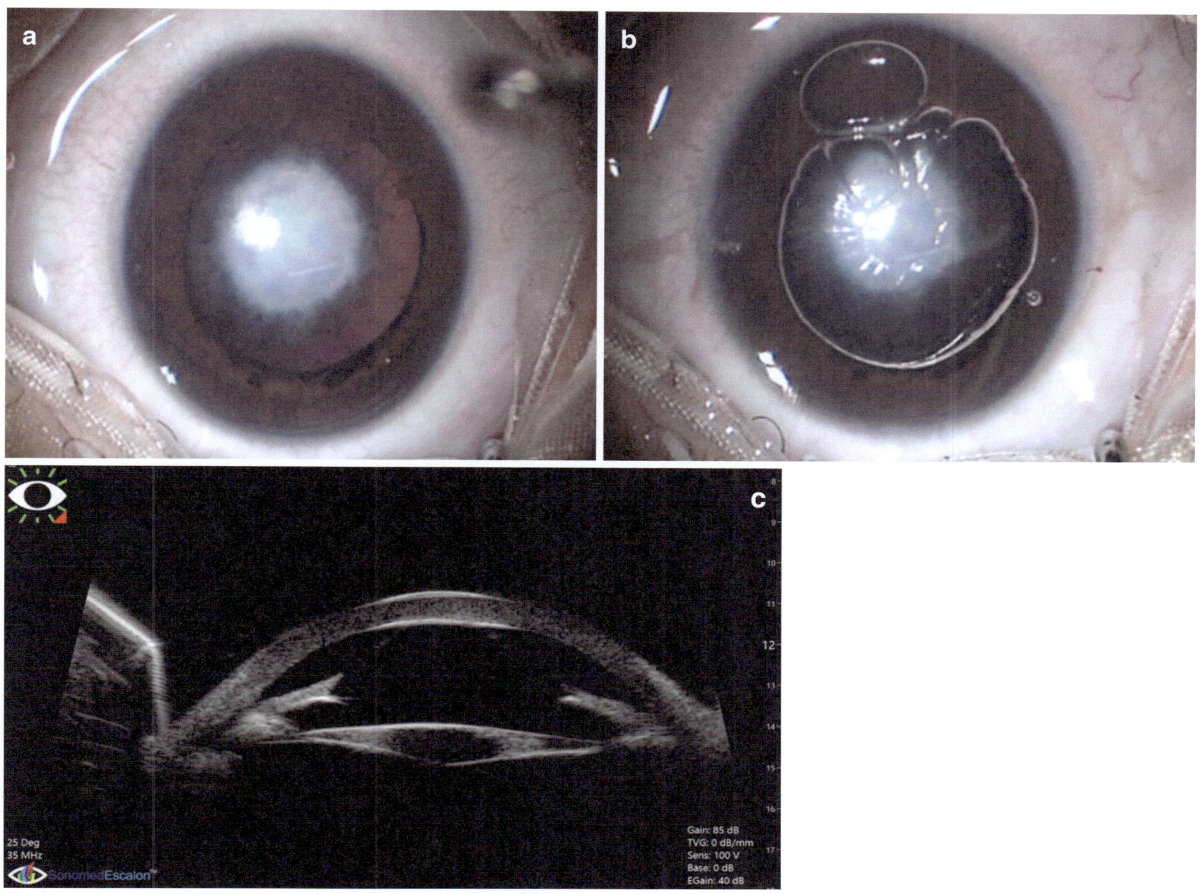

Fig. 11.10 Peter's anomaly type 1 in 2-month-old child. (**a**) Small corneal opacity with iridocorneal adhesions with cataract. (**b**) Intraoperative picture after injection of air in anterior chamber, irregular air bubble is seen due to iridocorneal adhesions. (**c**) Ultrasound biomicroscopy of the same showing fine central iridocorneal adhesions

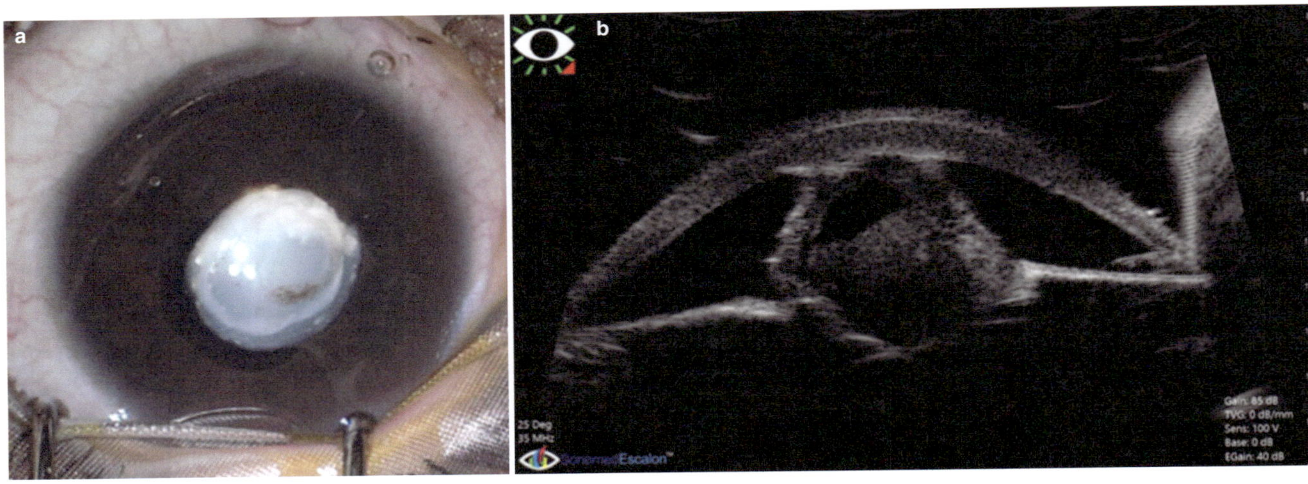

Fig. 11.11 Peter's anomaly type 2 in 4-month-old child. (**a**) Central corneal opacity with total cataract, (**b**) ultrasound biomicroscopy of the same showing iridolenticular adhesions with anterior displacement of lens

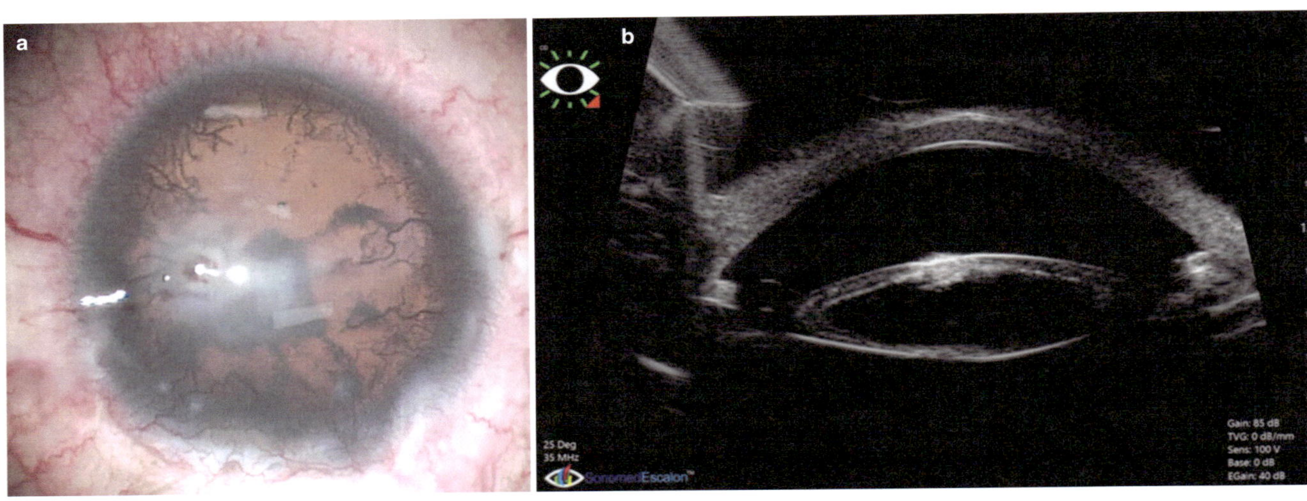

Fig. 11.12 Aniridia associated keratopathy with corneal opacity with 360° pannus. (**a**) Clinical picture, (**b**) ultrasound biomicroscopy of the same showing anterior subcapsular cataract, not clearly seen clinically

endothelial syndrome (Fig. 11.16), metabolic diseases like mucopolysaccharidosis, mucolipidoses, and tyrosinosis, congenital hereditary endothelial dystrophy, congenital hereditary stromal dystrophy, and dermoids.

11.2.5 Investigations

Apart from usual investigations ultrasound biomicroscopy may allow us to preoperatively assess the area beneath the corneal opacity. It helps us to determine the area of corneal opacity, depth of opacity, presence of iris adhesion, anterior chamber depth and angle details in the involved area. The lens can be visualized and observed for kerato-lenticular adhesion or presence of any tilting of the lens (Figs. 11.10b, 11.11b, and 11.13d, e). This can help us in the planning of the cataract surgery and expect a better outcome.

11.2.6 Surgical Pearls

Patients with ASD should be screened for glaucoma and managed appropriately. They require optimization of visual function which includes refractive error prescription and tinted contact lenses for photophobia. This is important for

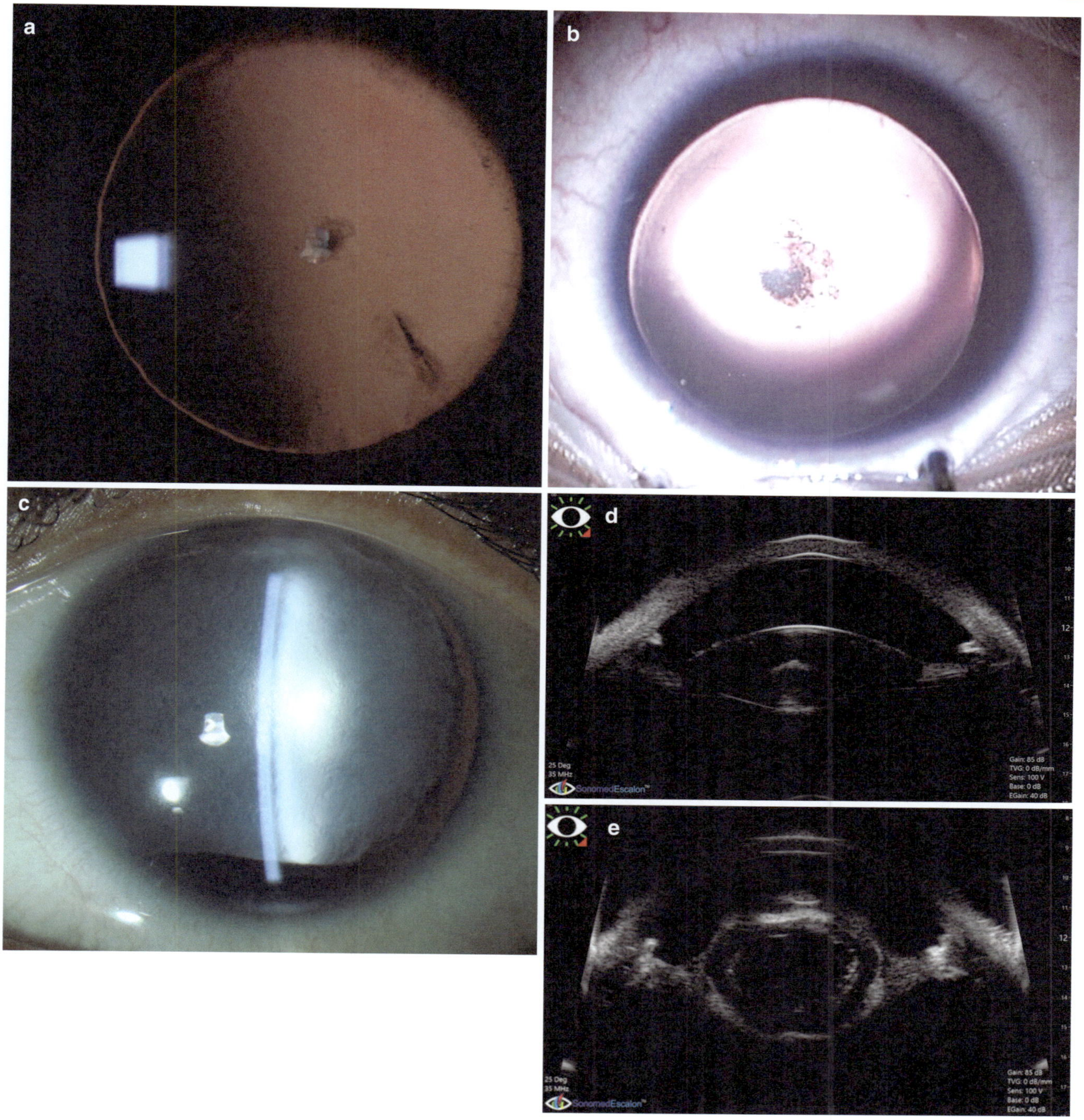

Fig. 11.13 Aniridia with cataract. (**a**) Clinical picture of insignificant anterior polar with cortical cataract. (**b**) Clinical picture of posterior subcapsular cataract. (**c**) Clinical picture of total cataract with inferior notching due to zonular laxity (Pseudo-lens coloboma). (**d**) UBM of aniridia patient showing minimal cataract and remnant of iris stump clearly with no subluxation. (**e**) UBM of aniridia patient with anterior polar and zonular cataract with zonular laxity causing increase in lens globularity

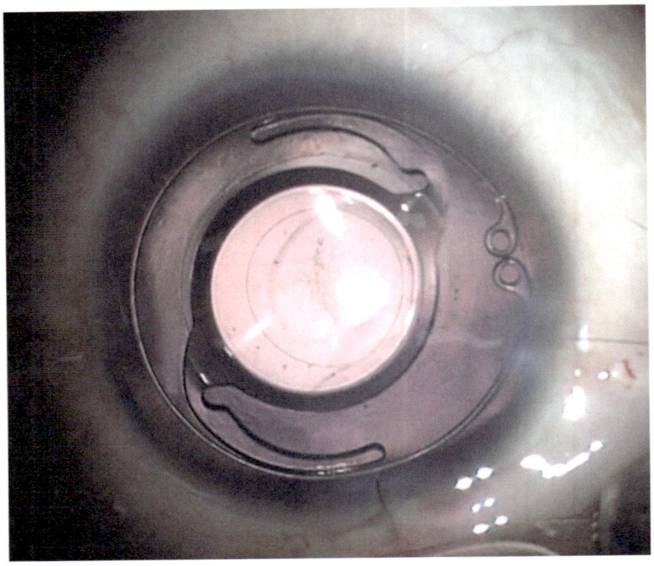

Fig. 11.14 Postoperative picture of aniridia with mild subluxation. Notice anterior and posterior capsulorhexis with well-centered IOL in bag with capsular tension ring

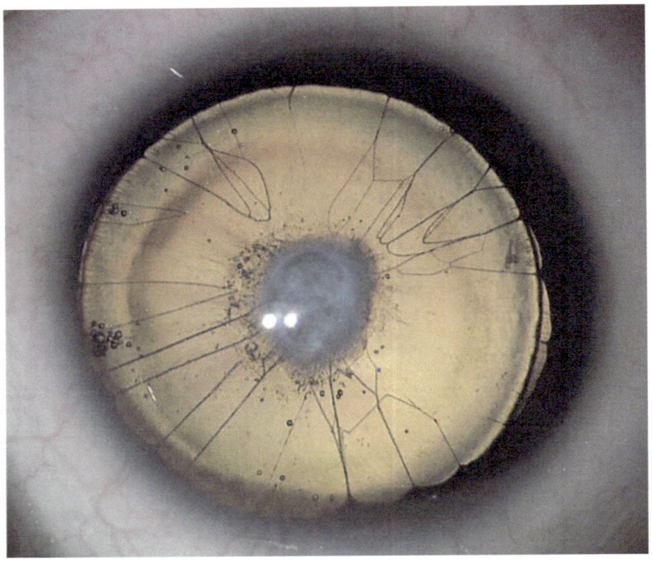

Fig. 11.15 Aniridia with anterior polar cataract with remnant of persistent fetal vasculature

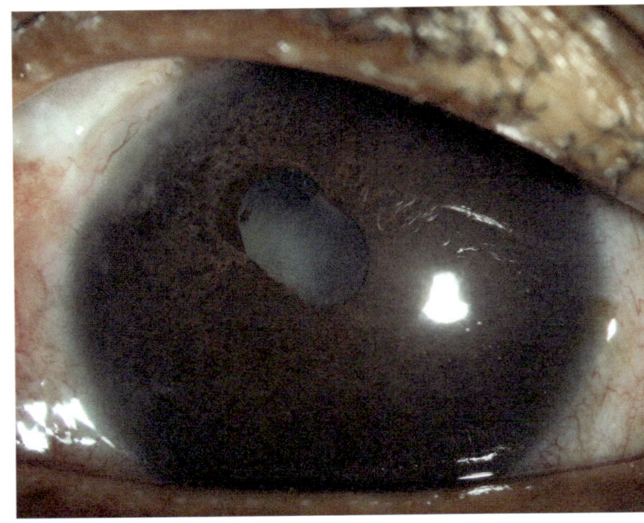

Fig. 11.16 A 16-year-old girl with Cogan Reese syndrome. Notice atrophic iris and corectopia with iris nodules

prevention and treatment of amblyopia. Few patients may also require surgery for corneal opacity, lens abnormality, or glaucoma management. Various challenges may be involved in the cataract surgery in cases with ASD.

- Corneal abnormalities: corneal opacity or aniridia associated keratopathy (AAK) may cause difficulty in anterior chamber visualization. Staining of the anterior capsule enhances its visualization during capsulorhexis. Other methods like use of illumination techniques like transcorneal oblique illumination or endoscope-assisted surgery can help in better visualization but are time-consuming methods with a greater learning curve [33–35]. Image-guided surgery using femtosecond laser for cataract surgery in Peter's syndrome has also been recently used [22]. However, the depth and height of the femtosecond laser should be cautiously adjusted to avoid damage to the endothelium.
- Presence of kerato-lenticular adhesion increases difficulty in surgical maneuvering. There may be risk of Descemet and endothelial damage during release of the keratolenticular adhesions and difficulty to achieve appropriate size regular capsulorhexis. We have also

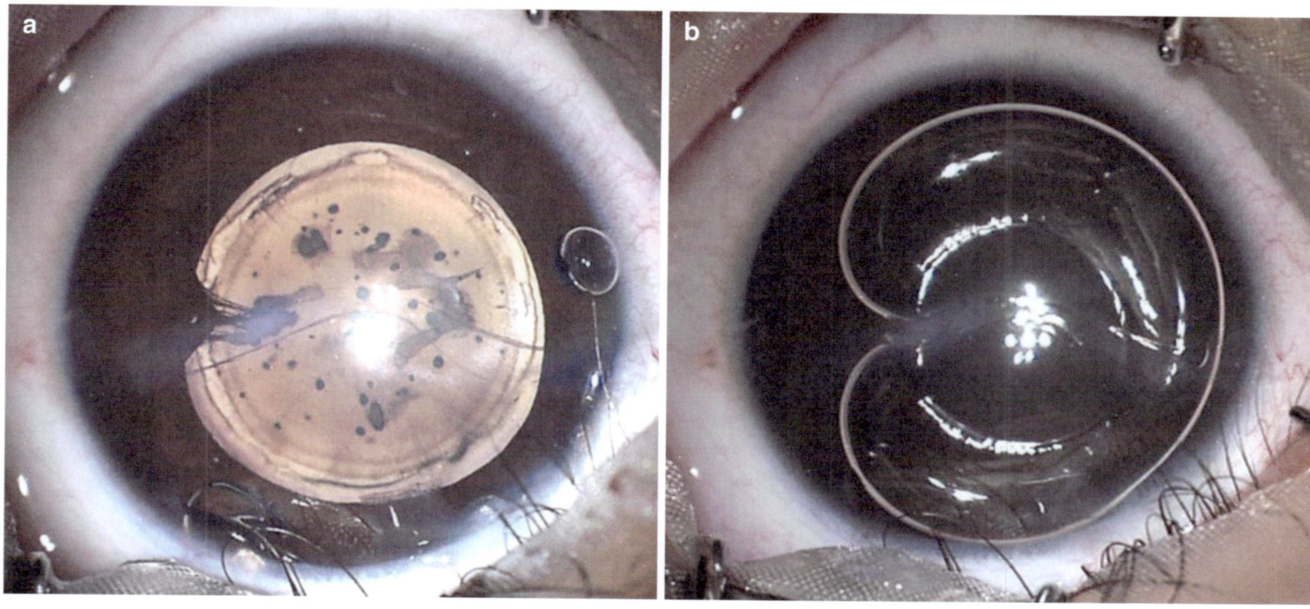

Fig. 11.17 Irregular air bubble sign in anterior segment dysgenesis with glaucoma. (**a**) Corneal opacity with iridocorneal adhesions with Haab striae with anterior capsular pigments and zonular cataract. (**b**) Intraoperative picture after ingestion of air in anterior chamber, irregular air bubble is seen. Iridocorneal adhesions which were not clearly seen preoperatively are enhanced

noticed "irregular air bubble" in anterior chamber as a sign of presence of adhesions when they are not clearly visible (Fig. 11.17a, b).

- Iris abnormalities like corectopia, polycoria, iridocorneal adhesion, posterior synechiae between iris and lens may require anterior segment reconstruction together with synechiae release, anterior chamber formation or pupilloplasty during cataract surgery. Aniridia patients require use of tinted glasses or contact lenses postoperatively. Iris prosthetic devices may be used [36]. There is risk of secondary glaucoma, corneal decompensation, band-shaped keratopathy and device displacement [37] (Fig. 11.18).
- Glaucoma management in cases with ASD is of importance and may include medical management, surgical management or both. Thus, a regular follow-up with monitoring of visual acuity and the intraocular pressure is crucial.

Challenges in surgery in patients with ASD have to be carefully dealt with in order to achieve satisfactory visual outcomes. In addition to cataract surgery, glaucoma management is of utmost importance in these cases.

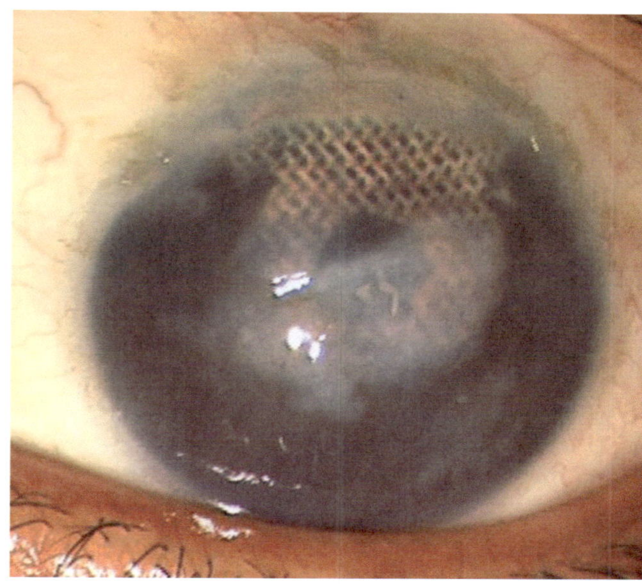

Fig. 11.18 One year postoperative picture of patient operated with iris implant (outside center) with acquired aniridia (traumatic) with band-shaped keratopathy and corneal decompensation

References

1. Wiggs JL, Damji KF, Haines JL, Pericak-Vance MA, Allingham RR. The distinction between juvenile and adult-onset primary open-angle glaucoma. Am J Hum Genet. Jan 1996;58(1):243–4.
2. Feroze KB, Patel BC. Buphthalmos. In: StatPearls [internet]. Treasure Island, FL: StatPearls Publishing; 2018.. http://www.ncbi.nlm.nih.gov/books/NBK430887/.
3. Yanoff M, Duker JS. Ophthalmology. 3rd ed. Philadelphia: Mosby Elsevier; 2009.
4. Basic and clinical science course (2011–2012). Glaucoma. American Academy of Ophthalmology.
5. Edmunds B, Thompson JR, Salmon J, Wornald RP. The national survey of trabeculectomy III. Early and late complications. Eye. 2002;16:297–303.
6. Adelman RA, Brauner SC, Afshari NA, Grosskreutz CL. Cataract formation after initial trabeculectomy in young patients. Ophthalmology. 2003;110:625–9.
7. Daugeliene L, Yamamoto T, Kitazawa Y. Cataract development after trabeculectomy with mitomycin C: a 1-year study. Jpn J Ophthalmol. 2000;44:52–7.
8. Khokhar SK, Pillay G, Agarwal E, Mahabir M. Innovations in pediatric cataract surgery. Indian J Ophthalmol. 2017; 65(3):210–6.
9. Hugkulstone CE. Changes in keratometry following trabeculectomy. Br J Ophthalmol. 1991;75(4):217–8.
10. Chan HHL, Kong YXG. Glaucoma surgery and induced astigmatism: a systematic review. Eye Vis [Internet]. 2017;4. https://www.ncbi.nlm.nih.gov/pmc/articles/PMC5691392/
11. Vaz FM, Osher RH. Cataract surgery and anterior megalophthalmos: custom intraocular lens and special considerations. J Cataract Refract Surg. 2007;33(12):2147–50.
12. Sukhija J, Kaur S, Pandav SS, Kaushik S, Raj S, Ram J. Cataract surgery in children with buphthalmos. Clin Exp Ophthalmol. 2016;44(8):739–40.
13. Dietlein TS, Jacobi PC, Krieglstein GK. Eyeball growth after successful glaucoma surgery in the 1st year of life--follow-up values for primary congenital glaucoma. Klin Monatsbl Augenheilkd. 1998;213(2):67–70.
14. Khokhar S, Yadav D, Gupta S, Chaurasia AK, Gupta A, Gupta V. Refractive outcomes of cataract surgery in primary congenital glaucoma. Eye (Lond). 2018; https://doi.org/10.1038/s41433-018-0253-6. [Epub ahead of print]
15. Waring GO, Rodrigues MM, Laibson PR. Anterior chamber cleavage syndrome. A stepladder classification. Surv Ophthalmol. 1975;20:3–27.
16. Shields MB, Buckley E, Klintworth GK, Thresher R. Axenfeld-Rieger syndrome. A spectrum of developmental disorders. Surv Ophthalmol. 1985;29:387–409.
17. Townsend WM, Font RL, Zimmerman LE. Congenital corneal leukomas. 2. Histopathologic findings in 19 eyes with central defect in Descemet's membrane. Am J Ophthalmol. 1974;77:192–206.
18. Beauchamp G, Knepper P. Role of the neural crest in anterior segment development and disease. J Pediatr Ophthalmol Strabismus. 1984;21:209–14.
19. Glaser T, Walton DS, Maas RL. Genomic structure, evolutionary conservation and aniridia mutations in the human PAX6 gene. Nat Genet. 1992;2:232–9.
20. Phillips JC, et al. A second locus for Rieger syndrome maps to chromosome 13q14. Am J Hum Genet. 1996;59:613–9.
21. Dahl E, Koseki H, Balling R. Pax genes and organogenesis. BioEssays. 1997;19:755–65.
22. Doward W, et al. A mutation in the RIEG1 gene associated with Peters' anomaly. 4.
23. Iseri SU, et al. Seeing clearly: the dominant and recessive nature of FOXE3 in eye developmental anomalies. Hum Mutat. 2009;30:1378–86.
24. Fitch N, Kaback M. The Axenfeld syndrome and the Rieger syndrome. J Med Genet. 1978;15:30–4.
25. Chang TC, Summers CG, Schimmenti LA, Grajewski AL. Axenfeld-Rieger syndrome: new perspectives. Br J Ophthalmol. 2012;96:318–22.
26. Bhandari R, Ferri S, Whittaker B, Liu M, Lazzaro DR. Peters anomaly: review of the literature. Cornea. 2011;30:939–44.
27. Harissi-Dagher M, Colby K. Anterior segment dysgenesis: Peters anomaly and sclerocornea. Int Ophthalmol Clin. 2008;48:35–42.
28. Nelson LB, Spaeth GL, Nowinski TS, Margo CE, Jackson L. Aniridia. A review. Surv Ophthalmol. 1984;28:621–42.
29. Eden U, Riise R, Tornqvist K. Corneal involvement in congenital aniridia. Cornea. 2010;29:1096–102.
30. Chang JW, Kim JH, Kim SJ, Yu YS. Congenital aniridia: long-term clinical course, visual outcome, and prognostic factors. Korean J Ophthalmol. 2010;28:479–85.
31. Singh B, Mohamed A, Chaurasia S, Ramappa M, Mandal AK, Jalali S, Sangwan VS. Clinical manifestations of congenital aniridia. J Pediatr Ophthalmol Strabismus. 2014;51:59–62.
32. Khokhar S, Sinha G, Sharma R, Patil B, Mahabir M, Nayak B. Anterior pyramidal Cataract. A rare association. JAMA Ophthalmol. 2015;133(4):e144626. https://doi.org/10.1001/jamaophthalmol.2014.4626.
33. Farjo AA, Meyer RF, Farjo QA. Phacoemulsification in eyes with corneal opacification. J Cataract Refract Surg. 2003;29:242–5.
34. Moore JE, Herath GD, Sharma A. Continuous curvilinear capsulorhexis with use of an endoscope. J Cataract Refract Surg. 2004;30:960–3.
35. Al Sabti K, Raizada S, Al Abduljalil T. Cataract surgery assisted by anterior endoscopy. Br J Ophthalmol. 2009;93:531–4.
36. Srinivasan S, Ting DS, Snyder ME, Prasad S, Koch HR. Prosthetic iris devices. Can J Ophthalmol. 2014;49(1):6–17.
37. Mostafa YS, Osman AA, Hassanein DH, Zeid AM, Sherif AM. Iris reconstruction using artificial iris prosthesis for management of aniridia. Eur J Ophthalmol. 2018;28(1):103–7.

12 Cataract in Retinal Pathology and Miscellaneous Conditions

Chirakshi Dhull, Sagnik Sen, and Sudarshan Kumar Khokhar

Pediatric cataract surgery in retinal pathology or other miscellaneous conditions require special attention. Associated comorbidities whether ocular or systemic disease may have an impact on outcome of cataract surgery. Hence, a thorough examination and preoperative clinical diagnosis of such pathology helps in better planning and prognostication in such children.

12.1 Cataract in Retinal Pathology

We shall discuss common retinal pathologies, which are found in association with cataract in pediatric age group. These include retinopathy of prematurity, iridofundal coloboma, retinal detachment, post retinal detachment (silicone oil-filled/gas-filled eyes), retinitis pigmentosa, and hereditary vitreo-retinopathies such as Stickler syndrome.

12.1.1 Retinopathy of Prematurity (ROP)

Cataract may be seen in children affected with ROP [1, 2]. It may be spontaneous or secondary to underlying pathology or intervention [3–8]. Cataracts have been reported post cryotherapy [8] and laser treatment [3–6]. After laser therapy, cataract may be visually insignificant [9] in the form of vacuolated or punctate opacities or visually significant diffuse or total cataract [3–6] (Fig. 12.1). After pars plana vitrectomy, cataract formation may be seen [7, 8]. Cataract may be associated *with* post intravitreal anti vascular endothelial growth factor (anti-VEGF) injection secondary to lens touch as seen in adults [10]. Spontaneous infantile cataract may also be seen which may be congenital or developmental (Fig. 12.2).

C. Dhull · S. K. Khokhar (✉)
Dr. Rajendra Prasad Centre for Ophthalmic Sciences, All India Institute of Medical Sciences, New Delhi, India

S. Sen
Aravind Eye Hospital, Madurai, India

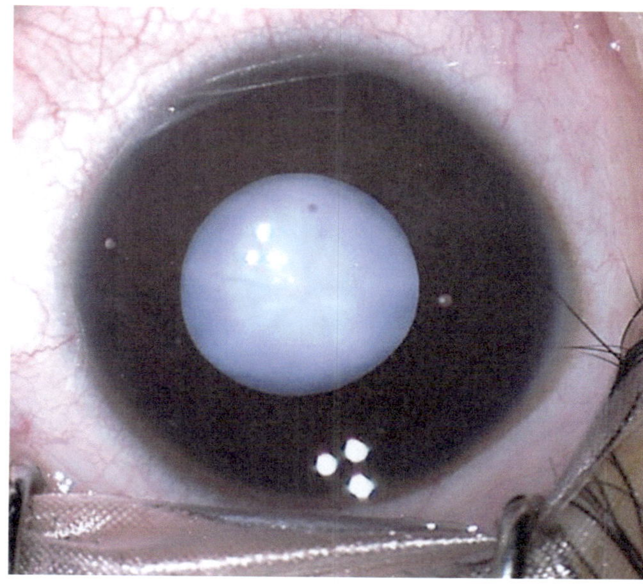

Fig. 12.1 40 weeks post gestational age patient with total cataract a 4 weeks following laser therapy for Zone 1 stage 3 ROP

Morphology may be total, zonular, nuclear, anterior/posterior subcapsular, or diffuse cataract.

Visually insignificant cataracts can be observed over a period of time. Simultaneous or sequential management of the underlying retinal pathology is required. If cataract is visually significant or causing hindrance in retinal treatment, cataract surgery may be required (Figs. 12.3 and 12.4). Cataract surgery in these cases may be more challenging due to presence of posterior capsular defect due to lens touch, zonular weakness or due to vitrectomized eye [12, 13]. Also, there are greater chances of associated comorbidities such as secondary glaucoma and retinal detachment in these cases [3, 4]. Overall results of cataract surgery in these patients without associated comorbidities have been satisfactory [12]. IOL implantation may be appropriate in cases where corneal diameter is >10 mm and results of IOL implantation have been encouraging [12–14]. Common postoperative

S. K. Khokhar, C. Dhull (eds.), *Atlas of Pediatric Cataract*, https://doi.org/10.1007/978-981-13-6939-1_12

complications include visual axis opacification, glaucoma, and retinal detachment and can be managed in similar fashion as cataract without ROP [14].

12.1.2 Ocular Coloboma

Ocular coloboma is a congenital anomaly caused by failure of closure of embryonal or choroidal fissure during fifth to seventh week of life [15]. It can involve iris, lens, ciliary body, choroid, retina, and optic disc (Fig. 12.5a–d) [16]. Cataract development may be seen earlier in these patients [16–18]. It may be associated with microphthalmos, retinal detachment, or glaucoma [16]. Typical iris coloboma is inferonasal but atypical coloboma may be seen rarely (Fig. 12.6a, b). Cataract may be visually insignificant in the form of isolated lenticular opacities or visually significant as diffuse or total cataract. Surgery in visually significant cataract requires special consideration due to smaller size of cornea, vitreous prolapse in anterior chamber, and zonular weakness [16–18]. Notching in lens may be seen in these patients due to defect in zonules (Fig. 12.7) [16]. IOL placement can be considered in eyes with adequate corneal diameter. Cataract surgery may be accompanied by placement of capsular tension ring in the bag to reduce chances of capsular phimosis and IOL displacement [19]. Iris repair may be considered using suture or implants although capsular phimosis and/or contact lens may be sufficient in most cases (Fig. 12.8) [20, 21]. Outcome depends on coexisting retinal pathology, type of coloboma, involvement of disc and macula, secondary glaucoma, and presence of amblyopia [16].

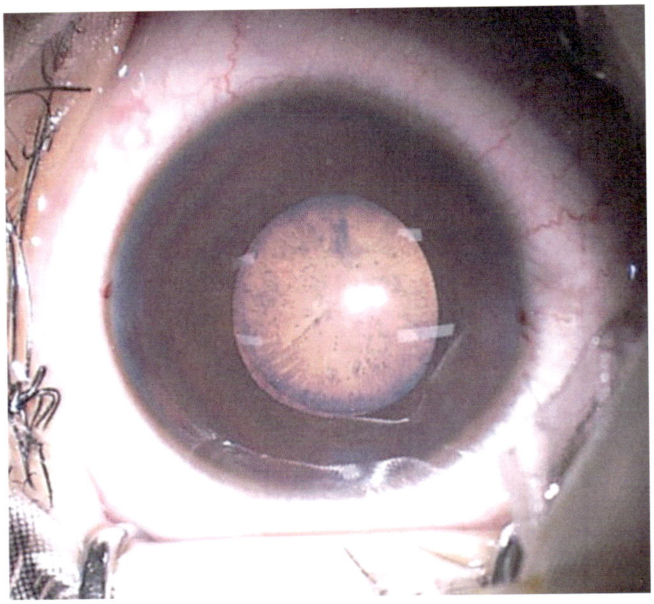

Fig. 12.2 52 weeks post gestation age patient with cataract pulverulenta, no treatment received, Zone 2 stage 1 regressed ROP

12.1.3 Retinal Detachment

Retinal detachment may be associated with trauma, myopia, retinopathy of prematurity, or hereditary conditions in pediatric age group [22, 23]. Cataract or subluxation may be associated in cases of retinal detachment with or without trauma [22]. Morphology may range from anterior/posterior subcapsular cataract with or without fibrosis to diffuse cataract, partially absorbed or total cataract

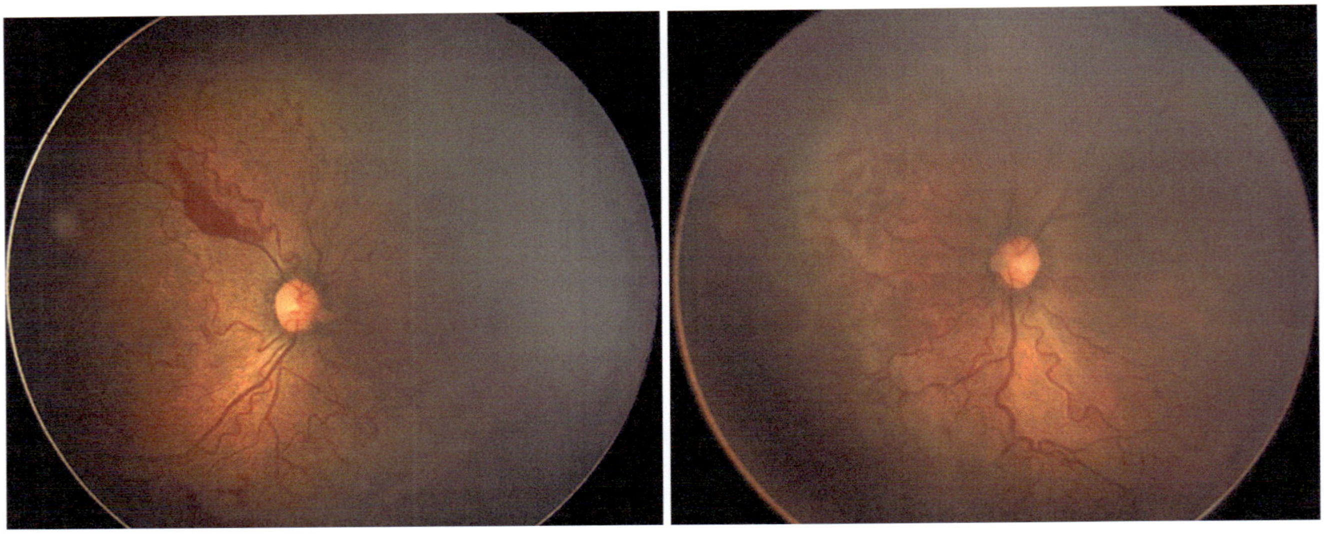

Fig. 12.3 28 week born patient with bilateral Zone 1 (Aggressive posterior retinopathy of prematurity) OD&OS [11]

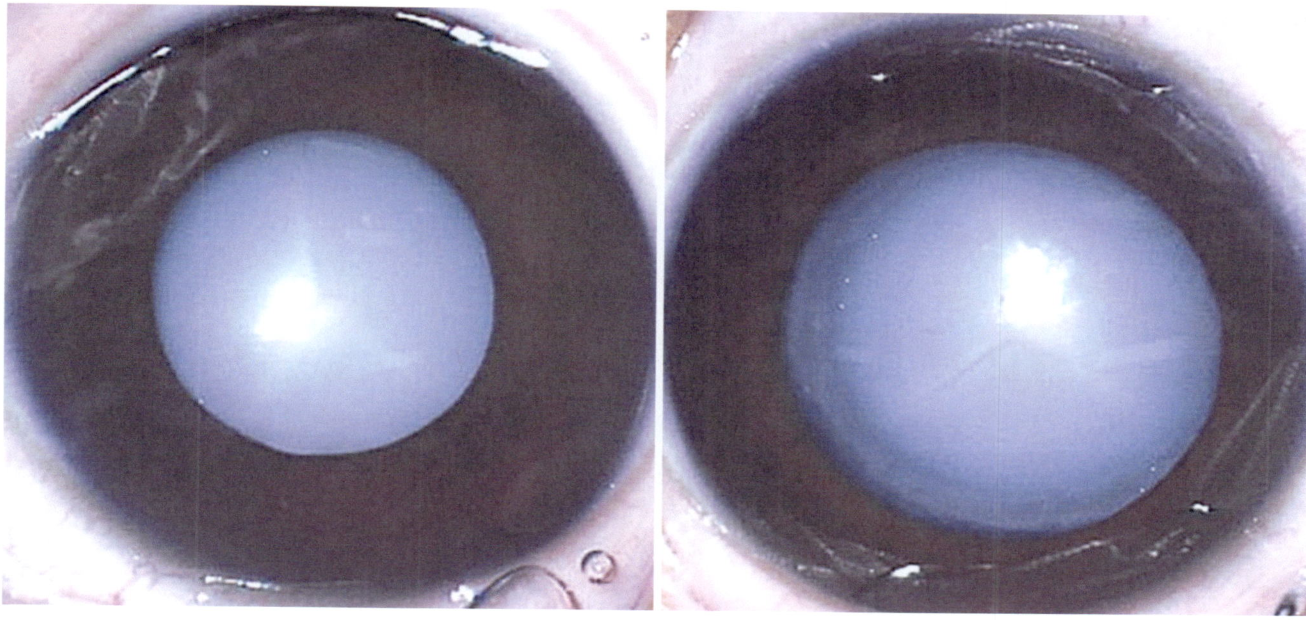

Fig. 12.4 Same patient as Fig. 12.3, developed bilateral total cataract in both eyes 6 weeks after anti-VEGF administration [11]

(Fig. 12.9a–d). Syndromes such as *Stickler syndrome* may be associated with distinctive type of cataract such as wedge-shaped cataract or fleck cataract (Fig. 12.10a, b) [24]. Cataract may also be seen after management of retinal detachment such as in *silicone oil-filled/gas-filled eyes* [25]. Such cataracts generally start as feathery cataract or posterior subcapsular cataract, later on total or intumescent cataracts may be seen in children (Fig. 12.11). Surgery may become difficult due to zonular weakness or subluxation, presence of anterior or posterior capsular plaques, lack of vitreous support, lack of normal fundal glow, or posterior chamber oil tamponade. Management for each case has to be individualized based on presentation. Before surgical intervention, ultrasonography should be performed in all cases to look for the configuration of detachment and prognostication (Fig. 12.10a, b).

12.1.4 Retinitis Pigmentosa

Cataract in association with retinitis pigmentosa is generally seen in adults but may be present in adolescents as well [26, 27]. Common morphology includes subcapsular cataract or diffuse cataract (Fig. 12.13) [26]. Special attention has been given for coexisting zonular weakness [28] and capsular tension ring placement may reduce postoperative complications such as anterior capsular phimosis (Fig. 12.14) [28, 29]. Prognosis depends on severity of the underlying disease and hence has to be explained in advance [26].

12.2 Miscellaneous Conditions

12.2.1 Drug Induced Cataract

Numerous drugs have been implicated with formation of cataract. Steroids are the commonest [30]. Other drugs include pilocarpine, oral contraceptives, tranquilizers, quinoline, methotrexate, ergot, streptozotocin, sulfanilamide, amiodarone, epinephrine, thiazide, thiazolidinediones, antipsychotic drugs, gold, allopurinol, tetracyclines, etc. [31–35]. List includes hundreds of medications; hence, a thorough history taking is of utmost importance as cataract may be reversible in many cases.

Steroid induced cataract may be seen secondary to systemic as well as topical or inhalational route. Morphology may be posterior subcapsular cataract (Fig. 12.15) (most common), diffuse cataract, or total cataract [36–38]. In children, commonly steroid induced cataract is seen in patients suffering from nephrotic syndrome [39]. Screening of such children on long-term steroids is recommended for cataract and glaucoma and alternately immunosuppressant can be considered in these cases [39].

12.2.2 Electric Cataract

Electric injury can be associated with numerous ocular and systemic complications [40]. Ocular associations could be cataract, corneal opacities, uveitis, retinal edema, choroidal

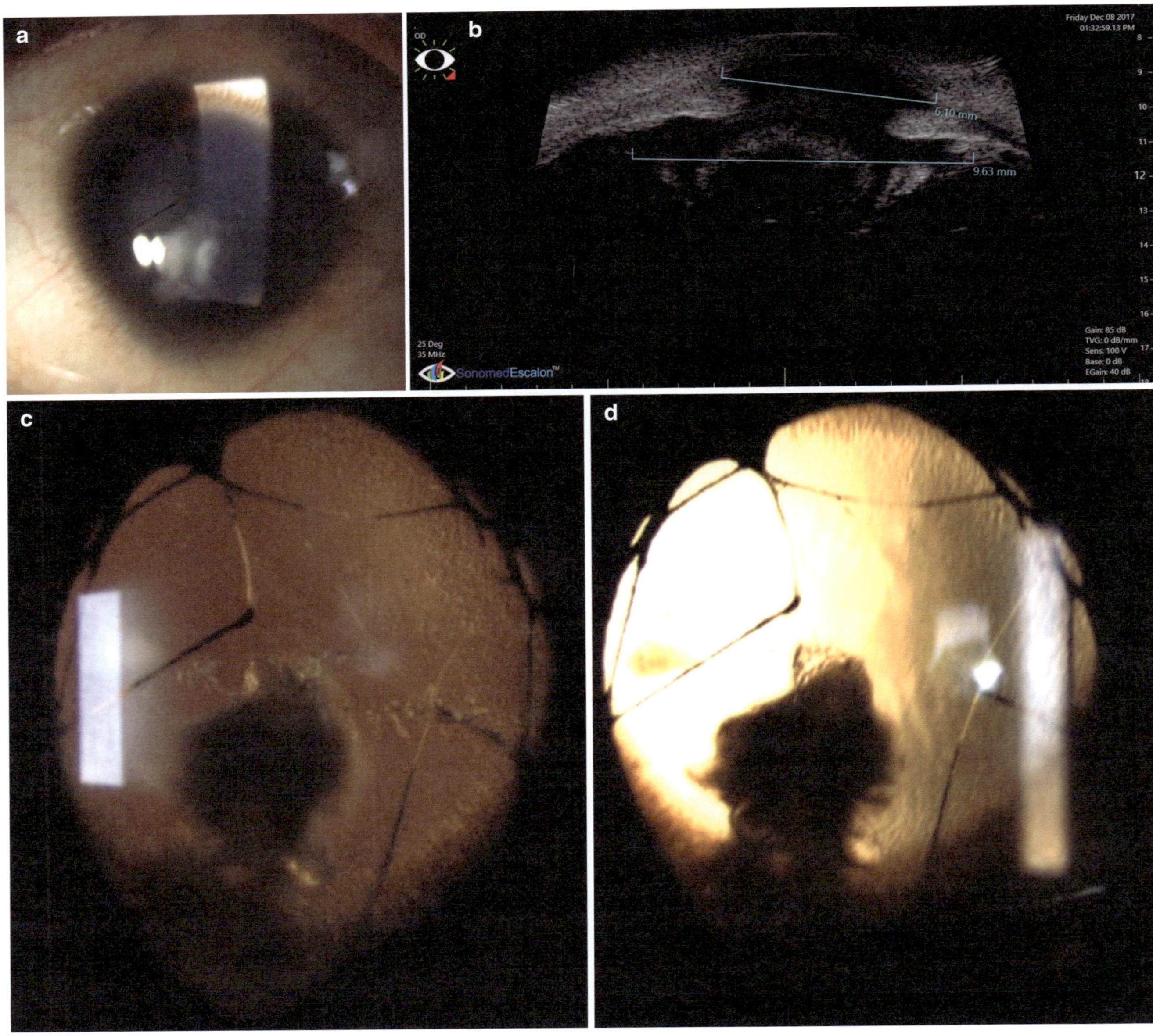

Fig. 12.5 Typical inferonasal iridofundal coloboma in a 12-year-old boy with pear-shaped microcornea, persistent pupillary membrane, and small lenticular opacity. (**a**) Slit illumination picture showing inferior lenticular opacity. (**b**) Ultrasound biomicroscopy (UBM) of the same showing small cornea (angle to angle distance 6.10 mm) and relatively normal size of lens (bag diameter 9.63 mm). (**c**) Retroillumination picture showing visually insignificant cataract against red glow (normal fundal glow). (**d**) Retroillumination picture showing visually insignificant cataract against yellow glow (due to coloboma). Notice coloboma can be detected before indirect ophthalmoscopy by distant direct examination

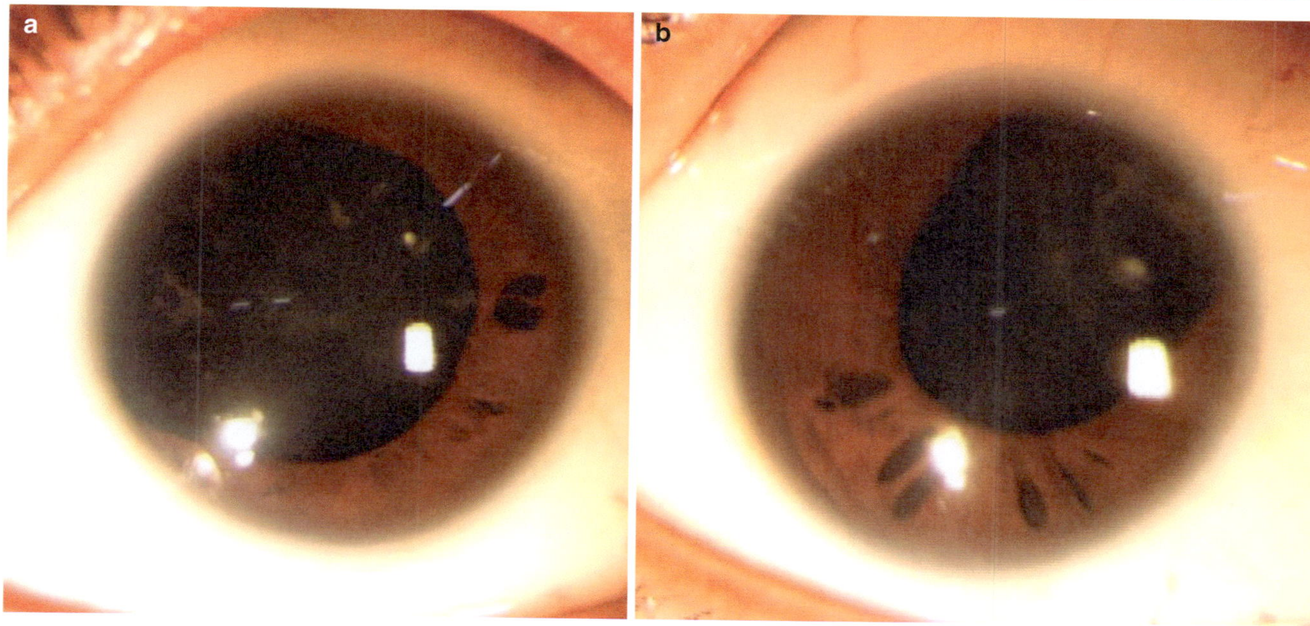

Fig. 12.6 (**a**, **b**) Atypical superotemporal bilateral iris coloboma in both eyes. Fine lenticular opacities are noted in both eyes

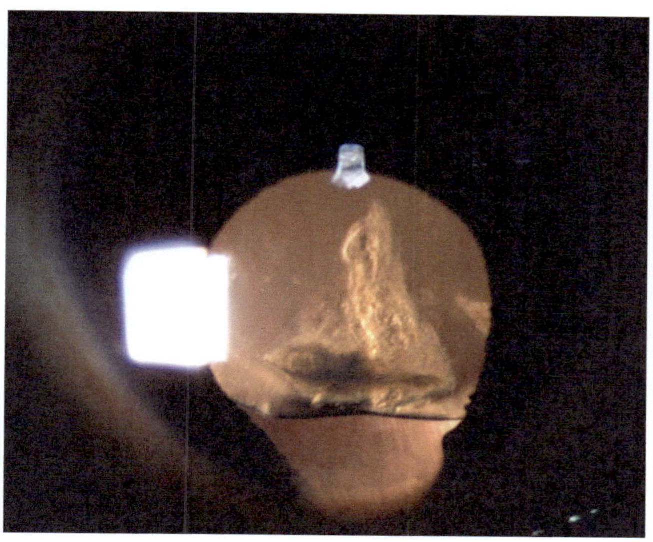

Fig. 12.7 Retroillumination picture of iridofundal coloboma with notching in the lens due to zonular defect. Mild cortical cataract is also seen

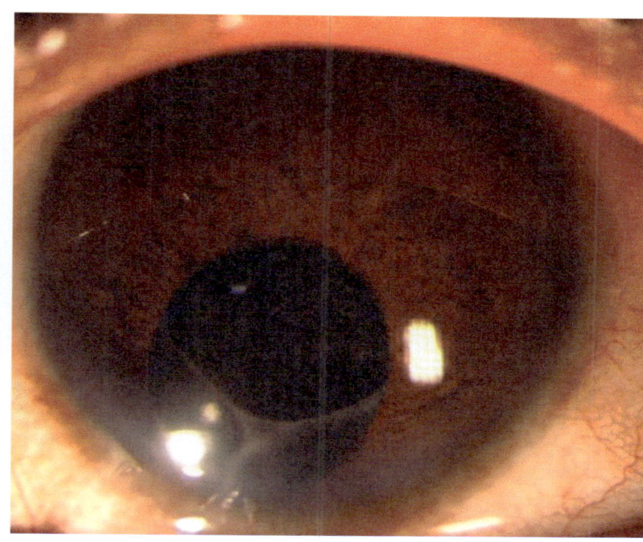

Fig. 12.8 Diffuse illumination picture of iridofundal coloboma with pseudophakia with inferior anterior capsular fibrosis. This reduces photophobia and excess light entry in the eye

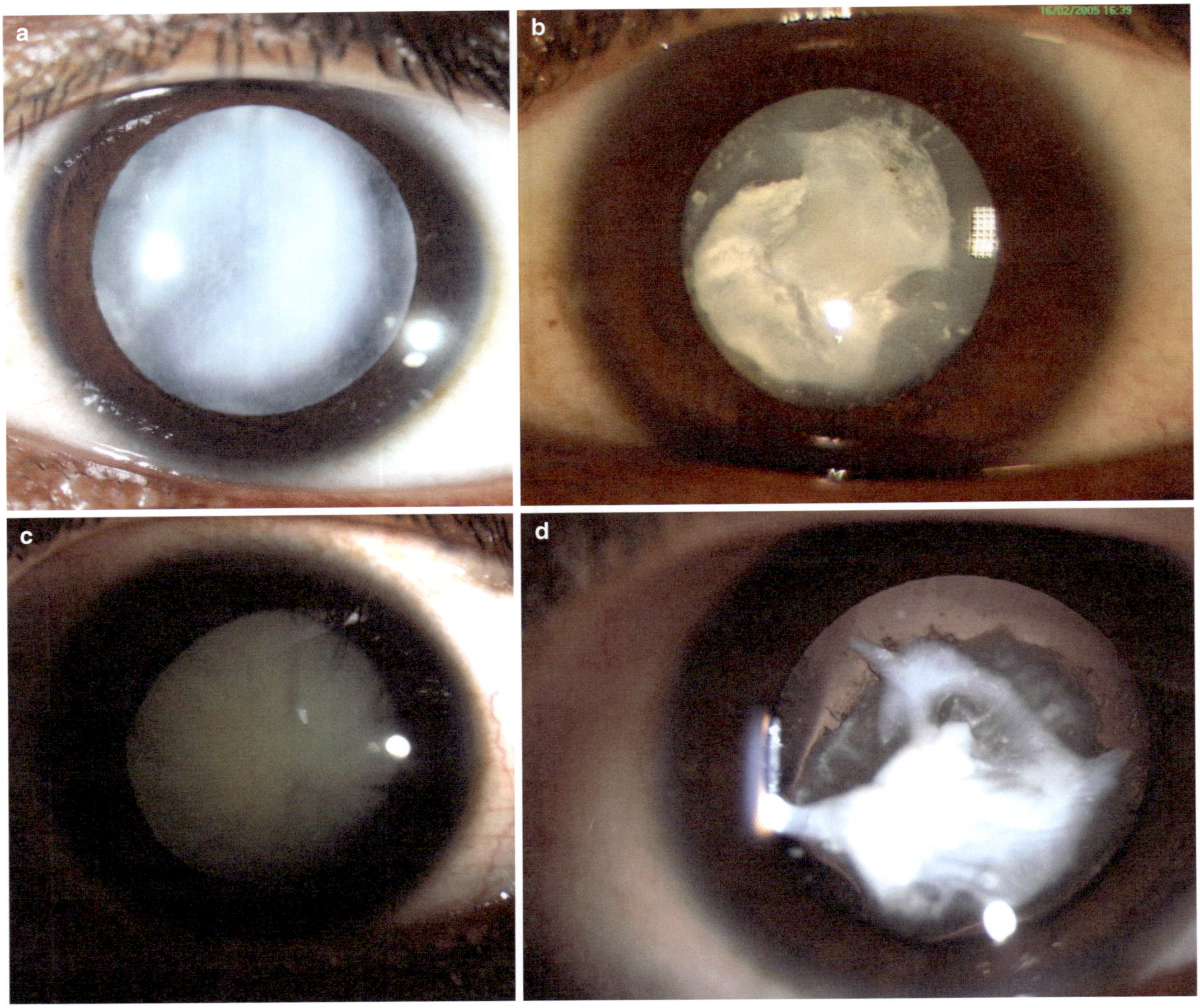

Fig. 12.9 Variable presentation of cataract with associated rhegmatogenous retinal detachment. (**a**) Total cataract. (**b**) Total cataract with anterior capsular plaque. (**c**) Total cataract with yellowish hue. Here cataract was seen in association with endophthalmitis with rhegmatogenous retinal detachment post scleral perforation. (**d**) Central cataract with anterior and posterior subcapsular cataract seen in a patient with X-linked retinoschisis with retinal detachment

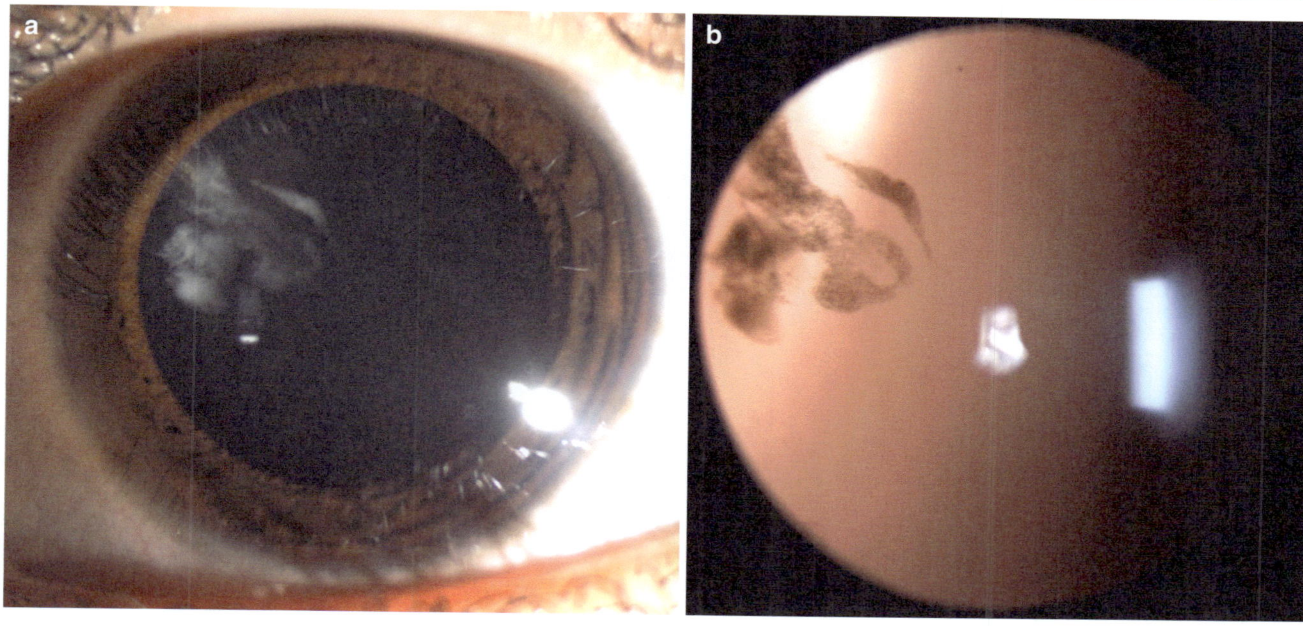

Fig. 12.10 Wedge-shaped cataract in an 8-year-old boy with Stickler syndrome. (**a**) Diffuse illumination picture, (**b**) retroillumination picture

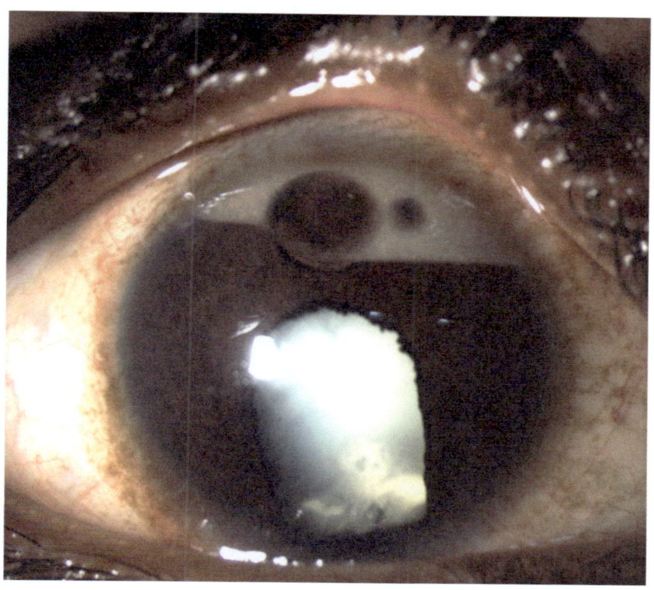

Fig. 12.11 Iridofundal coloboma with post silicone oil total cataract with fibrosis with hyperoleon

ruptures, chorioretinal necrosis, and optic neuritis [40–42]. Electric cataract is usually a late complication typically seen after a latent period [43]. Cataract is likely secondary to coagulation of proteins and damage to subcapsular epithelium. This is supported by the presence of anterior and posterior capsular fibrosis [44] which may progress to involve the remaining lens matter (Fig. 12.16a, b). Hypertrophic scars may be seen on skin at the area of contact (Fig. 12.17a, b). Cataract surgery is required in most cases and may involve cutting of plaques with microincision scissors and forceps. Prognosis depends on the associated retinal and optic nerve condition and favorable outcomes are seen in most cases with comorbidities.

12.2.3 Oculocutaneous Albinism

Oculocutaneous albinism is associated with refractive errors, decreased visual acuity, nystagmus, foveal and/or disc hypoplasia [45, 46]. Less commonly, it may be associ-

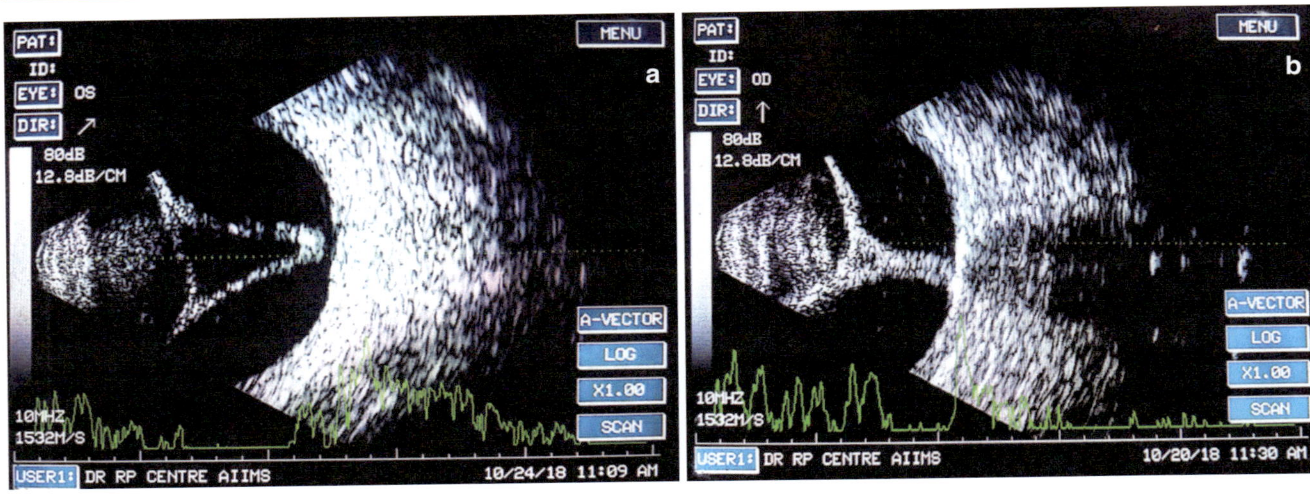

Fig. 12.12 Ultrasonography showing thick membrane attached to the disc. (**a**) Open configuration of retinal detachment. (**b**) Posteriorly closed configuration of retinal detachment suggestive of poor prognosis

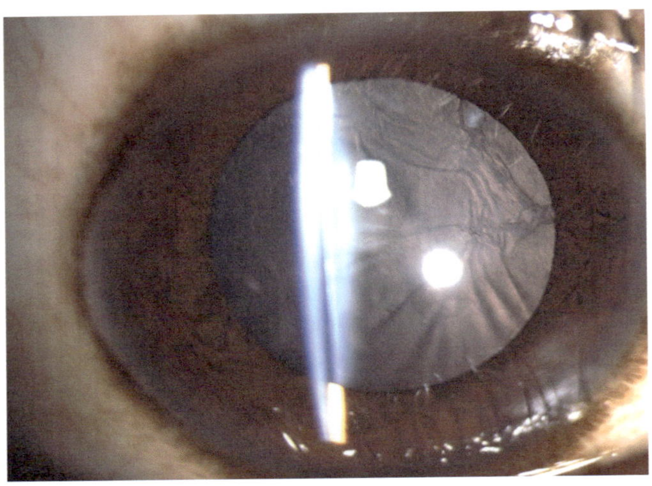

Fig. 12.13 A 13-year-old patient with retinitis pigmentosa with anterior and posterior subcapsular cataract with folds in the capsule and mild fibrosis

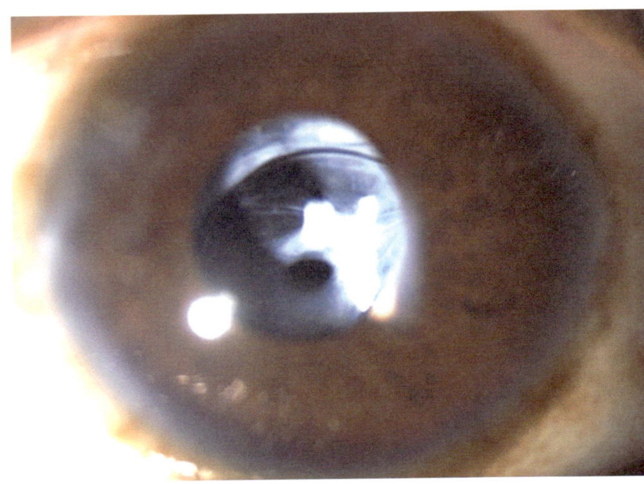

Fig. 12.14 Pseudophakia with severe anterior capsular phimosis 2 years after surgery in left eye of the same patient as Fig. 12.12. Note no capsular tension ring put in left eye

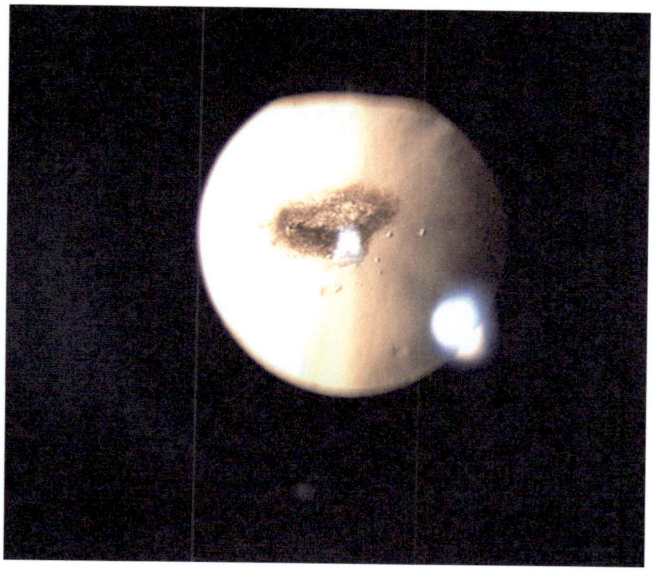

Fig. 12.15 Steroid induced posterior subcapsular cataract

ated with cataract [47]. These cataracts are generally age related; sometimes developmental cataract may be seen in association (Fig. 12.18a, b) [46, 47]. We are giving a special mention to this condition as in addition to cataract surgery, patient requires treatment for lack of iris pigmentation. This ranges from use of tinted glasses, contact lens to placement of aniridia ring [48]. We prefer conservative management for most children with use of tinted glasses or contact lens. Outcome of cataract surgery depends primarily on the presence or absence of foveal hypoplasia [47]. Presence of nystagmus with significant head posture may warrant intervention.

In conclusion, various retinal and miscellaneous pathologies have been discussed in this chapter to lay emphasis on holistic management of children with associated ocular/ systemic pathologies. Patient information, understanding and informed consent are of utmost importance in these challenging situations.

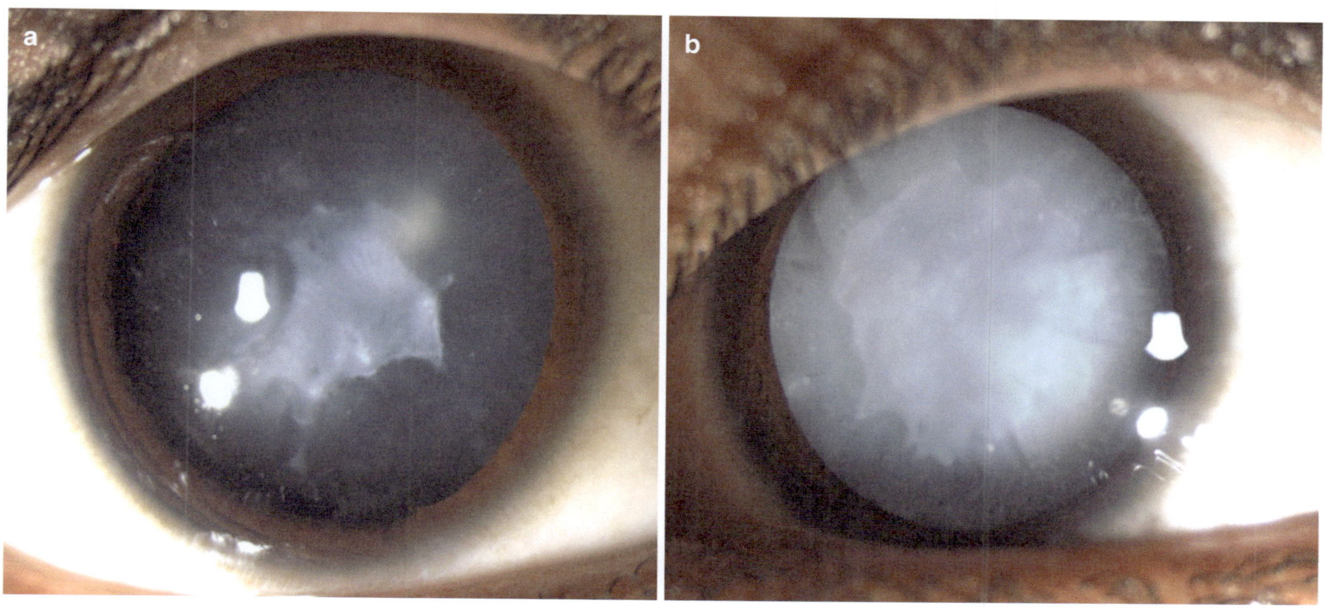

Fig. 12.16 Electric cataract in a 14-year-old boy, 10 months after injury. (**a**) Right eye diffuse illumination picture showing anterior subcapsular cataract with plaque and mild diffuse cataract. (**b**) Left eye diffuse illumination picture showing total cataract with anterior capsular plaque

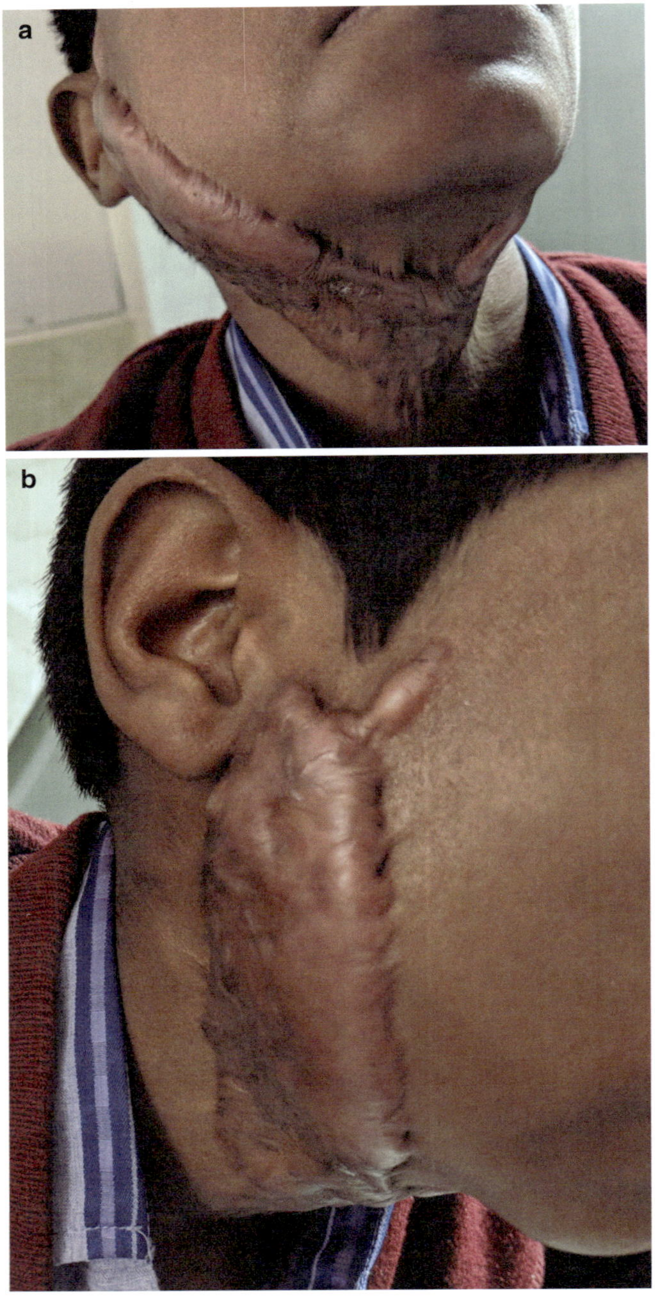

Fig. 12.17 Hypertrophic scar over neck and mandibular area of the same patient as Fig. 12.16

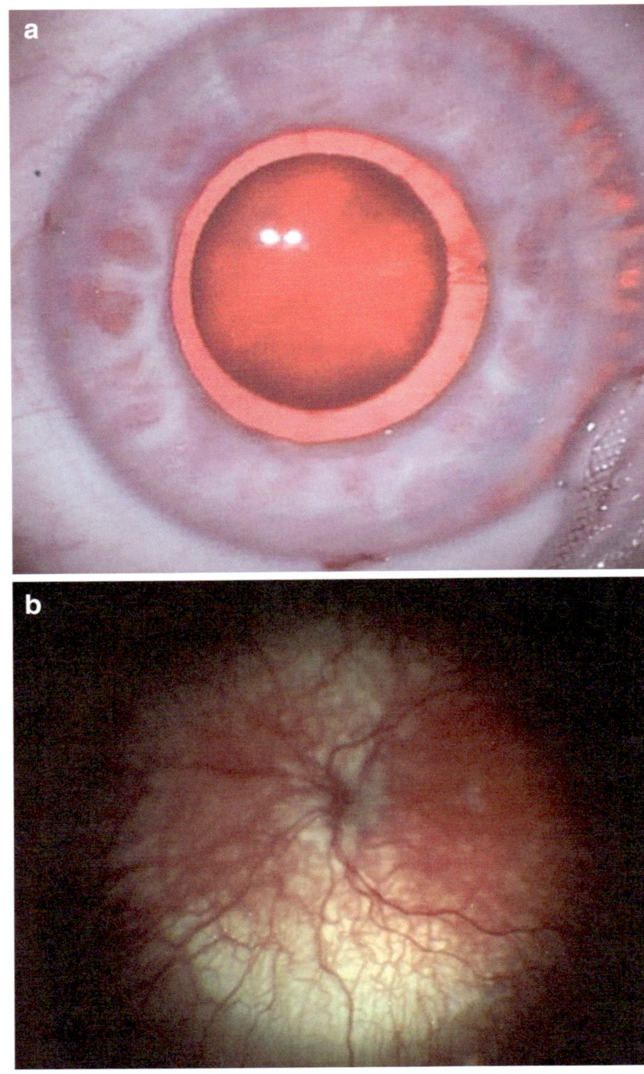

Fig. 12.18 A 3-year-old boy with oculocutaneous albinism (**a**) Retroillumination picture showing iris transillumination and zonular cataract. (**b**) Fundus picture of the same showing prominent choroidal vasculature and foveal hypoplasia

References

1. Cuthbertson F, Newsom R. UK retinopathy of prematurity treatment survey. Eye(Lond). 2007;21:156–7.
2. Davitt BV, Christiansen SP, Hardy RJ, et al. Early treatment for retinopathy of prematurity cooperative group. Incidence of cataract development by 6 months' corrected age in the early treatment for retinopathy of prematurity study. J AAPOS. 2013;17:49–53.
3. Lambert SR, Capone A Jr, Cingle KA, et al. Cataract and phthisis bulbi after laser photoablation for threshold retinopathy of prematurity. Am J Ophthalmol. 2000;129:585–91.
4. Salgado CM, Celik Y, VanderVeen DK. Anterior segment complications after diode laser photocoagulation for prethreshold retinopathy of prematurity. Am J Ophthalmol. 2010;150:6–9.
5. Chandra P, Khokhar S, Kumar A. Bilateral Total cataract after laser treatment of aggressive posterior retinopathy of prematurity. Indian Pediatr. 2016;53(Suppl 2):S157–8.

6. Lakhanpal RR, Davis GH, Sun RL, et al. Lens clarity after 3-port lens-sparing vitrectomy in stage 4A and 4B retinal detachments secondary to retinopathy of prematurity. Arch Ophthalmol. 2006;124:20–3.
7. Choi J, Kim JH, Kim SJ, et al. Long-term results of lens-sparing vitrectomy for stages 4B and 5 retinopathy of prematurity. Korean J Ophthalmol. 2011;25:305–10.
8. Repka MX, Summers CG, Palmer EA, et al. On behalf of the Cryotherapy for retinopathy of prematurity cooperative group. The incidence of ophthalmologic interventions in children with birth weights less than 1251 grams. Results through 51/2 years. Ophthalmology. 1998;105:1621–7.
9. Capone A Jr, Drack AV. Transient lens changes after diode laser retinal photoablation for retinopathy of prematurity. Am J Ophthalmol. 1994;118:533–5.
10. Meyer CH, Rodrigues EB, Michels S, Mennel S, Schmidt JC, Helb HM, et al. Incidence of damage to the crystalline lens during intravitreal injections. J Ocul Pharmacol Ther. 2010;26:491–5.
11. Khokhar S, et al. Bilateral total cataract after intravitreal bevacizumab injection in aggressive posterior retinopathy of prematurity. J Pediatr Ophthalmol Strabismus. 2019;56:e28–30. https://doi.org/10.3928/01913913-20190219-02.
12. Ezisi CN, Kekunnaya R, Jalali S, Balakrishnan D, Kumari PR, Mohamed A, et al. Cataract surgery in children with retinopathy of prematurity (ROP): surgical outcomes. Br J Ophthalmol. 2017;101:1128–31.
13. Krolicki TJ, Tasman W. Cataract extraction in adults with retinopathy of prematurity. Arch Ophthalmol. 1995;113:173–7.
14. Yu YS, Kim SJ, Chang BL. Cataract surgery in children with and without retinopathy of prematurity. J Cataract Refract Surg. 2004;30:89–94.
15. Chang L, Blain D, Bertuzzi S, Brooks BP. Uveal coloboma: clinical and basic science update. Curr Opin Ophthalmol. 2006;17(5):447–70.
16. Onwochei BC, Simon JW, Bateman JB, Couture KC, Mir E. Ocular colobomata. Surv Ophthalmol. 2000;45:175–94.
17. Nordlund ML, Sugar A, Moroi SE. Phacoemulsification and intraocular lens placement in eyes with cataract and congenital coloboma: visual acuity and complications. J Cataract Refract Surg. 2000;26:1035–40.
18. Chaurasia S, Ramappa M, Sangwan VS. Cataract surgery in eyes with congenital iridolenticular choroidal coloboma. Br J Ophthalmol. 2012;96(1):138–40.
19. Mizuno H, Yamada J, Nishiura M, Takahashi H, Hino Y, Miyatani H. Capsular tension ring use in a patient with congenital coloboma of the lens. J Cataract Refract Surg. 2004;30:503–6.
20. Cionni RJ, Karatza EC, Osher RH, Shah M. Surgical technique for congenital iris coloboma repair. J Cataract Refract Surg. 2006;32:1913–6.
21. Olali C, Mohammed M, Ahmed S, Gupta M. Contact lens for failed pupilloplasty. J Cataract Refract Surg. 2008;34:1995–6.
22. Khokhar S, Agarwal T, Kumar G, Kushmesh R, Tejwani LK. Lenticular abnormalities in children. J Pediatr Ophthalmol Strabismus. 2012;49:32–7.
23. Memon MN, Narsani AK, Nizamani NB. Visual outcome of unilateral traumatic cataract. J Coll Physicians Surg Pak. 2012;22:497–500.
24. Seery CM, Pruett RC, Liberfarb RM, et al. Distinctive cataract in the stickler syndrome. Am J Ophthalmol. 1990;110:143–8.
25. Borislav D. Cataract after silicone oil implantation. Doc Ophthalmol. 1993;83:79–82.
26. Heckenlively J. The frequency of posterior subcapsular cataract in the hereditary retinal degenerations. Am J Ophthalmol. 1982;93:733–8.
27. Jackson H, Garway-Heath D, Rosen P, et al. Outcome of cataract surgery in patients with retinitis pigmentosa. Br J Ophthalmol. 2001;85:936–8.
28. Bayyoud T, Bartz-Schmidt KU, Yoeruek E. Long-term clinical results after cataract surgery with and without capsular tension ring in patients with retinitis pigmentosa: a retrospective study. BMJ Open. 2013;3:e002616.
29. Dikopf MS, Chow CC, Mieler WF, Tu EY. Cataract extraction outcomes and the prevalence of zonular insufficiency in retinitis pigmentosa. Am J Ophthalmol. 2013;156:82–88 e2.
30. Urban RC Jr, Cotlier E. Corticosteroid-induced cataracts. Surv Ophthalmol. 1986;31:102–10.
31. Lerman S, Balasubramanian D, Bansal AK, Basti S, Bhatt KS, Murthy JS, Rao CM, editors. Potent ocular complications of psoralen UVA therapy. The biology of cataract. The Hyderabad cataract resear group. Indian J Ophthalmol. 1993;41:153–71.
32. Michael DA, Colleen MD, Kimberly AN. Ciglitazone induced lenticular opacities in rats: in vivo an whole lens explant culture evaluation. J Pharmacol Exp Ther. 2005;312:1027–33.
33. Steven P, Steven K, Robert H, Judy H. Amiodarone corneal topography. Digital J Ophthalmol. 1997;3:03.
34. Alexender LJ, Bowerman L, Thompson LR. The prevalance of the ocular side effects of chlorpromazine in the Tuscaloosa Veterens administration patient population. J Am Optom Assoc. 1985;56:872–6.
35. Greiner AC, Berry K. Skin pigmentation and corneal and lens opacities with prolonged chlorproma therapy. Can Med Assoc J. 1964;90:663–5.
36. Jobling AI, Augusteyn RC. What causes steroid cataracts? A review of steroid induced posterior subcapsular cataracts. Clin Exp Optom. 2002;85:61–75.
37. Spencer R, Andelman S. Steroids are bad cataracts. Posterior subcapsular cataract formation in rheumatoid arthritis patients on long term steroid therapy. Arch Ophthalmol. 1965;74:38–41.
38. Urban RC, Cotlier E. Corticosteroid-induced cataracts. Surv Ophtalmol. 1986;31:102–10.
39. Brocklebank JT, Harcourt RB, Meadow SR. Corticosteroid induced cataracts in idiopathic nephrotic syndrome. Arch Dis Child. 1982;53:30–4.
40. Boozalis GT, Purdu GF. Ocular changes from electric burn injuries: a literature review and report of cases. J Burn Care Rehabil. 1991;12:458.
41. Grewal DS, Jain R, Brar GS, Grewal SPS. Unilateral electric cataract: Scheimpflug imaging and review of the literature. J Cataract Refract Surg. 2007;33(6):1116e1119.
42. Riaz Khan M, El Faki HMA. Acute cataract and optic atrophy after high-voltage electrical injury. Eur J Plast Surg. 2008;31:73e74.
43. Saffle JR, Crandall A. Cataracts a long term complication of electrical injury. J Trauma. 1985;25(1):17e21.
44. Hashemi H, Jabbarvand M, Mohammadpour M. Bilateral electric cataracts: clinicopathologic report. J Cataract Refract Surg. 2008;34(8):1409–12.
45. Summers CG. Albinism: classification, clinical characteristics, and recent findings. Optom Vis Sci. 2009;86:659–862.
46. Kirkwood BJ. Albinism and its implications with vision. Insight. 2009;34:13–6.
47. Hayasaka S, Noda S, Setogawa T. Posterior chamber intraocular lens implantation in a patient with oculocutaneous albinism. J Cataract Refract Surg. 1992;18:527–9.
48. Farahi A, Hashemi H, Mehravaran S. Combined cataract surgery and aniridia ring implantation in oculocutaneous albinism. J Cataract Refract Surg. 2015;41(11):2438–43.

Preoperative Workup and Investigations in Pediatric Cataract Surgery

13

Chirakshi Dhull, Sagnik Sen, and Sudarshan Kumar Khokhar

Preoperative evaluation has a major role to play in the postoperative outcomes of cataract surgery in children. The age of detection, morphology of cataract, unilateral/bilateral, time of presentation, best-corrected distance visual acuity, presence of strabismus, nystagmus, and glaucoma all may predict the postoperative visual outcome of surgery [1]. The delay in presentation for surgery is generally associated with poor outcome.

13.1 Visual Acuity Assessment

The initial part of ocular examination of any child is visual acuity assessment. Fixation is to be checked; central fixation suggests fovea as the fixing point, steady fixation suggests absence of nystagmus, and maintained fixation suggests that there is no squint [2]. Preoperative good best-corrected distance visual acuity is a good prognostic factor as it rules out amblyopia in these eyes, whereas cataract associated with strabismus generally indicates poor visual acuity in that eye [3]. More specialized tests have been developed to test for visual acuity in preverbal children, e.g., visual-evoked response (VER), Catford drum, optokinetic nystagmus, and Teller's acuity cards. In 1–2 years of age, Worth's ivory ball test, Boeck's candy test, the Screening Test for Young Children and Retards (STYCAR), and Cardiff's acuity test (Fig. 13.1) can be done. In 2–3 years age, miniature toy test, coin test, and LEA symbols® test are used. In children aged 3–5 years, Allen's picture card, Lippman's HOTV test, and letter test are used. In ages more than 5 years, Tumbling E, Landolt's broken ring, Snellen's chart, and LogMAR chart can be used [4].

C. Dhull (✉) · S. Sen · S. K. Khokhar
Dr. Rajendra Prasad Centre for Ophthalmic Sciences, All India Institute of Medical Sciences, New Delhi, India

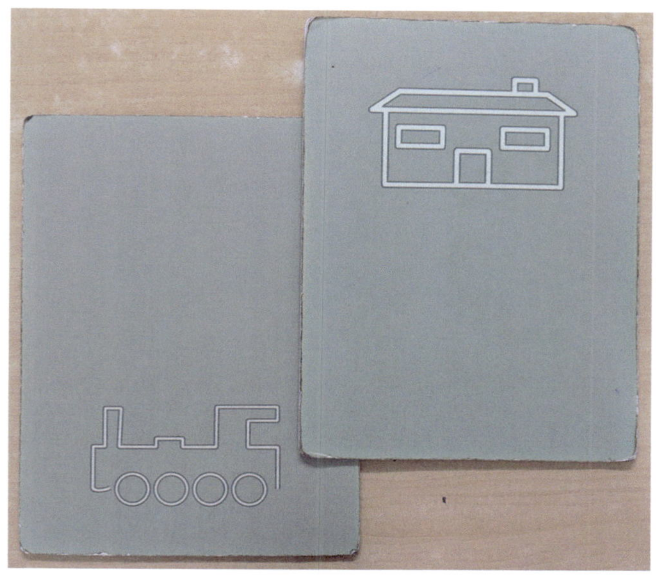

Fig. 13.1 Cardiff visual acuity cards

13.2 Screening for Cataract

A child is most comfortable in his mother's lap/shoulder hold. Hence, the child can be examined with child's head on the parent's shoulder, which is convenient for ophthalmic examination (Fig. 13.2). After assessing the visual acuity and pupillary response, a distant direct examination is performed to look for anterior segment changes like corneal opacity, shallow anterior chamber, peripheral anterior synechiae (Peter's anomaly), microcornea (microcornea-cataract syndrome), posterior synechiae (uveitis), key-hole pupil (iridofundal coloboma), and enlarged ciliary processes with vessels on lens (persistent fetal vasculature). The red reflex screening with direct ophthalmoscope kept at 30 cm and focused on each pupil separately (Bruckner's test) helps in the identification of lenticular opacity (Fig. 13.3). If the diagnosis is not clear, a dilated pupil

S. K. Khokhar, C. Dhull (eds.), *Atlas of Pediatric Cataract*, https://doi.org/10.1007/978-981-13-6939-1_13

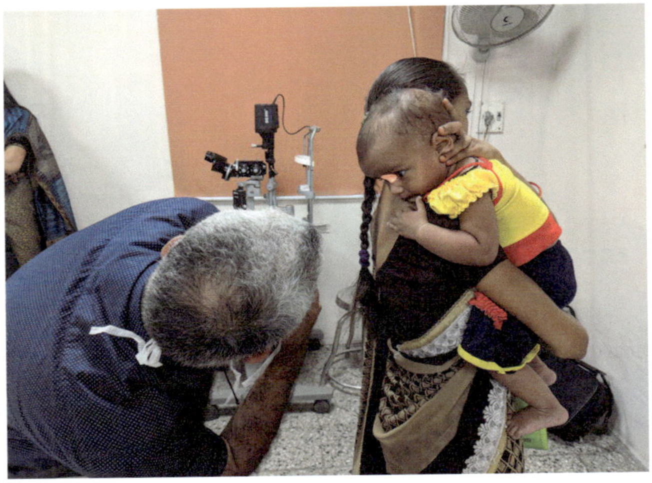

Fig. 13.2 Examination of patient with distant direct in shoulder hold by parent

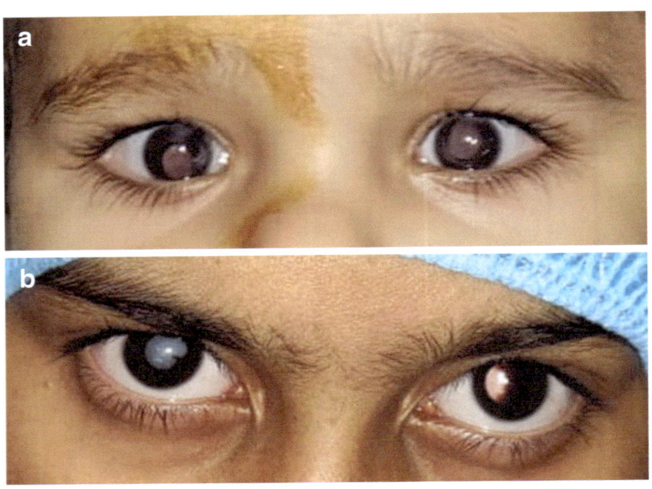

Fig. 13.3 Red reflex. (**a**) Both eyes show red glow with no media opacity. (**b**) White reflex seen in right eye and red glow in the left eye

examination with mydriatic agent can be done. Viewing both the eyes simultaneously with direct ophthalmoscope from 3 feet may help in identifying anisometropia based on the difference in the two glows. Strabismus and asymmetric cataract may also be detected with this method and also by checking the fixation pattern [5]. If a child has poor fixation and cannot follow objects after 2 months of age, an urgent referral to an ophthalmologist is warranted.

13.3 Systemic Evaluation

Most Unilateral cataracts and a large number of bilateral cataracts are idiopathic in nature; however, this diagnosis is made after excluding other causes. In this regard, systemic investigations include fasting blood sugar, urine for reducing substance for galactosemia after milk feeding, and urine amino acids for Lowe's syndrome. Plasma phosphorus, red blood cells transferase and galactokinase levels and calcium evaluation for hypothyroidism are also performed. Titers for toxoplasma, rubella, cytomegalovirus, and herpes simplex (TORCH) are ordered to rule out these respective disorders. Genetic testing may be carried out for children with congenital cataract. Echocardiography is to be done in cases of Marfan's syndrome and Rubella cataract to detect aortic regurgitation, aortic root dilation, patent ductus arteriosus, and atrial septal defect. In cases of juvenile idiopathic arthritis needing immunosuppressant medications, a rheumatology opinion is needed. In cases of seizure and gross developmental delay, child is referred to a neurologist. Nephrology opinion is sought in cases of nephrotic syndrome and Lowe syndrome. Systemic investigationns should be performed based on clinical suspicion.

13.4 Ocular Imaging

Ultrasonography (USG), apart from helping in intraoperative management, also helps in prognostication, especially in unilateral cataract cases with dense cataracts and poor glow, where the posterior segment in not properly visible with funduscopy. USG helps in ruling out retinal detachment, fundal coloboma, persistent fetal vasculature (PFV), and retinoblastoma (Fig. 13.4a–d) [6]. PFV, which may be missed on USG, can be detected using magnetic resonance imaging (MRI) scans [7]. Flow inside a PFV may be picked on a Color Doppler. X-ray and/or Computed Tomography (CT) scan in cases of traumatic cataract are used to localize any intraocular foreign body [8].

13.5 Axial Length

An important challenge in pediatric cataract surgery is assessing axial length growth and hence, predicting the refractive outcome. Axial length increases rapidly in the first 6 months (0.62 mm/month), then becomes relatively slow (infantile phase growth) (0.19 mm/month) till 18 months, followed by a slower (juvenile phase growth) increase (0.01 mm/month) [9, 10]. Axial length increase postoperatively varies among children. Axial length increases more rapidly in pseudophakic children than in unilateral cases compared to bilateral cases [11]. Immersion A-scan is more accurate than contact A-scan because it avoids compression of the anterior surface of the cornea. Axial length measurements made using contact technique give 0.24–0.32 mm lesser average measurements as compared to immersion technique. Nevertheless, indentation method is performed more commonly (Fig. 13.5a). Hence, if immersion scan is not possible, A-scan reading with maximum anterior cham-

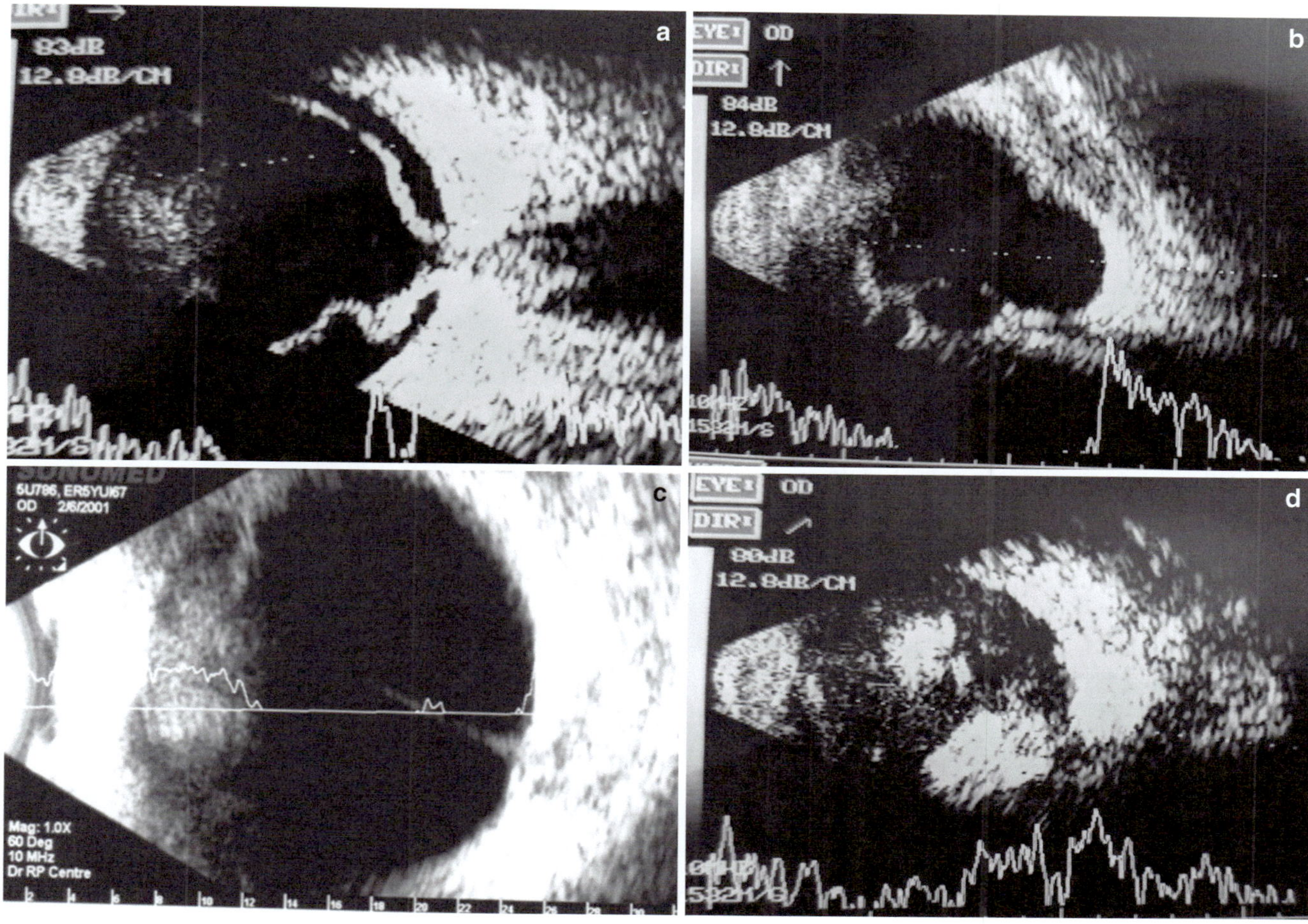

Fig. 13.4 Ultrasonography for posterior segment evaluation with pathology. (**a**) Retinal detachment, (**b**) fundal coloboma, (**c**) persistent fetal vasculature, (**d**) mass lesion with calcification—retinoblastoma in this case

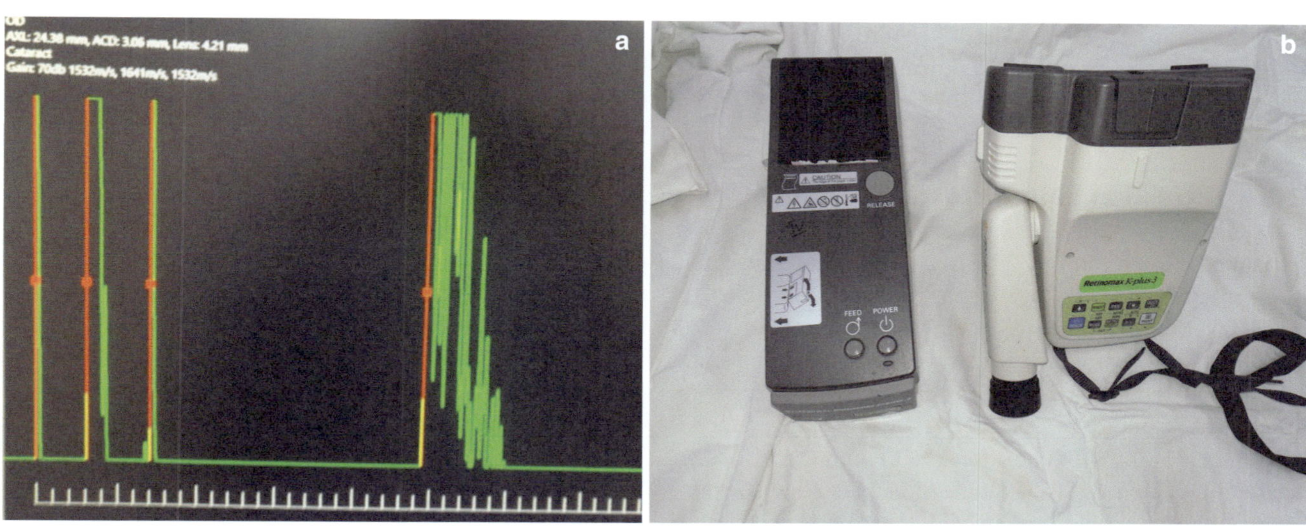

Fig. 13.5 (**a**) Contact Ascan for axial length measurement. Note all spikes are 100% suggesting good scan. (**b**) Hand held auto-keratometer

ber depth should be taken. However, all of these scans may not pass through the fovea as the child does not always fixate towards the probe; hence, there is a need for a device which may be able to track the axial length across the fovea.

13.6 Keratometry

Keratometry data is generally obtained under general anesthesia using a handheld auto-keratometer (Fig. 13.5b). However, it can also be measured with a manual keratometer in older children. Keratometry steeply reduces in the first 6 months (−0.40 D/month), at −0.14 D/month in the second half of first year, and at −0.08 D/month in the second year [12]. Adult corneal curvature is achieved at around 3 years of age [13]. It has been observed that keratometry is steeper in eyes with monocular cataracts than those of bilateral cataracts [14]. Also, keratometry is steeper in cataractous eyes as against the fellow eyes. The mean preoperative keratometry is also higher in congenital (47.78 D) than in the developmental cataract (44.35 D) 15. Keratometry readings should be taken without the speculum as there may be erroneous readings due to deforming effect of the speculum on the globe.

13.7 Intraocular Pressure Determination

Pediatric cataract eyes with cataract may be associated with preoperative or postoperative pseudophakic glaucoma. Rubella cataracts, post-traumatic and uveitic cataracts may also be associated with raised IOP. Intraocular pressure documentation before surgery is of paramount importance both in terms of preoperative control of glaucoma and also for prognosticating the outcome, depending on the optic nerve status. In this regard, preoperatively, Perkins tonometer may be used during examination under general anesthesia.

13.8 Ultrasound Biomicroscopy (UBM)

Ultrasound biomicroscopy (UBM) is used to image the anterior segment of an eye using higher frequencies of 35 MHz, and 50 MHz as compared to conventional USG. UBM can be used for ocular biometry including anterior chamber depth (ACD), lens thickness (LT), angle to angle (ATA), sulcus to sulcus (STS), and bag diameter (BD) (Fig. 13.6). With the increase in frequency, ocular penetration decreases [16, 17]. UBM can also be used preoperatively to assess the sulcus and assessment of anterior capsule for secondary intraocular lens (IOL) (Fig. 13.7a–f).

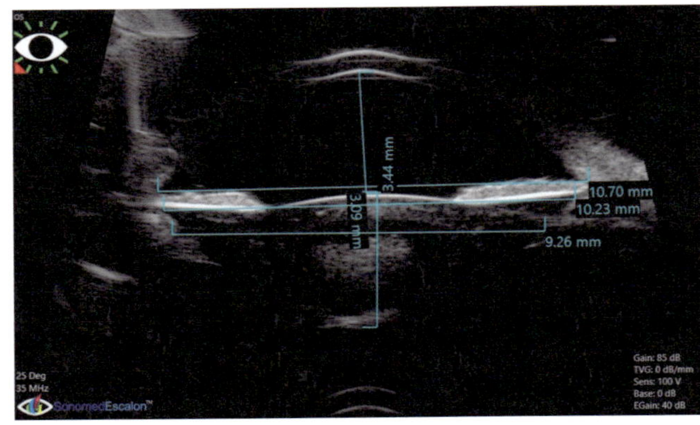

Fig. 13.6 Ocular biometry using UBM anterior chamber depth (ACD), lens thickness (LT), angle to angle (ATA), sulcus to sulcus (STS), and bag diameter (BD)

It is also used in evaluation of morphology of lens and detection of abnormalities like capsular plaque, posterior lenticonus, persistent fetal vasculature (PFV), buphalmic eyes, etc. which helps in better planning and management (Fig. 13.8a–f) [17–19]. UBM may also help evaluate for subluxation, iridodialysis, cyclodialysis, foreign body localization in anterior segment, lens evaluation in corneal opacity, posterior capsular dehiscence (Fig. 13.9a–d) and postoperative IOL centration and tilt (Fig. 13.10a, b) [20].

13.9 Optical Coherence Tomography (OCT)

OCT is a state-of-the-art noninvasive, noncontact technique for imaging the anterior and posterior segment of the eye with high resolutions of up to 1 μm [21]. Swept-source OCT using a wavelength of 1060 nm [22] can image the choroid also with good resolution [23]. The retinal nerve fiber layer thickness (RNFL) on OCT has been found to be negatively correlated to axial length [24]. Macular edema which is sometimes missed on clinical examination in children can be captured on OCT in around 25% of children operated for complicated cataract in uveitic eyes (e.g., JIA) [25]. Besides these, anterior segment OCT is used to check vaulting of phakic intraocular lenses [26], placement of anterior chamber IOL (ACIOL), and also to assess angle structures and look for anomalies.

13.10 Intraocular Lens Power Calculation

Since axial length and keratometry are constantly changing in children both naturally and after surgery, predicting the right power of intraocular lens for a child's eye is difficult

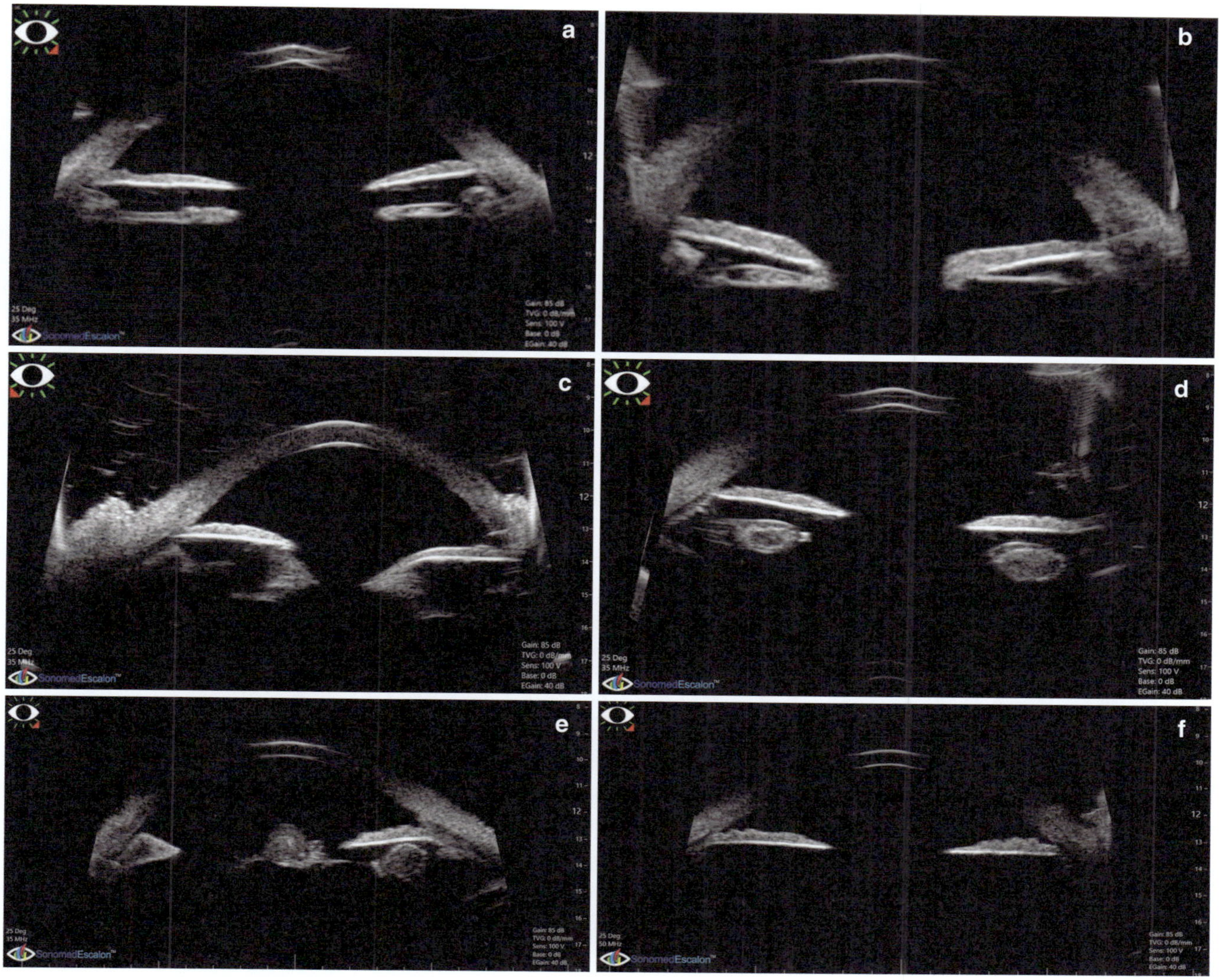

Fig. 13.7 Rim of sulcus (ROS) assessment and surgical planning. (**a**) Fibrosed ROS with clear separation from iris—IOL can be placed with minimum manipulation. (**b**) Fibrosed ROS adhered to iris—requires release of synechiae before IOL placement. (**c**) Fleshy ROS with adequate support, can be opened for IOL placement in bag. (**d**) Fleshy ROS in the periphery, IOL cannot be placed in bag, optic capture not possible, IOL placed in sulcus. (**e**) ROS seen less than 180°, IOL cannot be safely placed in sulcus. (**f**) No ROS seen, plan for ACIOL/iris claw/scleral fixation

and may often lead to postoperative IOL surprises. Implantation of IOL in aphakic eyes of young children and infants is always preferred especially in the developing countries where postoperative care and follow-up are difficult, as compared to leaving them aphakic with correction using glasses/contact lenses as is commonly practiced in the West, with a secondary IOL implantation at a later date [27]. More so in monocular cataract eyes, primary IOL implantation at the time of cataract surgery is of extreme importance to avoid postoperative aniseikonia from glasses and prevent onset of amblyopia. IOL power determination is done taking into account various factors like age of presentation, morphology of cataract, visual acuity at presentation, time of development of cataract (congenital/developmental), biometry at presentation, unilateral or bilateral cataract, and refractive status of the fellow eye [28]. IOL should preferably be implanted in eyes with axial length > 17 mm and corneal diameter > 10 mm. A postoperative hypermetropia is desirable to avoid excessive myopic shift during growth. Dahan et al. had suggested under correction of 20% in children <2 years and 10% for ages between 2 years and 8 years [29]. Prost suggested 20% under correction between 1 year and

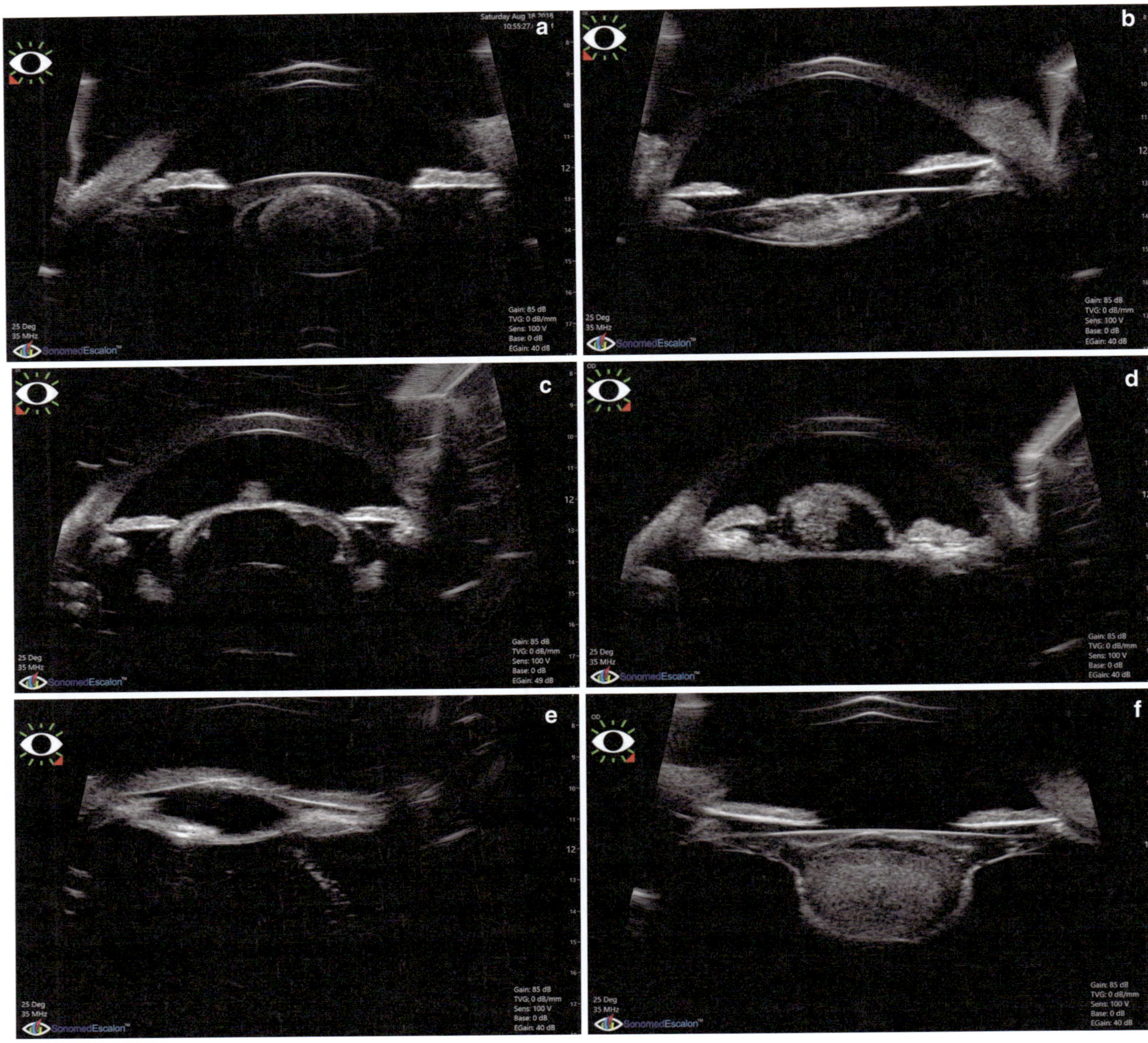

Fig. 13.8 Morphology of pediatric cataract. (**a**) Zonular cataract, (**b**) membranous cataract with anterior capsular plaque, (**c**) Morgagnian cataract with anterior pyramidal cataract, (**d**) anterior PFV with elongated ciliary processes, (**e**) mixed PFV with elongated ciliary processes and stalk of PFV seen behind the lens, (**f**) total cataract with posterior lenticonus

2 years of age, 15% under correction between 2 years and 4 years, and 10% between 4 years and 8 years of age [30]. Enyedi et al. suggested the sum of age and postoperative refraction be kept equal to 7 [31]. Intraoperative aphakic refraction can also be used to calculate the IOL power now using measurement of intraoperative aberrometry [32]. Various IOL formulae have been used in adult eyes for IOL power prediction. However, they have not shown to be that predictable and accurate in pediatric eyes. Although SRK-II formula is the most commonly used, SRK/T and the Holladay 2 formulae have been shown to have the least predictive error in children [33]. We have devised a formula for Indian eyes which has been in use for quite some time. We have observed relatively less growth in our population compared to western eyes. We use 20 % undercorrection for children <3 months, 10% at 1 year, 5% at 2 years and only 2% at 5 years. Beyond 5 years, minimal growth is seen (IJO-accepted for publication).

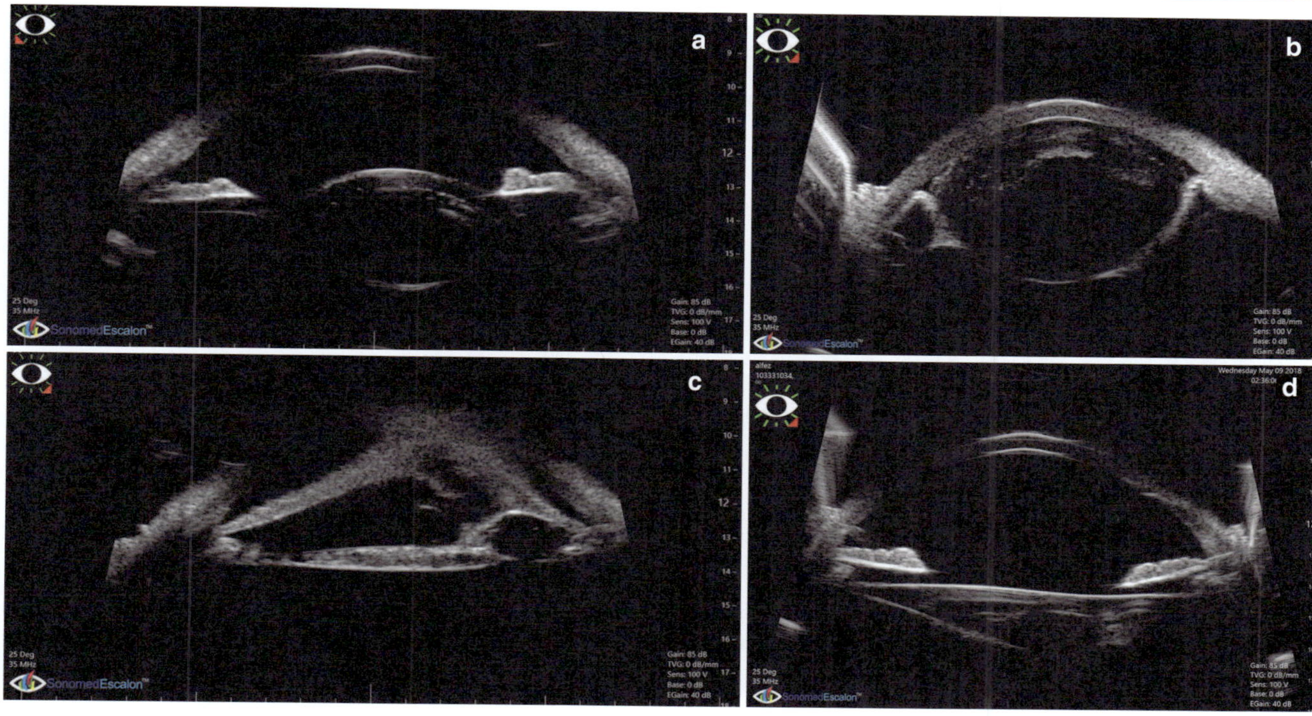

Fig. 13.9 Complex situations. (**a**) Subluxated lens, no tilt, (**b**) anteriorly dislocated cataractous lens, (**c**) adherent leukoma with partially absorbed cataract, (**d**) post vitrectomy posterior capsular dehiscence secondary to lens touch

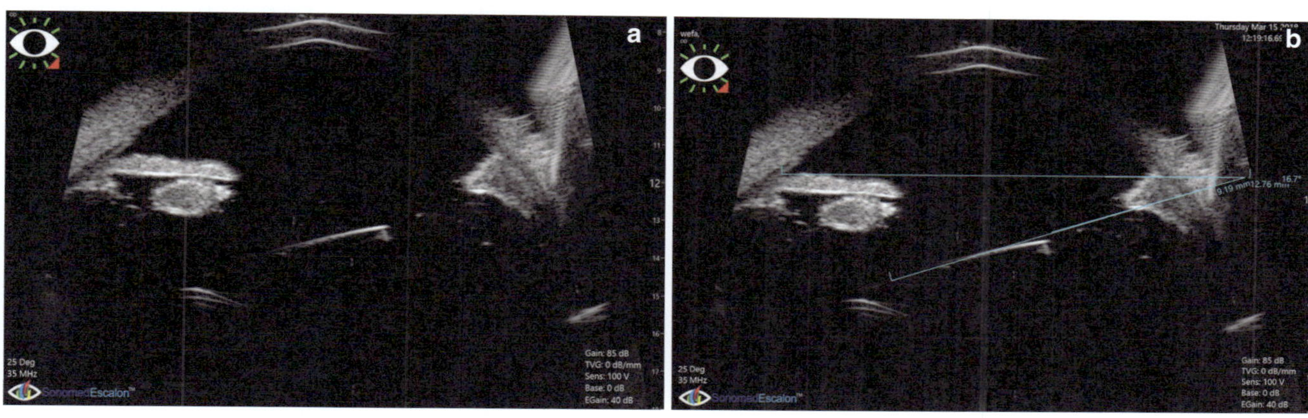

Fig. 13.10 IOL tilt. (**a**) Scleral fixated IOL with significant tilt post trauma with fist. (**b**) Objectively degree of tilt can be measured, here it is 16.7° (Up to 12° is considered tolerable)

References

1. Bonaparte LA, Trivedi RH, Ramakrishnan V, Wilson ME. Visual acuity and its predictors after surgery for bilateral cataracts in children. Eye (Lond). 2016;30:1229–33.
2. Lin AA, Buckley EG. Update on pediatric cataract surgery and intraocular lens implantation. Curr Opin Ophthalmol. 2010;21:55–9.
3. Spanou N, Alexopoulos L, Manta G, Tsamadou D, Drakos H, Paikos P. Strabismus in pediatric lens disorders. J AAPOS. 2011;48:163–6.
4. Gole G. Visual acuity assessment in children. Clin Exp Ophthalmol. 1989;17:1–2.
5. Anker S, Atkinson J, Braddick O, Ehrlich D, Hartley T, Nardini M, et al. Identification of infants with significant refractive error and strabismus in a population screening program using noncycloplegic videorefraction and orthoptic examination. Invest Ophthalmol Vis Sci. 2003;44:497–504.

6. Kaya A. Preoperative usage of ultrasound biomicroscopy in pediatric cataract. Arq Bras Oftalmol. 2016;79:62.
7. Khokhar S, Jose CP, Sihota R, Midha N. Unilateral congenital cataract: clinical profile and presentation. J Pediatr Ophthalmol Strabismus. 2018;55(2):107–12. doi:10.3928/01913913-20170703-11change numbers accordingly.
8. Qi Y, Zhang YF, Zhu Y, Wan MG, Du SS, Yue ZZ, et al. Prognostic factors for visual outcome in traumatic cataract patients. J Ophthalmol. 2016;2016:1748583.
9. Wilson ME, Trivedi RH. Axial length measurement techniques in pediatric eyes with cataract. Saudi J Ophthalmol. 2012;26:13–7.
10. Gordon R.A., Donzis P.B. Refractive development of the human eye. Arch Ophthalmol. 1985;103:785–9.
11. Vasavada AR, Raj SM, Nihalani B. Rate of axial growth after congenital cataract surgery. Am J Ophthalmol. 2004;138:915–24.
12. Capozzi P, Morini C, Piga S, Cuttini M, Vadalà P. Corneal curvature and axial length values in children with congenital/infantile cataract in the first 42 months of life. Invest Ophthalmol Vis Sci. 2008;49:4774–8.
13. Ehlers N, Sorensen T, Bramsen T, Poulsen EH. Central corneal thickness in newborns and children. Acta Ophthalmol. 1976;54:285–90.
14. Trivedi RH, Wilson ME. Keratometry in pediatric eyes with cataract. Arch Ophthalmol. 2008;126:38–42.
15. Flitcroft DI, Knight-Nanan D, Bowell R, Lanigan B, O'Keefe M. Intraocular lenses in children: changes in axial length, corneal curvature, and refraction. Br J Ophthalmol. 1999;83:265–9.
16. Pavlin CJ, Harasiewicz K, Sherar MD, Foster FS. Clinical use of ultrasound biomicroscopy. Ophthalmology. 1991;98:287–95.
17. Silverman RH. High-resolution ultrasound imaging of the eye – a review. Clin Exp Ophthalmol. 2009;37:54–67.
18. Xiang D, Chen L, Hu L, Song S, Xie W, Long J. Image features of lens opacity in pediatric cataracts using ultrasound biomicroscopy. J AAPOS. 2016;20(6):519–22.
19. Gupta V, Jha R, Srinivasan G, Dada T, Sihota R. Ultrasound biomicroscopic characteristics of the anterior segment in primary congenital glaucoma. J AAPOS. 2007;11:546–50.
20. Kucukevcilioglu M, Hurmeric V, Ceylan OM. Preoperative detection of posterior capsule tear with ultrasound biomicroscopy in traumatic cataract. J Cataract Refract Surg. 2013;39:289–91.
21. Fujimoto JG. Optical coherence tomography for ultrahigh resolution in vivo imaging. Nat Biotechnol. 2003;21:1361–7.
22. Hirata M, Tsujikawa A, Matsumoto A, Hangai M, Ooto S, Yamashiro K, et al. Macular choroidal thickness and volume in normal subjects measured by swept-source optical coherence tomography. Invest Ophthalmol Vis Sci. 2011;52:4971–8.
23. Fujiwara T, Imamura Y, Margolis R, Slakter JS, Spaide RF. Enhanced depth imaging optical coherence tomography of the choroid in highly myopic eyes. Am J Ophthalmol. 2009;148:445–50.
24. Pang Y, Goodfellow GW, Allison C, Block S, Frantz KA. A prospective study of macular thickness in amblyopic children with unilateral high myopia. Invest Ophthalmol Vis Sci. 2011;52:2444–9.
25. Paroli MP, Spinucci G, Fabiani C, Pivetti-Pezzi P. Retinal complications of juvenile idiopathic arthritis-related uveitis: a microperimetry and optical coherence tomography study. Ocul Immunol Inflamm. 2010;18:54–9.
26. Baikoff G, Lutun E, Wei J, Ferraz C. Contact between 3 phakic intraocular lens models and the crystalline lens: an anterior chamber optical coherence tomography study. J Cataract Refract Surg. 2004;30:2007–12.
27. Wilson ME, Pandey SK, Thakur J. Paediatric cataract blindness in the developing world: surgical techniques and intraocular lenses in the new millennium. Br J Ophthalmol. 2003;87:14–9.
28. Magli A, Forte R, Carelli R, Rombetto L, Magli G. Long-term outcomes of primary intraocular lens implantation for unilateral congenital cataract. Semin Ophthalmol. 2016;31:548–53.
29. Dahan E, Drusedau MU. Choice of lens and dioptric power in pediatric pseudophakia. J Cataract Refract Surg. 1997;23(Suppl 1):618–23.
30. Prost ME. IOL calculations in cataract operations in children. Klin Ocz. 2004;106:691–4.
31. Enyedi LB, Peterseim MW, Freedman SF, Buckley EG. Refractive changes after pediatric intraocular lens implantation. Am J Ophthalmol. 1998;126:772–81.
32. Zhang Z, Thomas LW, Leu SY, Carter S, Garg S. Refractive outcomes of intraoperative wavefront aberrometry versus optical biometry alone for intraocular lens power calculation. Indian J Ophthalmol. 2017;65:813–7.
33. Vasavada V, Shah SK, Vasavada VA, Vasavada AR, Trivedi RH, Srivastava S, et al. Comparison of IOL power calculation formulae for pediatric eyes. Eye (Lond). 2016;30:1242–50.

Surgical Management of Pediatric Cataract

14

Sudarshan Kumar Khokhar, Chirakshi Dhull, and Yogita Gupta

The aim of surgery is not just to clear visual axis but also to maintain clear visual axis for a long time. Success of pediatric cataract surgery depends on meticulous surgery, close follow-up, and compliance to visual rehabilitation aids. Surgery is not required in all cases of cataract. It is recommended in visually significant cataract >3 mm [1], dense nuclear or posterior cataracts, cataracts not permitting fundus evaluation, and those associated with nystagmus or strabismus.

14.1 Timing of Surgery

The ideal time to perform cataract surgery is when optimal visual outcome can be achieved with minimum risk of complications. Delay in surgery increases risk of stimulus deprivation amblyopia while early surgery is associated with higher risks of complications. There is evidence that risk of glaucoma reduces if cataract surgery is performed at older age [2, 3]. Visual outcome has been observed to be better in surgery at earlier age especially in cases of unilateral cataract [4, 5]. Birch et al. [4] identified a 6 week latent period for unilateral cataract where there was no difference in visual outcome in this period. We have identified the ideal time for surgery in unilateral and bilateral cataract to be by 6 weeks and 8 weeks, respectively [6]. In case of bilateral cataract, we prefer to perform sequential surgery within a week's time [6]. Simultaneous surgery is not recommended for most cases. After IOL placement in one eye, fine tuning of IOL power can be done at the time of second eye surgery based on retinoscopy of first eye.

14.2 Anesthesia

General anesthesia team plays an essential role in management of pediatric cataract. Considerations in facilitating surgery include control of intraocular pressure, eye movements including Bell's phenomena, understanding risk of apnea in infants, and control of postoperative pain, nausea, and vomiting [7].

14.3 Surgical Steps for Cataract Surgery

14.3.1 Head Positioning and Proper Exposure

Pediatric cases require proper head positioning to ensure good exposure and ease of surgery as the child is under general anesthesia. Head ring of correct size can be used according to the age along with shoulder support. Size of the speculum in relation to palpebral aperture has to be taken into consideration (Fig. 14.1a–c).

14.3.2 Incision

Two paracentesis incision almost 180° apart give access to whole of the anterior chamber and lens with ease. They can be used for bimanual surgery along with injecting viscoelastic devices. Main incision can be clear corneal or scleral tunnel. Both incision techniques are acceptable and are shown to similar surgically induced astigmatism (SIA) [8]. Superior incision is preferable in small children as it protects from inadvertent trauma. Incision can be placed in steepest axis in older children for reducing SIA [9].

14.3.3 Anterior Capsulorhexis

Staining of anterior capsule is required in cases of total cataract or in cases where good glow is absent. High molecular weight ocular viscoelastic devices (OVDs) should be used to flatten the anterior capsule [10]. Manual capsulorhexis is considered gold standard although it is more difficult in children due to elastic nature of capsule [11]. Steps of manual

S. K. Khokhar · C. Dhull (✉) · Y. Gupta
Dr. Rajendra Prasad Centre for Ophthalmic Sciences, All India Institute of Medical Sciences, New Delhi, India

S. K. Khokhar, C. Dhull (eds.), *Atlas of Pediatric Cataract*, https://doi.org/10.1007/978-981-13-6939-1_14

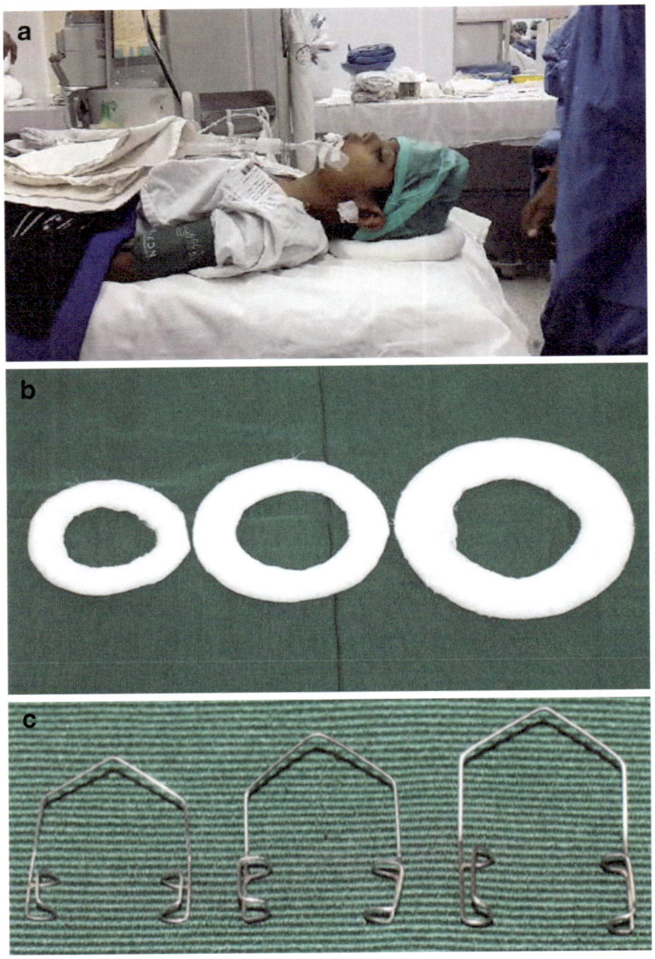

Fig. 14.1 (**a**) Ideal head position after intubation with head ring and shoulder roll for appropriate exposure. (**b**) Various size of head rings. (**c**) Various size of eyelid speculum

capsulorhexis are shown in (Fig. 14.2a–d). During manual capsulorhexis, aim should be to pull the capsulorhexis to center with frequent regrasps near the tearing edge to avoid extension. The anterior capsulotomy shape, size, and edge integrity are very important for the long-term centration of intraocular lens (IOL). In cases where manual capsulorhexis is not possible, vitrectomy cutter can be used to create capsulorhexis [12, 13] referred to as vitrectorhexis. Various other methods including use of diathermy, Fugo blade, femtosecond laser, etc. for creation of capsulorhexis are also available and can be selected for specific cases [14–19]. Tools for measurement of rhexis size accurately can be used. These include internal rings or external devices. Capsulorhexis size assesment and intruments which can be used to perform rhexis are shown in (Fig. 14.3a–f).

14.3.4 Hydrodissection and Lens Aspiration

Gentle hydrodissection in all quadrants can help in reducing surgical duration and improve cortical clean up [20]. Coaxial and bimanual techniques are available for lens matter removal. Bimanual technique of lens matter removal helps in complete removal of lens matter including subincisional cortex. It also allows for better chamber stability and more controlled lens aspiration. We prefer using wider gauze (20 gauze) bimanual instrument for irrigation and aspiration (Fig. 14.4a, b). Vitrectomy cutter can be used for lens aspiration in special cases such as preexisting posterior capsular defect, which have been discussed before.

14.3.5 Posterior Capsulorhexis and Anterior Vitrectomy

As mentioned earlier, aim of pediatric surgery includes maintaining clear visual axis for a long time. Visual axis opacification (VAO) remains the commonest complication post pediatric cataract surgery. Posterior capsulorhexis with or without anterior vitrectomy has been used to reduce VAO formation since 1980s [21]. This has been advocated over and again and is now considered standard of care for pediatric cataract surgery [22–25]. We recommend posterior capsulorhexis in children up to 8 years of age and anterior vitrectomy in children up to 6 years of age [6, 26].

Posterior capsulorhexis can be performed manually or with vitrectomy cutter. Technique of manual posterior capsulorhexis (PCC) differs from anterior capsulorhexis (Fig. 14.5). In PCC, underfill of the bag is required to prevent extension of PCC. OVD is injected in the anterior chamber but not the capsular bag to prevent convexity of capsule. Afterwards, PCC is performed after giving nick and grasping with forceps (Fig. 14.6a–d). Size should be 4–4.5 mm about 1 mm smaller than anterior capsulorhexis (Fig. 14.7a, b).

Anterior vitrectomy should be performed in smaller children to remove scaffold for proliferation of epithelial cells. High cut rate and low aspiration should be used to avoid traction on retina. Current vitrectomy systems have better control and high cut rate. Vitrectomy can be performed using same machine as that for lens aspiration like centurion or separate machine like constellation (Fig. 14.8a, b).

Vitrectomy can be done before or after IOL placement depending on surgeon's preference. Triamcinolone can be used at the end of vitrectomy for better visualization [27].

14.3.6 IOL insertion

IOL can be implanted in eyes with AL >17 mm and white to white distance >10 mm [6]. Insertion of IOL in smaller eyes is associated with more complications.

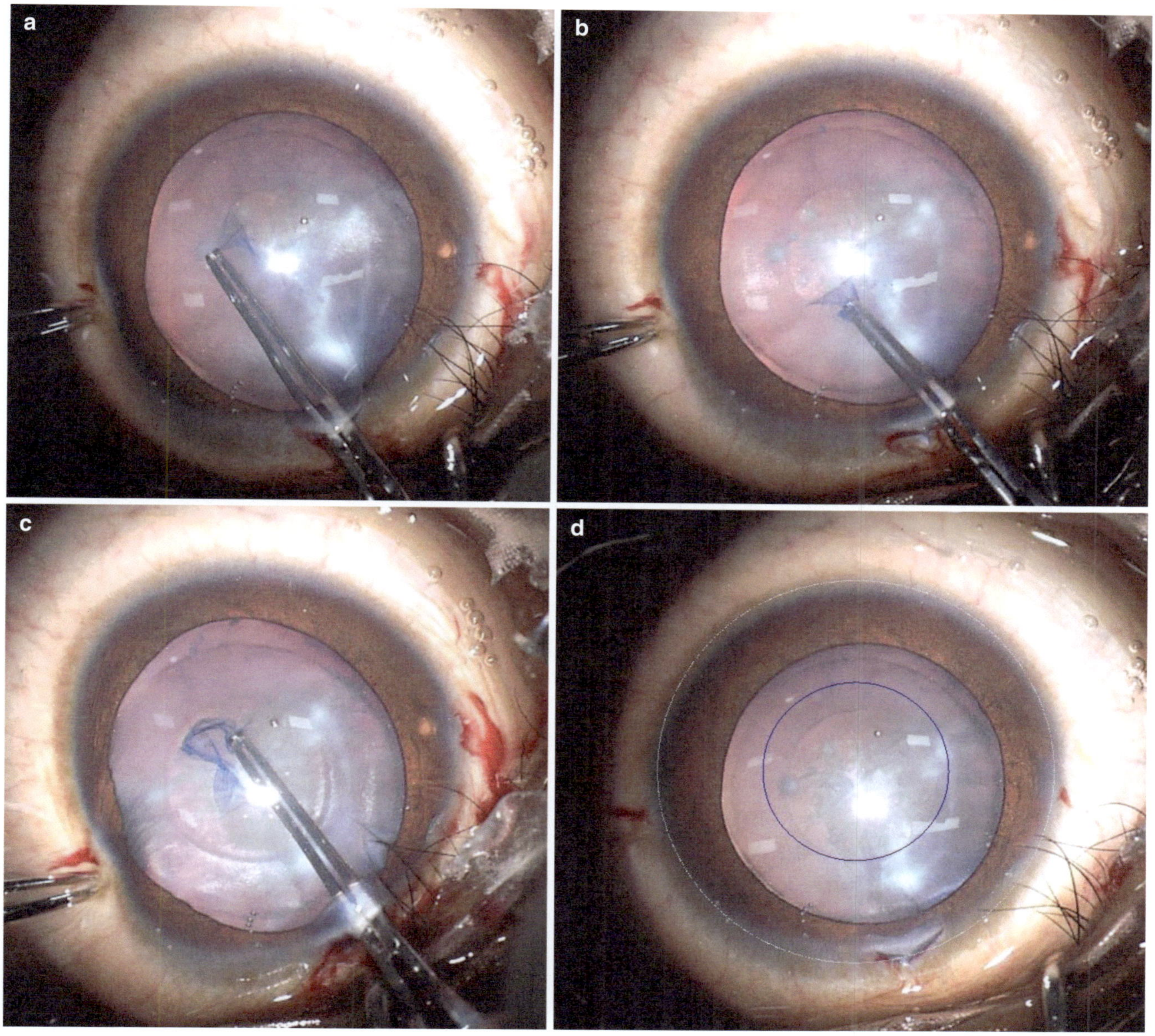

Fig. 14.2 Steps of anterior capsulorhexis. (**a**, **b**) After nick of capsule, sheering edge of the capsulorhexis is held with capsulorhexis forceps with frequent regrasp. (**c**) Capsulorhexis is completed in circular fashion. (**d**) Relative size and centration in relation to limbus using capsulorhexis assist of Zeiss Lumera 700 microscope

Placement of IOL in the bag is considered standard for all cataract surgery. Insertion of IOL is challenging in cases of open posterior capsule. We have described a safe technique of IOL insertion in pediatric cases [28]. Incision of 2.75 mm size is made (slightly larger than the IOL insertion system). Leading haptic of the IOL is gently inserted in the bag against the back surface of the anterior capsule. Once optic of IOL goes in the bag, trailing haptic is tucked into the bag without the need of dialing it (Fig. 14.9a–d).

Alternately, technique of optic capture [29] can be used in pediatric cataract. This has been used for reducing VAO formation as well [30, 31].

14.3.7 Viscoelastic Removal and Suturing

Viscoelastic should be removed at the end. Since high molecular weight OVD is used in most cases, removal is generally easy and quick. Main incision can be sutured with nonabsorbable or absorbable suture. Leaving the main wound sutureless may be associated with anterior chamber collapse or increased risk of infection especially in younger children who may rub their eyes. Hydration of paracentesis is generally adequate for stability of anterior chamber but they should be sutured if leak is suspected.

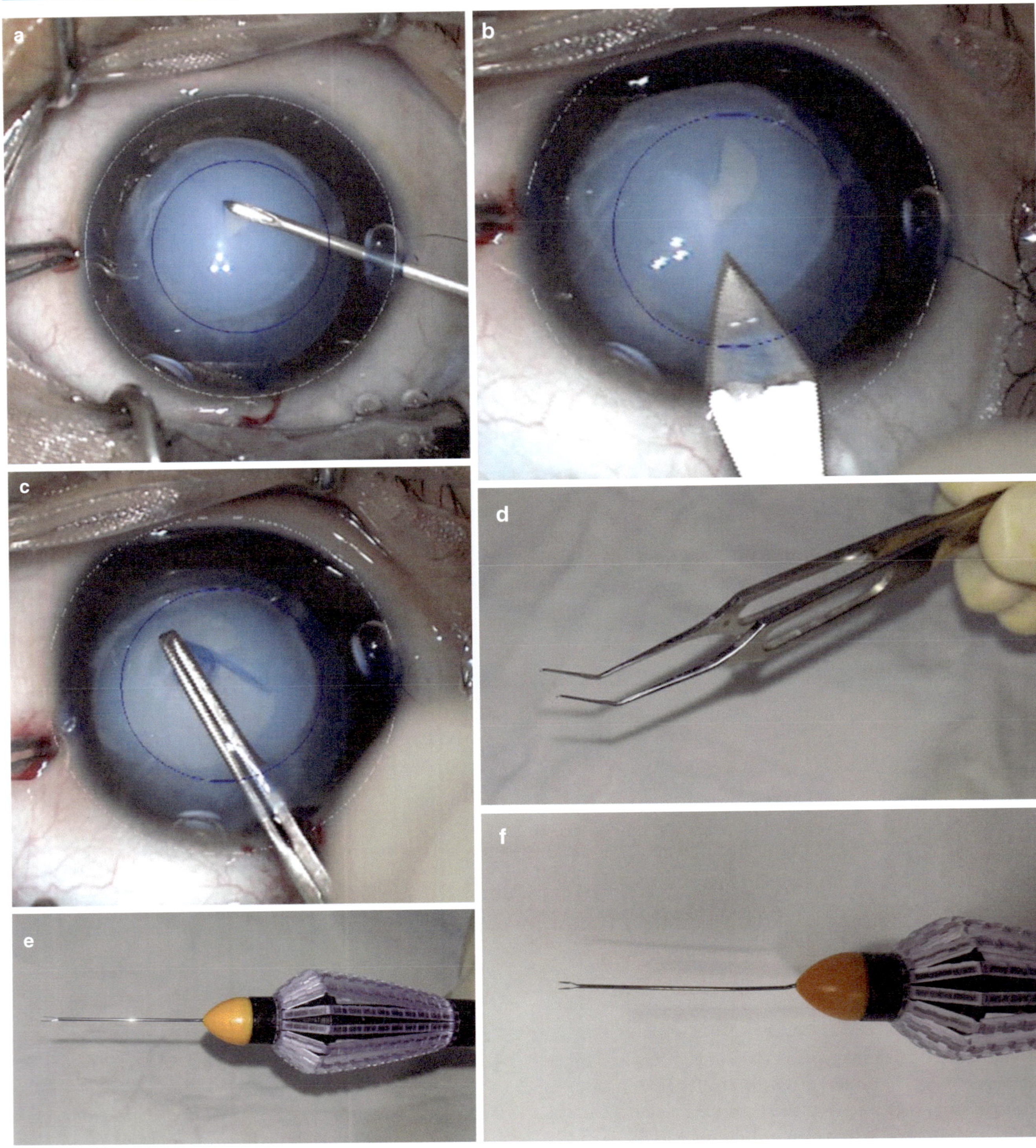

Fig. 14.3 Anterior capsulorhexis using capsulorhexis assist of Zeiss Lumera 700 microscope. (**a**) Nick is given to anterior capsule. (**b**) Nick is extended to 1 mm short of intended rhexis size and wound is extended. (**c**) Capsulorhexis is completed using Utrata capsulorhexis forceps. (**d**) Utrata capsulorhexis forceps. (**e**) Intravitreal forceps which can be used in place of microincision capsulorhexis forceps. (**f**) Serrated forceps (also known as Alligator forceps) generally used in scleral fixation of IOLs

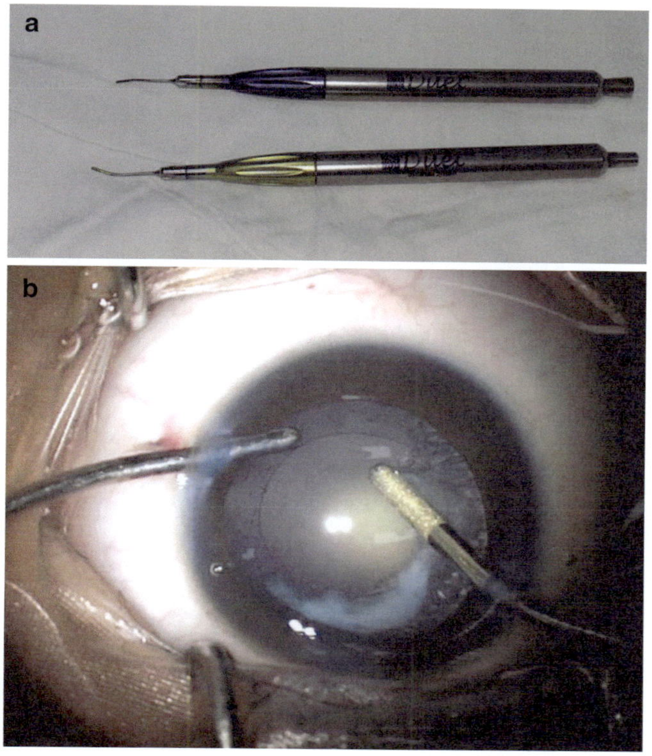

Fig. 14.4 (**a**) Bimanual Irrigation and aspiration instrument. (**b**) Intraoperative picture of bimanual Irrigation and aspiration in total cataract

14.4 Secondary IOL Implantation

In children, where primary implantation of IOL is not feasible due to age, smaller size of eye, or associated problems, secondary IOL implantation can be performed after considering a number of factors.

- Age of the patient—IOL can be implanted after 2 years of age as maximum growth of eye happens in the first 2 years of life [32].
- Best corrected visual acuity helps in guiding about patient's prognosis.
- Specular count should be performed whenever possible for objective assessment of corneal endothelium.
- Associated ocular pathology such as uveitis should be taken into consideration.
- Rim of sulcus should be assessed clinically. Ultrasound biomicroscopy can be used to assess details of rim, not otherwise clinically visible as discussed in previous chapter.

Technique of IOL placement depends on adequacy of rim. If adequate rim is present IOL can be placed in the bag or sulcus depending on the nature and size of rim [33–35] (Fig. 14.10). Formation and separation of rim of sulcus may be challenging in cases with extensive fibrosis. Each case requires unique approach (Fig. 14.11). Optic capture can help in better centration and VAO reduction (Fig. 14.12). If rim is inadequate, IOL can be placed in anterior chamber or iris fixated or scleral fixated IOL may be placed [36–38] (Fig. 14.13). Scleral fixated IOL is preferably avoided in small children with thin sclera as there is risk of haptic extrusion (Fig. 14.14).

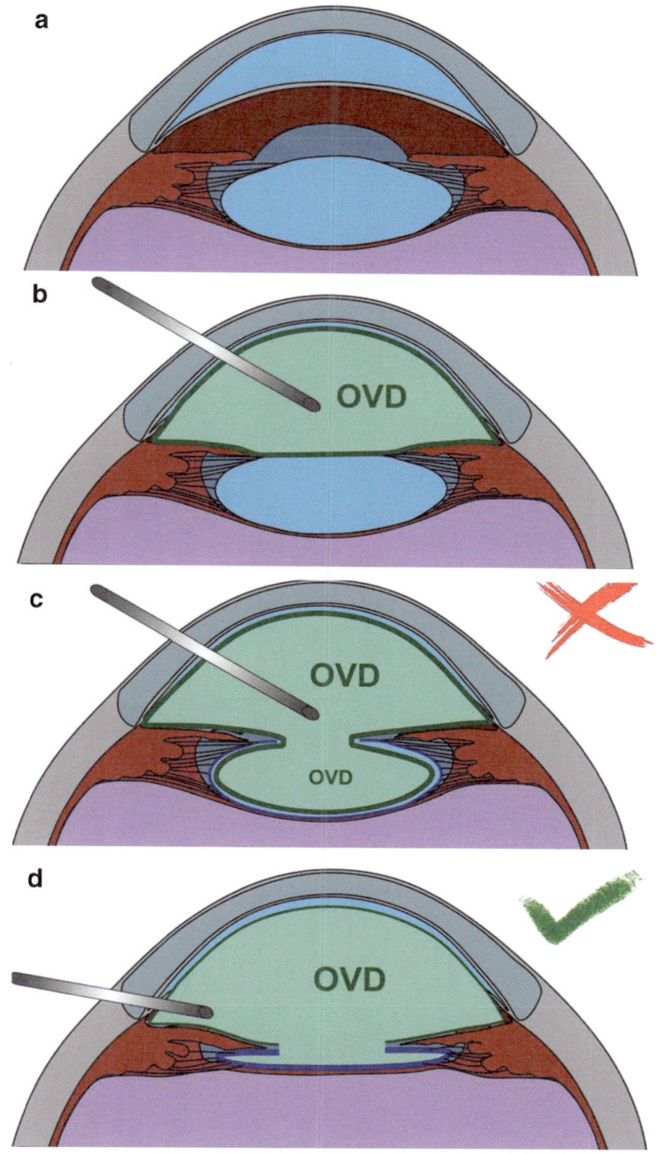

Fig. 14.5 Tricks for anterior and posterior capsulorhexis. (**a**) Sketch diagram showing lens and its capsule before capsulorhexis. (**b**) anterior chamber showing flattening of anterior lens capsule after insertion of OVD (ophthalmic viscosurgical device) for anterior capsulorhexis. (**c**) For posterior capsulorhexis, OVD, if filled inside the capsular bag would lead to bulging of posterior capsule (PC), which may lead to run out of posterior capsulorhexis. (**d**) For posterior capsulorhexis, OVD should be filled in anterior chamber only, to avoid posterior bulging of posterior capsule (PC). A flat PC maintained by just adequate vitreous pressure is desirable for good posterior capsulorhexis

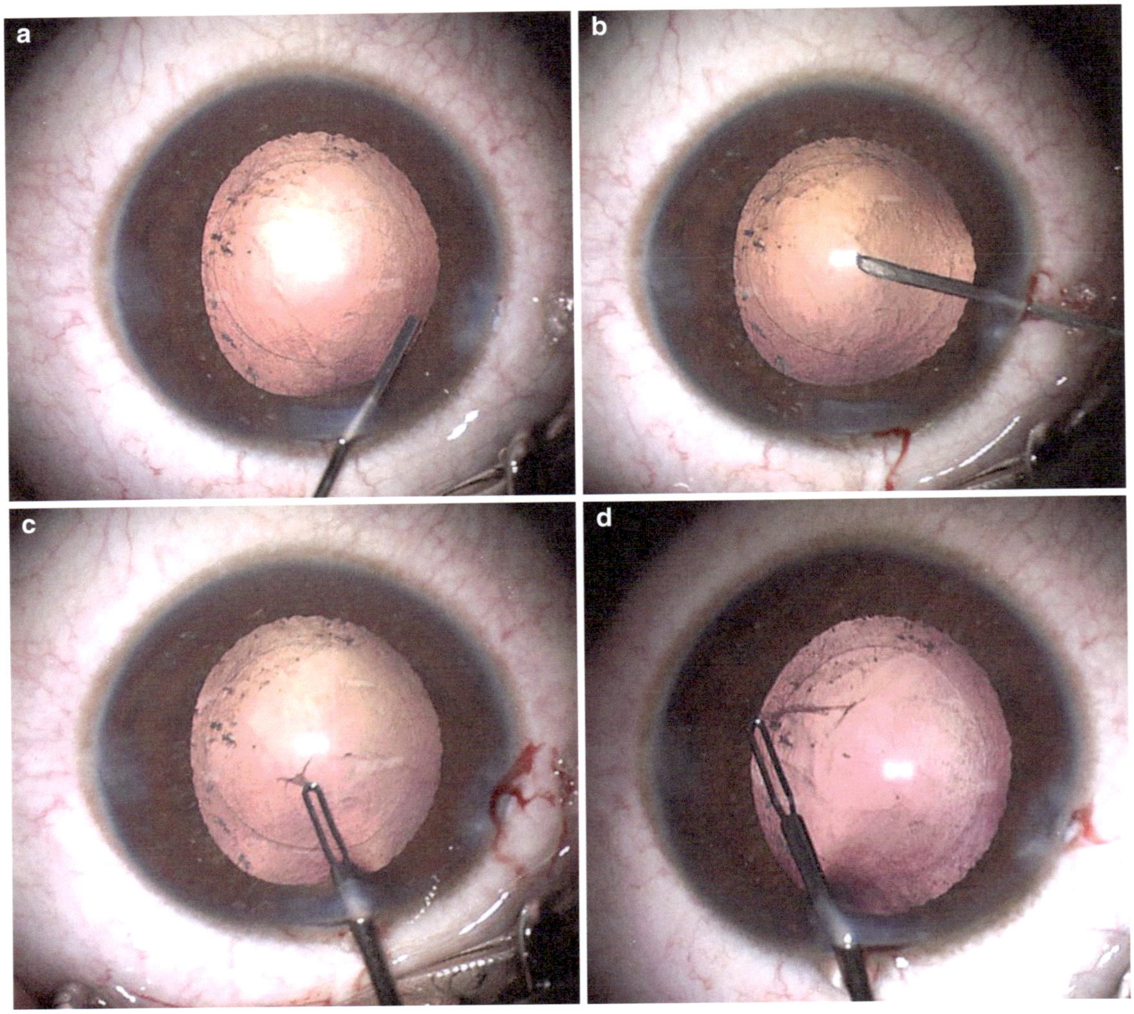

Fig. 14.6 Posterior capsulorhexis. (**a**) Anterior chamber is formed with viscoelastic devices. (**b**) Nick is given to posterior capsule. (**c**) Capsulorhexis started using microincision forceps. (**d**) Capsulorhexis is completed

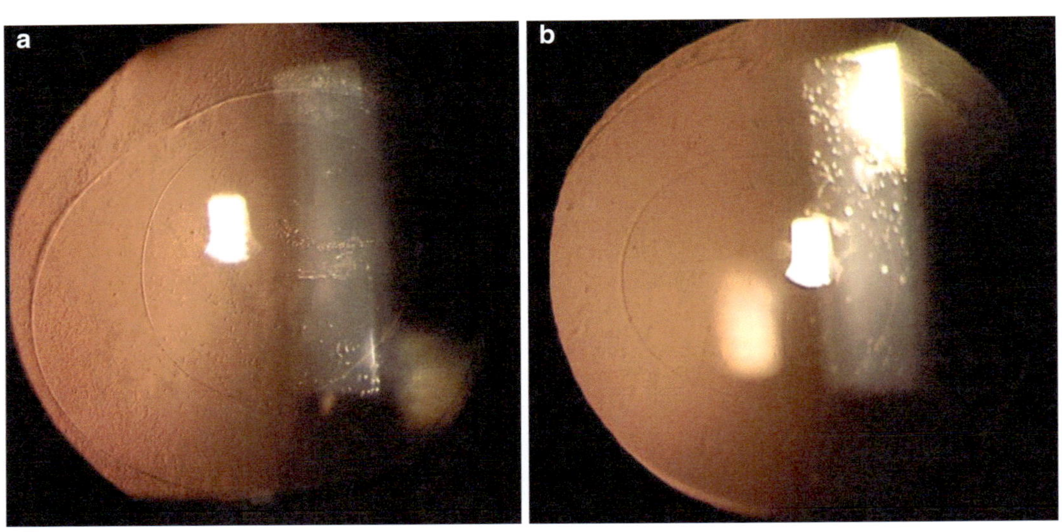

Fig. 14.7 (**a**, **b**) 5 months Postoperative picture of a 3-year-old boy with anterior and posterior capsulorhexis with IOL in bag in right and left eye, respectively. Note the sizing and centration of capsulorhexis. Slightly nasal posterior capsulorhexis is preferred

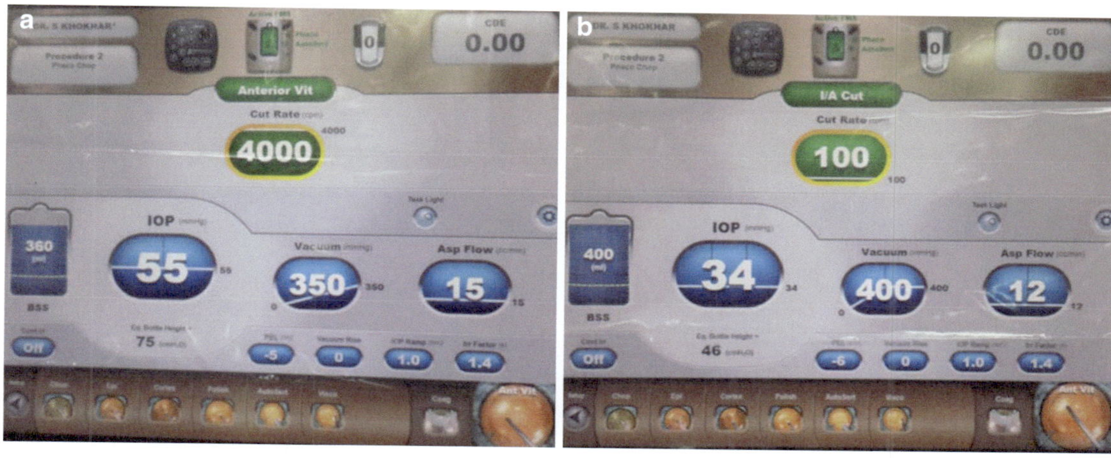

Fig. 14.8 Setting for vitrectomy machine (Centurion system @Alcon). (**a**) For anterior vitrectomy, use high cut rate and low vacuum. (**b**) For lens matter or viscoelastic removal keep low cut rate and more vacuum

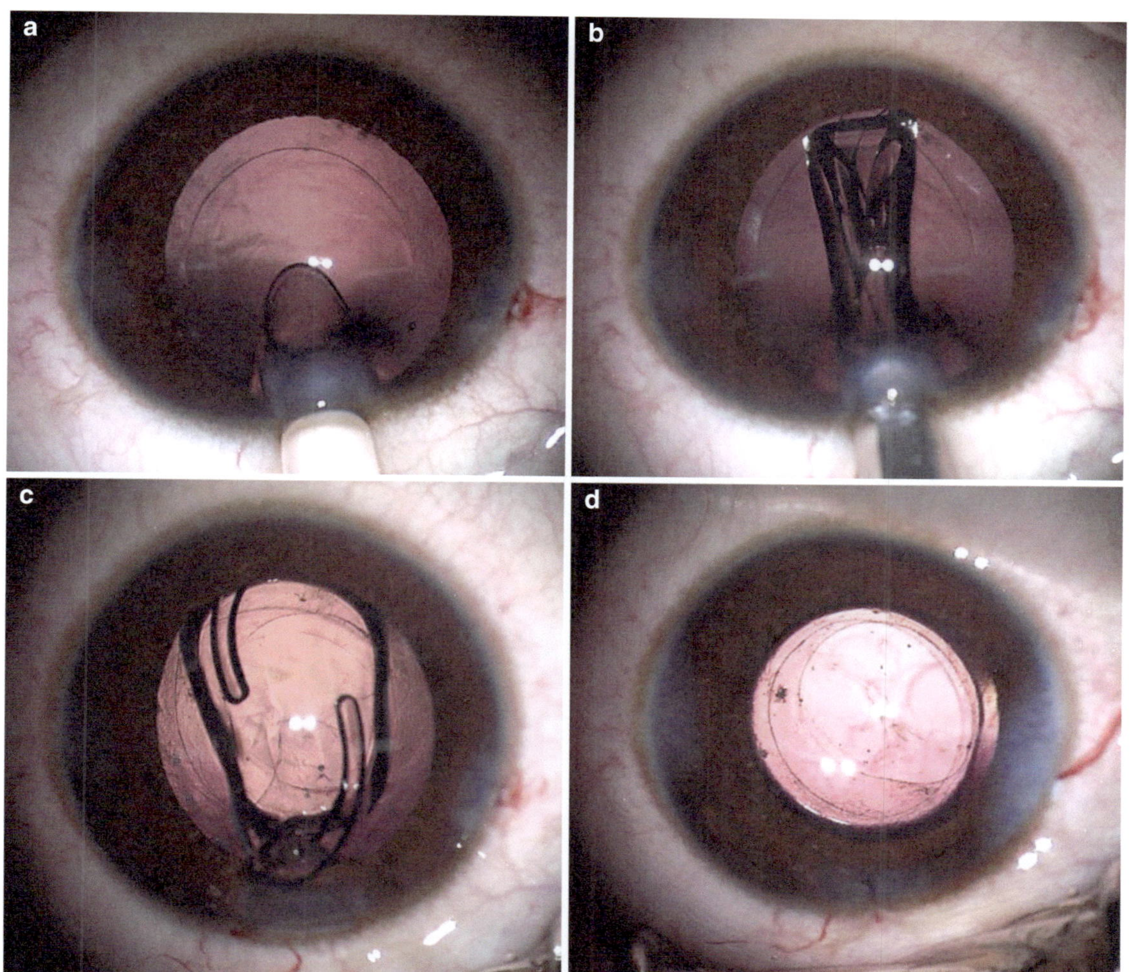

Fig. 14.9 Safe technique of IOL insertion in bag with posterior capsule opening. (**a**) Tip of IOL cartridge is inserted in anterior chamber via slightly larger incision. (**b**) Leading haptic of the IOL is gently inserted in the bag against the bag surface of the anterior capsule. (**c**) Allow IOL to open. (**d**) Final position of IOL after tucking trailing haptic

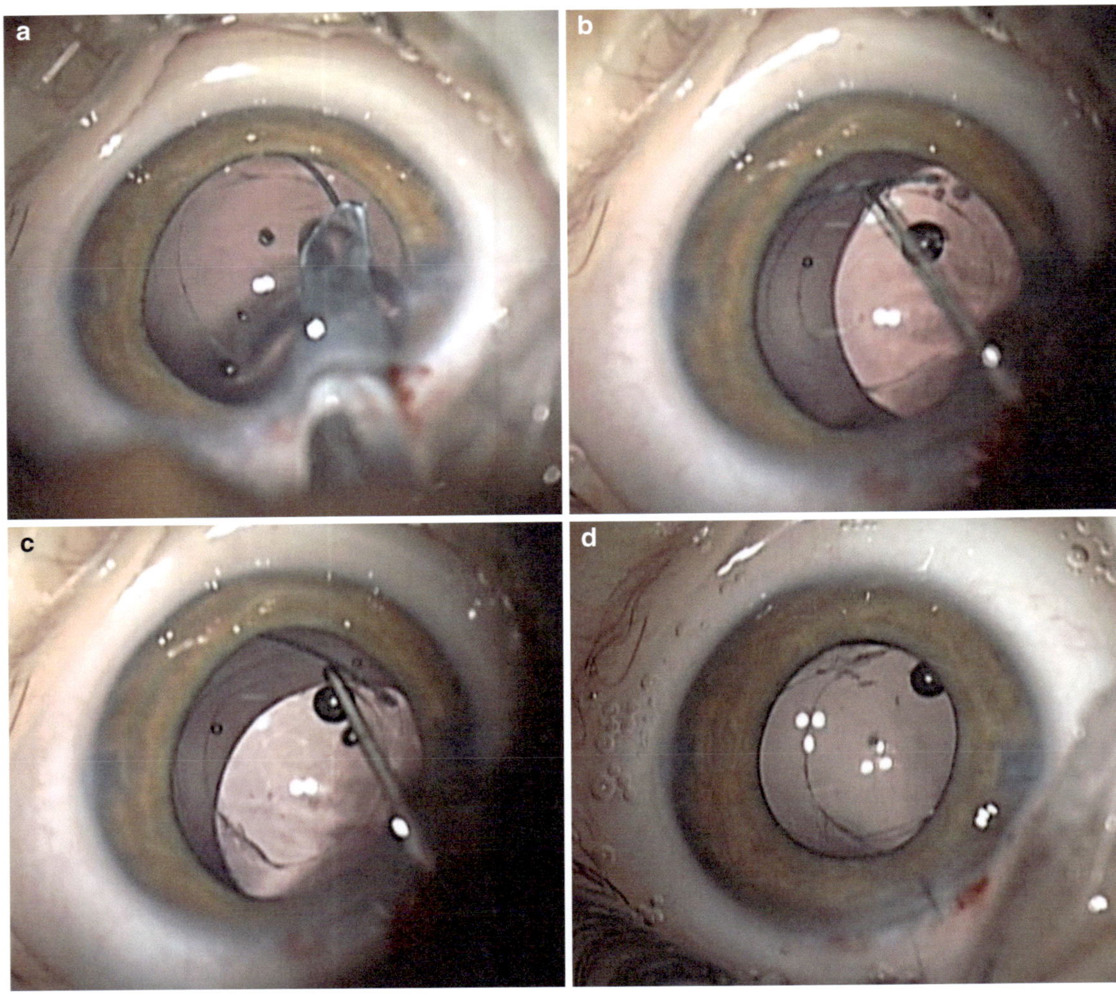

Fig. 14.10 Secondary IOL insertion. (**a**) Leading haptic of multipiece IOL is opened in the sulcus while rotating the IOL insertion system. (**b**) IOL is inserted in the sulcus and dialed. (**c**) IOL captured with anterior capsulorhexis. (**d**) Final position and centration of IOL

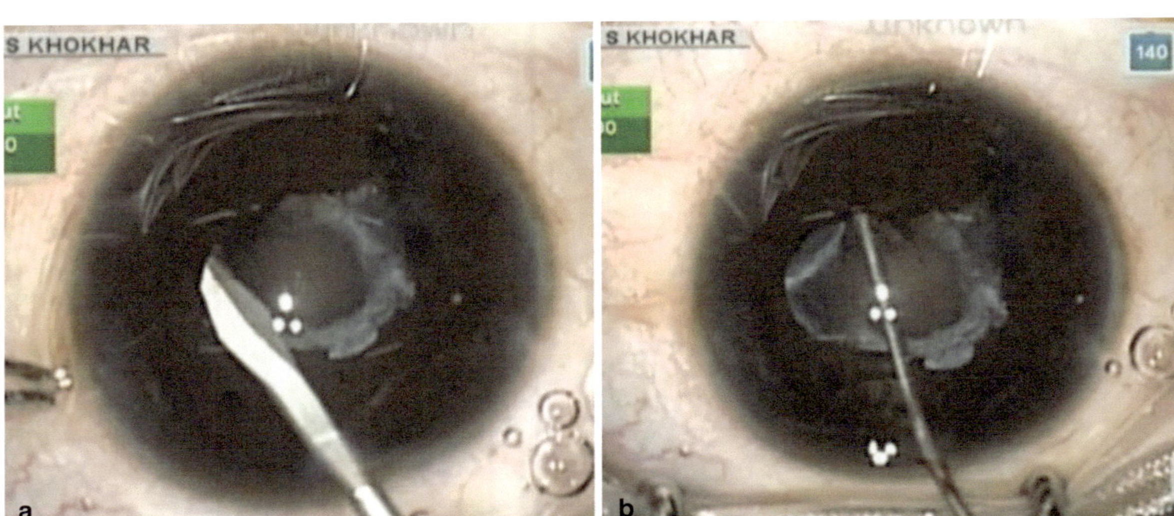

Fig. 14.11 Sulcus formation for difficult secondary IOL insertion. (**a**) Sharp dissection with 1 mm blade is used to make a first point of separation between capsule and iris. (**b**) Viscoelastic assisted separation is done once a plane is formed by sharp dissection, rest of the technique is similar

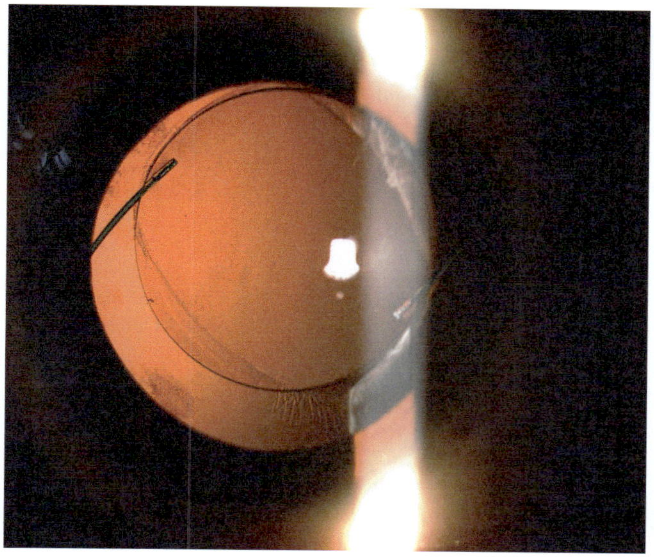

Fig. 14.12 1 year postoperative picture of a 5-year-old boy operated for secondary IOL with optic capture. IOL is well centered and visual axis is clear

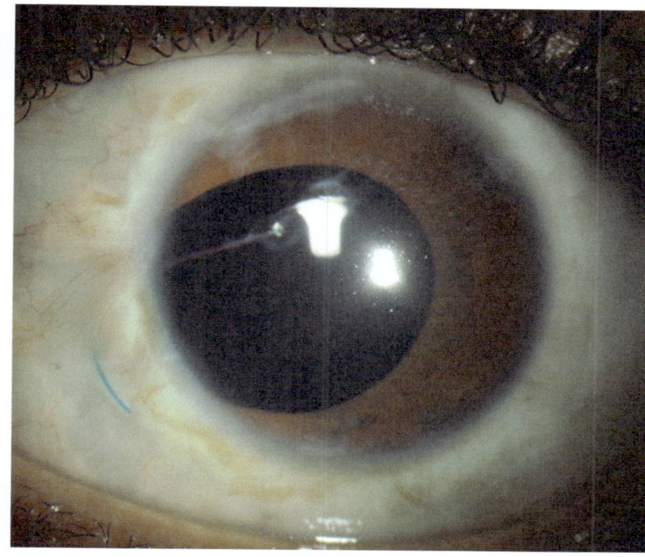

Fig. 14.14 5 months postoperative picture of 12-year-old girl with haptic extrusion of scleral fixated IOL with IOL decentration and tilt

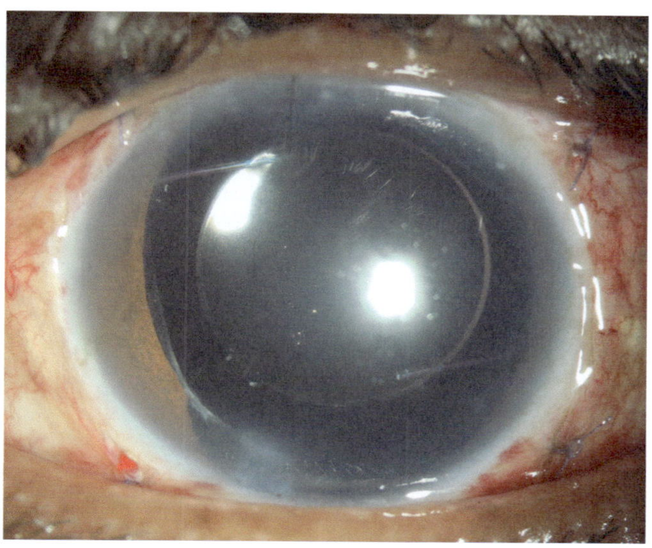

Fig. 14.13 Postoperative picture of scleral fixated IOL in a 10-year-old patient. Notice well-centered IOL, large iris defect (post trauma), and peripheral inadequate rim of sulcus in inferonasal quadrant

To summarize, cataract surgery in children poses greater surgical challenge as compared to adults due to difference in anatomy and higher risk of complications. Special considerations and meticulous surgical technique for primary surgery as well as secondary IOL implantation helps in achieving optimal outcome.

References

1. Vasavada AR, Nihalani BR. Pediatric cataract surgery. Curr Opin Ophthalmol. 2006;17:54–61.
2. Beck AD, Freedman SF, Lynn MJ, Bothun E, Neely DE, Lambert SR. Glaucoma-related adverse events in the infant Aphakia treatment study: 1-year results. Arch Ophthalmol. 2012;130:300–5.
3. Freedman SF, Lynn MJ, Beck AD, et al. Glaucoma-related adverse events in the first 5 years after unilateral cataract removal in the infant Aphakia treatment study. JAMA Ophthalmol. 2015;133:907–14.
4. Birch EE, Stager DR. The critical period for surgical treatment of dense congenital unilateral cataract. Invest Ophthalmol Vis Sci. 1996;37:1532–8.
5. Hartmann EE, Lynn MJ, Lambert SR. Infant Aphakia treatment study G. Baseline characteristics of the infant aphakia treatment study population: predicting recognition acuity at 4.5 years of age. Invest Ophthalmol Vis Sci. 2015;56:388–95.
6. Khokhar SK, Pillay G, Dhull C, Agarwal E, Mahabir M, Aggarwal P. Pediatric cataract. Indian J Ophthalmol. 2017;65(12):1340–9.
7. Gayer S, Tutiven J. Anesthesia for pediatric ocular surgery. Ophthalmol Clin North Am. 2006;19(2):269–78.
8. Bar-Sela SM, Spierer A. Astigmatism outcomes of scleral tunnel and clear corneal incisions for congenital cataract surgery. Eye (Lond). 2006;20:1044–8.
9. Matsumoto Y, Hara T, Chiba K, et al. Optimal incision sites to obtain an astigmatism-free cornea after cataract surgery with a 3.2 mm sutureless incision. J Cataract Refract Surg. 2001;27:1615–9.
10. Wilson ME Jr. Anterior lens capsule management in pediatric cataract surgery. Trans Am Ophthalmol Soc. 2004;102:391–422.
11. Krag S, Olsen T, Andreassen TT. Biomechanical characteristics of the human anterior lens capsule in relation to age. Invest Ophthalmol Vis Sci. 1997;38:357–63.
12. Taylor D. Choice of surgical technique in the management of congenital cataract. Trans Ophthalmol Soc U K. 1981;101:114–7.

13. Wilson ME, Saunders RA, Roberts EL, et al. Mechanized anterior capsulectomy as an alternative to manual capsulorhexis in children undergoing intraocular lens implantation. J Pediatr Ophthalmol Strabismus. 1996;33:237–40.
14. Comer RM, Abdulla N, O'Keefe M. Radiofrequency diathermy capsulorhexis of the anterior and posterior capsules in pediatric cataract surgery: preliminary results. J Cataract Refract Surg. 1997;23(Suppl 1):641–4.
15. Kloti R. Anterior high frequency capsulotomy. I. Experimental study. Klin Monbl Augenheilkd. 1992;200:507–10.
16. Fugo RJ, Delcampo DM. The Fugo blade: the next step after capsulorhexis. Ann Ophthalmol. 2001;33:13–20.
17. Khokhar S, Tejwani LK, Kumar G, Kushmesh R. Approach to cataract with persistent hyperplastic primary vitreous. J Cataract Refract Surg. 2011;37:1382–5.
18. Palanker DV, Blumenkranz MS, Andersen D, et al. Femtosecond laser assisted cataract surgery with integrated optical coherence tomography. Sci Transl Med. 2010;2:58–85.
19. Toropygin SG, Krause M, Akkaya A, et al. Experimental femtosecond laser-assisted nanosurgery of anterior lens capsule. Eur J Ophthalmol. 2011;21:237–42.
20. Vasavada AR, Trivedi RH, Apple DJ, et al. Randomized, clinical trial of multiquadrant hydrodissection in pediatric cataract surgery. Am J Ophthalmol. 2003;135:84–8.
21. Parks MM. Management of the posterior capsule in congenital cataracts. J Pediatr Ophthalmol Strabismus. 1984;21:114–7.
22. BenEzra D, Cohen E. Posterior capsulectomy in pediatric cataract surgery the necessity of a choice. Ophthalmology. 1997;104:2168–74.
23. Vasavada A, Desai J. Primary posterior capsulorhexis with and without anterior vitrectomy in congenital cataracts. J Cataract Refract Surg. 1997;23(Suppl 1):645–51.
24. Alexandrakis G, Peterseim MM, Wilson ME. Clinical outcomes of pars plana capsulotomy with anterior vitrectomy in pediatric cataract surgery. J AAPOS. 2002;6:163–7.
25. Guo S, Wagner RS, Caputo A. Management of the anterior and posterior lens capsules and vitreous in pediatric cataract surgery. J Pediatr Ophthalmol Strabismus. 2004;41:330–7.
26. Lin AA, Buckley EG. Update on pediatric cataract surgery and intraocular lens implantation. Curr Opin Ophthalmol. 2010;21:55–9.
27. Burk SE, Da Mata AP, Snyder ME, et al. Visualizing vitreous using Kenalog suspension. J Cataract Refract Surg. 2003;29:645–51.
28. Khokhar S, Sharma R, Patil B, Sinha G, Nayak B, Kinkhabwala RA, et al. A safe technique for in-the-bag intraocular lens implantation in pediatric cataract surgery. Eur J Ophthalmol. 2015;25:57–9.
29. Gimbel HV, DeBroff BM. Intraocular lens optic capture. J Cataract Refract Surg. 2004;30:200–6.
30. Raina UK, Gupta V, Arora R, et al. Posterior continuous curvilinear capsulorhexis with and without optic capture of the posterior chamber intraocular lens in the absence of vitrectomy. J Pediatr Ophthalmol Strabismus. 2002;39:278–87.
31. Zhou HW, Zhou F. A meta-analysis on the clinical efficacy and safety of optic capture in pediatric cataract surgery. Int J Ophthalmol. 2016;9:590–6.
32. Nihalani BR, Vanderveen DK. Secondary intraocular lens implantation after pediatric aphakia. J AAPOS. 2011;15:435–40.
33. Kim DH, Kim JH, Kim SJ, et al. Long-term results of bilateral congenital cataract treated with early cataract surgery, aphakic glasses and secondary IOL implantation. Acta Ophthalmol. 2012;90:231–6.
34. Wilson ME Jr, Hafez GA, Trivedi RH. Secondary in-the-bag intraocular lens implantation in children who have been aphakic since early infancy. J AAPOS. 2011;15:162–6.
35. Grewal DS, Basti S. Modified technique for removal of Soemmering ring and in-the-bag secondary intraocular lens placement in aphakic eyes. J Cataract Refract Surg. 2012;38:739–42.
36. Epley KD, Shainberg MJ, Lueder GT, et al. Pediatric secondary lens implantation in the absence of capsular support. J AAPOS. 2001;5:301–6.
37. Dureau P, de Laage de Meux P, Edelson C, et al. Iris fixation of foldable intraocular lenses for ectopia lentis in children. J Cataract Refract Surg. 2006;32:1109–14.
38. Bardorf CM, Epley KD, Lueder GT, et al. Pediatric transscleral sutured intraocular lenses: efficacy and safety in 43 eyes followed an average of 3 years. J AAPOS. 2004;8:318–24.

15 Visual Axis Opacification (VAO)

Sudarshan Kumar Khokhar, Yogita Gupta, and Chirakshi Dhull

Visual axis opacification (VAO) after cataract surgery is commonly encountered in children, at a higher rate than that in adults. It may lead to amblyopia and hinders with the achievement of visual rehabilitation in pediatric cataract. For this reason, distant direct examination and retroillumination examination in the postoperative follow-up period becomes an important tool for early detection of any media opacification.

Commonest cause of VAO is posterior capsular opacification (PCO) in children. Other causes are listed in Table 15.1. In this chapter, we will discuss VAO related to PCO in detail.

Table 15.1 Causes of VAO in children

I. Early media opacification
Corneal edema
Vitreous hemorrhage (e.g., bleed going posteriorly from iris vessels)
Inflammatory reaction in anterior or posterior segment/inflammatory pupillary membrane formation (viz. secondary to iris manipulation, flare up of uveitis) (Fig. 15.1)
Acute onset endophthalmitis
Remnant cortical matter coming into visual axis
II. Delayed media opacification
Posterior capsular opacification (PCO) (Fig. 15.2)
Hyaloid face opacification
Glistening of intraocular lens (IOL) (Fig. 15.3)
Debris, pigments deposition on IOL
Delayed-onset endophthalmitis

15.1 Etiopathogenesis

15.1.1 Mechanism of PCO Development

The growth of lens epithelial cells (LECs) on the posterior capsule or anterior hyaloid face leads to PCO formation. LECs proliferate, migrate, and differentiate into myofibroblasts [1] by the process of epithelial-to-mesenchymal differentiation (EMT) [1–3]. Fibrotic PCO is formed primarily by EMT of LECs causing fibrous metaplasia and leading to formation of folds and wrinkles in the posterior capsule [2]. Proliferative PCO by regeneration of lenticular fibers which express crystallins from equatorial LECs [3]. Anterior hyaloid face acts as a scaffold for deposition of cells, debris, and pigments which leads to PCO formation.

15.1.2 Predisposing Factors for VAO

PCO is the most common complication following pediatric cataract surgery. Its incidence may be as high as 95% in pediatric cataracts [4]. Pediatric cataract surgeons, worldwide, consider primary management of posterior capsule during surgery by performing posterior continuous curvilinear capsulorrhexis (PCCC), with or without anterior vitrectomy (AV), with or without IOL implantation to delay the PCO formation (Table 15.2). The incidence of PCO has been reported to be: 9.2% [5] in cases left aphakic within first 18 months of life.

Researchers have analyzed various risk factors predisposing for PCO development, even despite PCCC and AV such as:

- Younger age of child: more intense inflammation has been noted in children operated at a younger age [6, 7].
- Surgical trauma or complicated cataract surgery (Fig. 15.4).
- Smaller capsulorrhexis size: an anterior capsulorrhexis should be adequately sized while performing cataract surgery. A 5 mm opening in anterior capsulorrhexis is considered as adequate. Smaller capsulorhexis may be associated with anterior capsular phimosis (Fig. 15.5).
- Traumatic cataracts: traumatic cataracts after cataract extraction lead to more PCO formation than congenital or developmental cataracts.
- Uveitic cataracts: postoperative inflammation may result into faster and higher rate of PCO formation in uveitic

S. K. Khokhar · Y. Gupta · C. Dhull (✉)
Dr. Rajendra Prasad Centre for Ophthalmic Sciences, All India Institute of Medical Sciences, New Delhi, India

S. K. Khokhar, C. Dhull (eds.), *Atlas of Pediatric Cataract*, https://doi.org/10.1007/978-981-13-6939-1_15

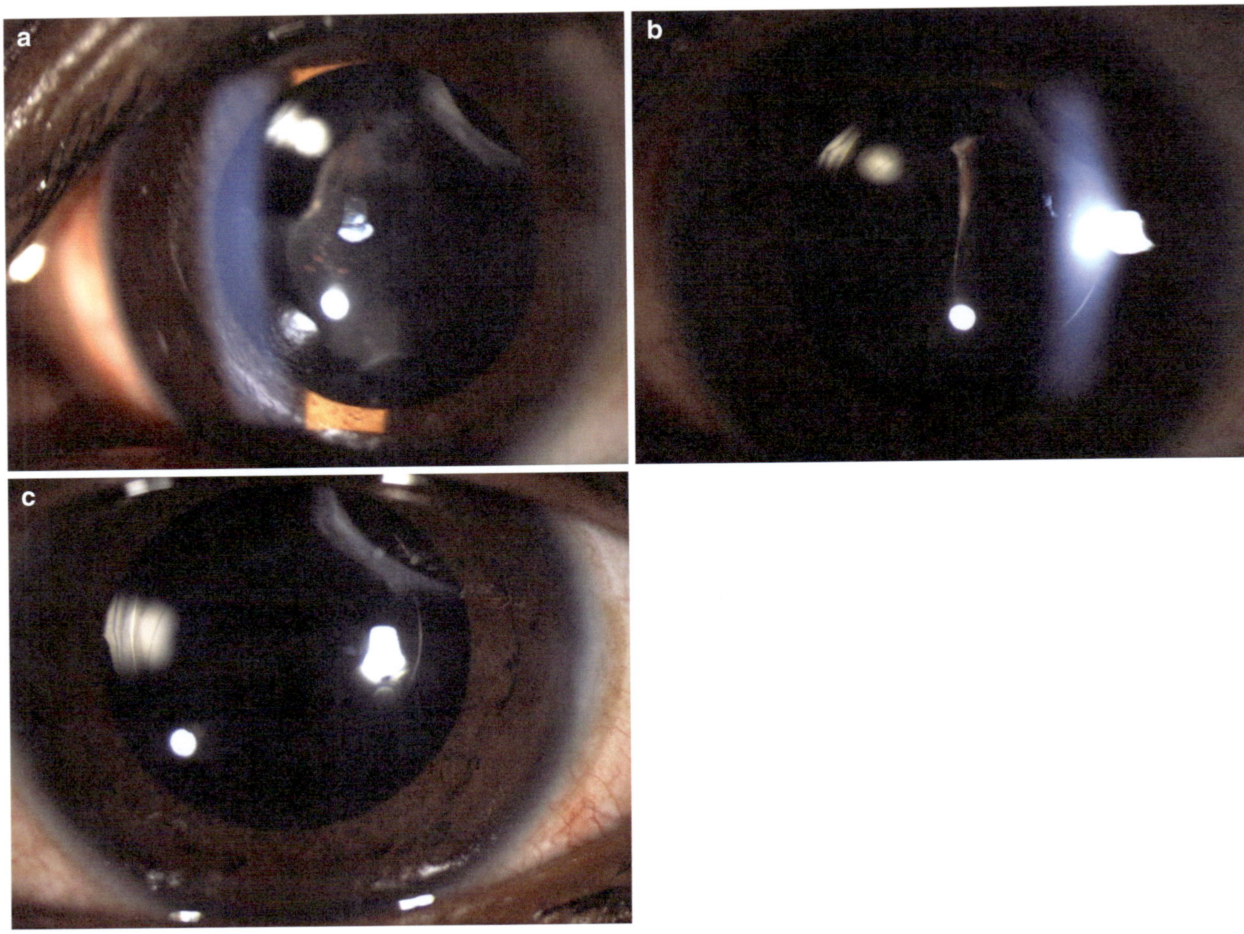

Fig. 15.1 Postoperative serial picture of a 12-year-old boy with post-traumatic cataract. (**a**) Day 1: dense fibrinous membrane in AC. (**b**) Day 2: size of the membrane reduced with intensive anti inflammatory therapy. (**c**) Day 3: fibrinous membrane almost completely disappeared

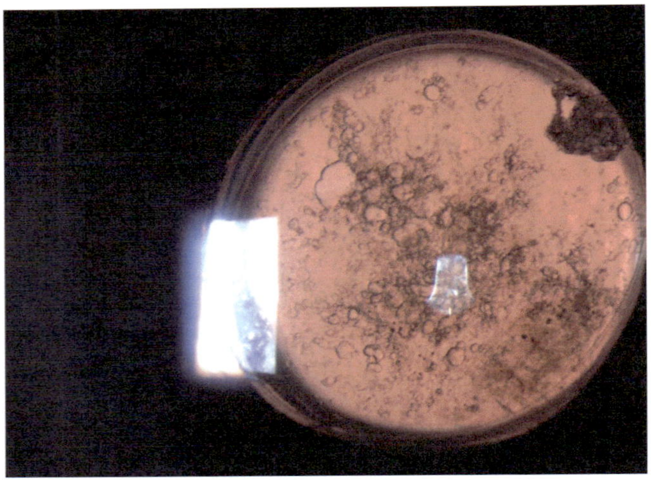

Fig. 15.2 Posterior capsular opacification seen 4 months post surgery in an 8-year-old child (posterior capsule intact)

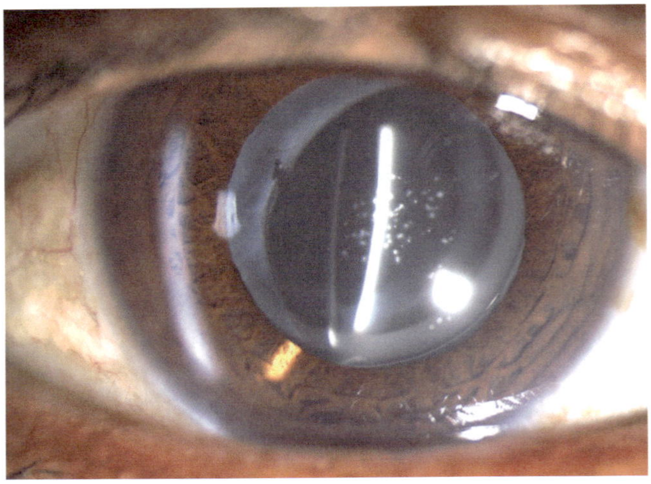

Fig. 15.3 IOL glistening seen with anterior capsular fibrosis 4 years after surgery

Table 15.2 Incidence of VAO according to management of posterior capsule and/or anterior vitrectomy

PCCC with AV without IOL implantation[a]	9.2% [5]
PCCC with AV with IOL implantation[b]	22.5% [6]
PCCC only[c]	42.9% [6]
No PCCC/AV[d]	78.6% [6]

[a]Study by Kuli et al. in children up to 18 months of age with mean follow-up of 39 months
[b]Study by Hosal and Biglan with median age of subjects as 27 months with mean postoperative follow-up of 65 months in those with intact posterior lens capsule
[c]Study by Hosal and Biglan with median age of subjects as 27 months with mean postoperative follow-up of 87 months in eyes with posterior capsulectomy
[d]Study by Hosal and Biglan with median age of subjects as 27 months with mean postoperative follow-up of 77 months in eyes with posterior capsulectomy and anterior vitrectomy

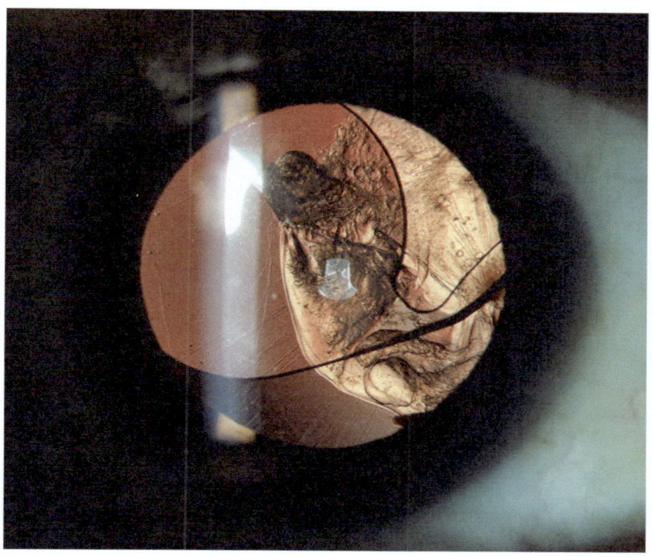

Fig. 15.4 Complicated cataract surgery with PCO formation. Note single piece foldable IOL in sulcus, superonasally decentered. Anterior capsular extension with zonular defect with proliferative and membranous VAO seen

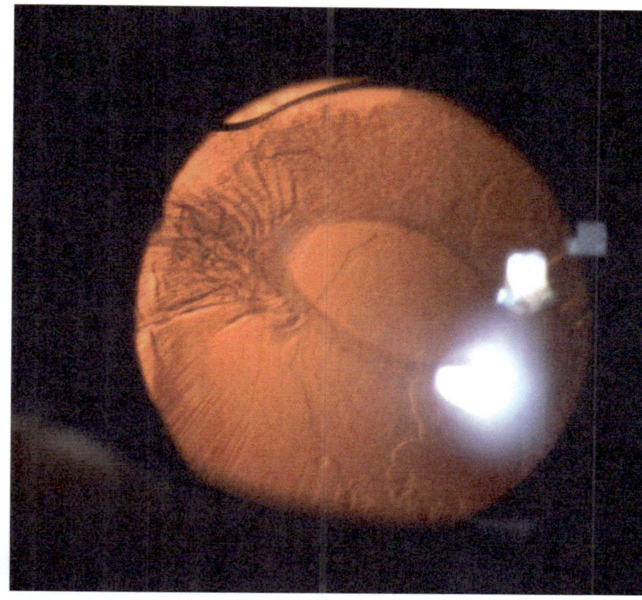

Fig. 15.5 Anterior capsular phimosis noted 1 year postoperatively. Small capsulorhexis was noted intraoperatively

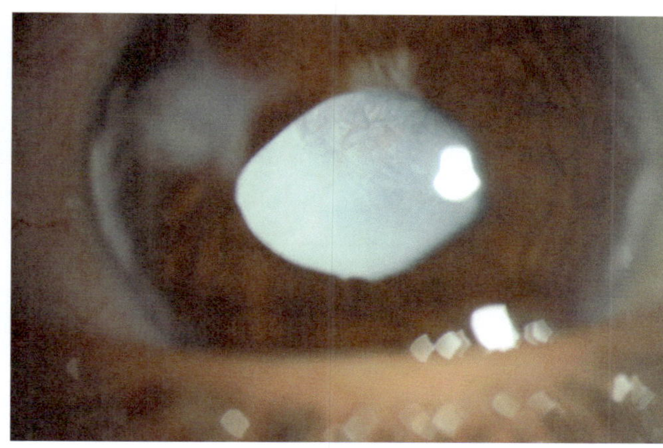

Fig. 15.6 An 8-year-old JIA patient with aphakia with vascularized visual axis opacification 1 year after surgery. Band-shaped keratopathy is also seen

cataracts. Membranes may be thick and vascularized in severe cases (Fig. 15.6). Capsular phimosis/anterior capsular contraction syndrome may result as early as few weeks in these cases [8].

- IOL biomaterial: studies comparing the acrylic material prove that hydrophilic acrylic material accelerates PCO formation more than hydrophobic material [9]. Heparin surface coating on polymethyl methacrylate (PMMA), i.e., heparin surface modified IOLs (HSM-IOLs) also cause less PCO formation and are used for uveitic cataracts [10].

(Hydrophilic acrylic IOL > PMMA IOL > hydrophobic IOL)

- IOL design: a capsular bend with sharp and square optic edge induce contact inhibition to migrating LECs, thus reducing PCO formation [11].
- Extent of cortical cleanup: vigorous cortical cleanup should be avoided as it may cause remnant lens matter to migrate to the posterior capsule during the surgery and LECs may rapidly proliferate to form VAO.
- Site of IOL fixation: in the bag fixation of posterior chamber IOL after PCCC and AV is currently the most accepted surgical choice to achieve excellent IOL centration and good visual outcomes. Other options of IOL fixation

which are equally effective in reducing PCO formation include: optic capture [12] of IOL behind the posterior capsule opening and bag-in-the-lens [13] fixation. Sulcus fixation of IOL may also result in higher PCO formation than bag fixation.

- Besides these, poorly centered anterior capsulorrhexis with IOL in the bag may also accelerate PCO formation if it does not cover all the edges of IOL (Figs. 15.7 and 15.8).

15.2 Clinical Presentation

Detection of VAO is challenging in pediatric patients. Often, parents will complain of noticing child's inability to follow objects, which they could earlier do after surgery. In unilateral cataracts where patching is being followed with good compliance, the child may now be noted to resist occlusion of the good eye. Clinician may find poor visual acuity on Cardiff's tests and a poor glow

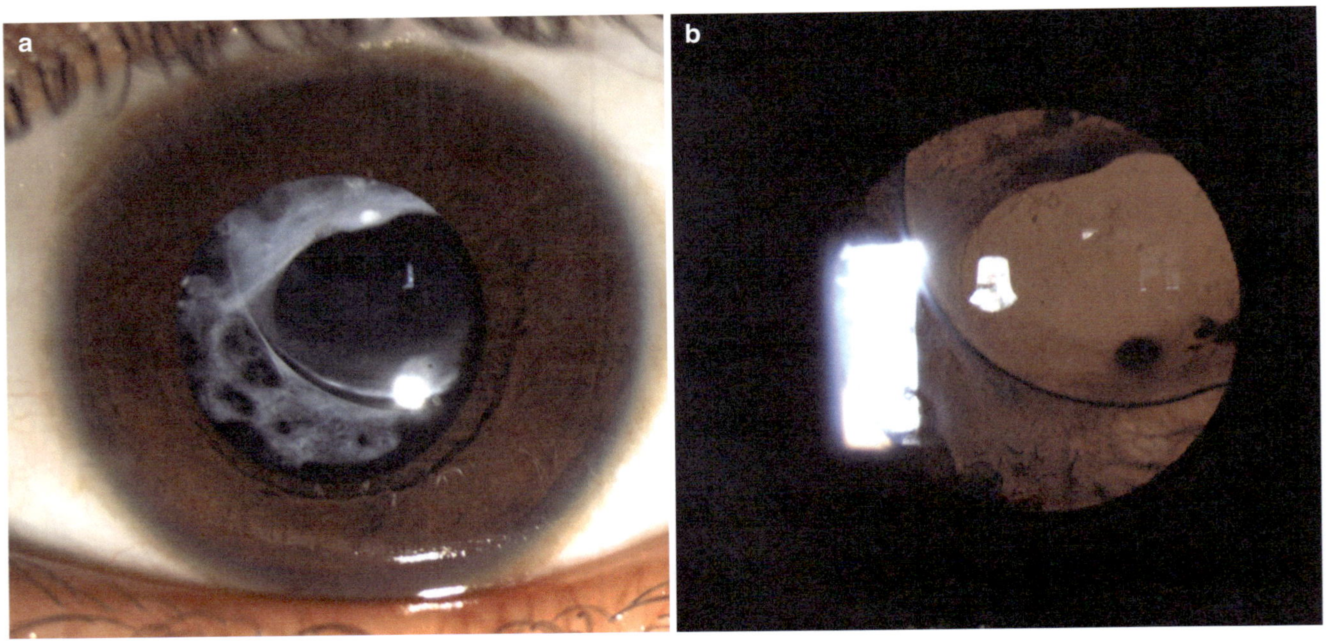

Fig. 15.7 VAO formation in eccentric anterior capsulorhexis and decentered IOL. (**a**) Diffuse illumination picture, (**b**) retroillumination picture. Note predominantly fibrotic type of PCO, anterior and posterior capsulorhexis adhesion is seen inferiorly with IOL optic outside capsular bag

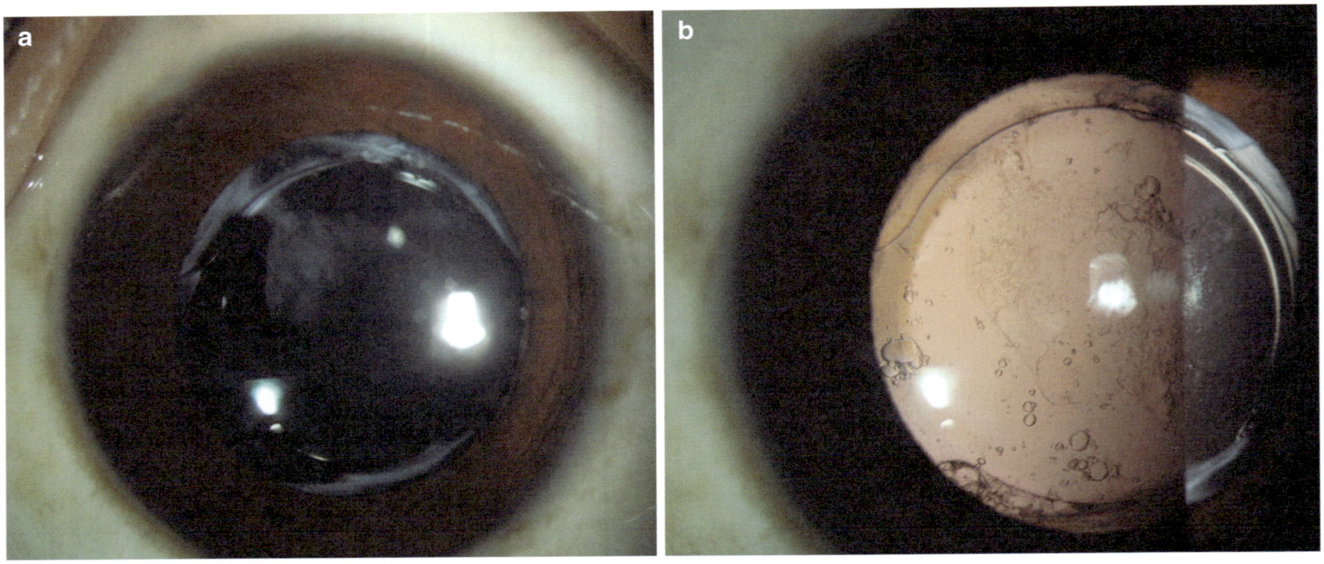

Fig. 15.8 PCO formation in case of larger capsulorhexis not covering IOL completely. (**a**) Diffuse illumination picture, (**b**) retroillumination picture. Note both fibrotic and pearl-like PCO formation

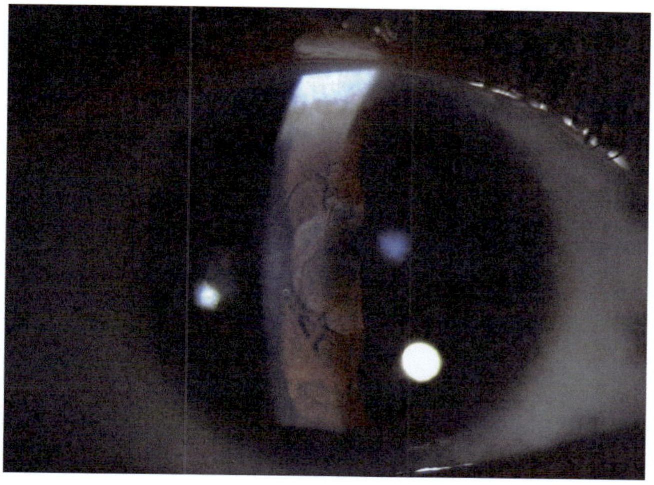

Fig. 15.9 Anterior pigmentation and membrane covering IOL in uveitic patient

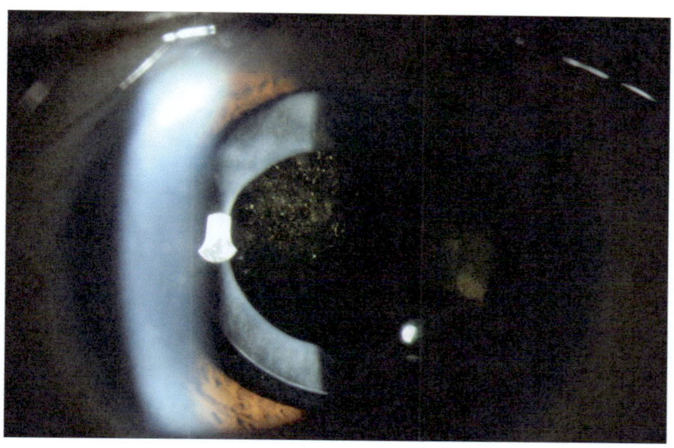

Fig. 15.10 Superotemporal Elschnig pearl formation, peripheral fibrosis. Patient kept on close follow as this may progress with time

(Bruckner reflex) through direct ophthalmoscope. A child presenting to clinic with a poor glow should be assessed through the corrective spectacles as high refractive error may show dull glow. VAO may be predominantly posterior to lens, anterior to lens, or combination of both (Fig. 15.9).

It may be visually insignificant when central visual axis is clear (Fig. 15.10).

It is classified as:

- Fibrotic type where capsule is thickened and fibrosed with folds and wrinkling in the capsule (Fig. 15.11a, b).
- Proliferative type which include both Elschnig pearls (Fig. 15.12a, b) and Soemmering ring (Fig. 15.13a, b).

15.3 Investigation

Ultrasonography should be performed preoperatively to rule out posterior segment pathology such as retinal detachment. Ultrasound biomicroscopy (UBM) can be performed in cases of severe VAO or non-dilating pupil. In addition to assessment of location and severity of VAO, it can provide information regarding IOL position and associated pathology such as persistent fetal vasculature. This can aid in surgical planning preoperatively (Fig. 15.14).

15.4 Treatment

PCO is amblyogenic in the critical period of visual development and causes stimulus deprivation in a child, thereby interfering with the goal of a successful cataract surgery.

VAO must be managed promptly and child may often have to be taken up for resurgery under general anesthesia. An informed consent must be obtained from caretakers/parents in these cases, with clinician explaining them the risk of recurrent PCO. Surgical options to manage VAO include: membranectomy via limbal route or pars-plana route (23 G or 25 G), posterior capsulotomy (Fig. 15.15) (if primary PCCC was not done) with or without anterior vitrectomy. If the VAO is predominantly anterior and/or fibrosis is limited, limbal approach may be preferred. In case of posterior capsular opacification with fibrosis around IOL, pars plana route may help in reducing surgical manipulation. Combined approach in difficult situations may give optimal outcome. Nd:YAG laser has also been used to perform posterior capsulotomy in bigger and cooperative children. However, with the use of Nd:YAG capsulotomy, two limitations remain: (1) the anterior hyaloid still remains intact, which may again act as scaffold for recurrent PCO formation and (2) a very thick fibrous PCO may not be easily cut with laser. An opening of at least 5 mm should be done when treating secondary posterior capsular membranes [14]. Risks of retreatment with Nd:YAG laser include: cystoid macular edema (CME) [15, 16] and low risk of retinal detachment [16]. IOL pitting can happen in uncooperative children especially with thick PCO (Fig. 15.16). VAO associated with complicated surgery or malpositioned IOL may require IOL exchange, repositioning or explant which may be surgically challenging due to extensive fibrosis and/or vascularization (Fig. 15.17).

Refractive correction after surgery is a must for early visual rehabilitation. Amblyopia therapy should be initiated as soon as media is rendered clear.

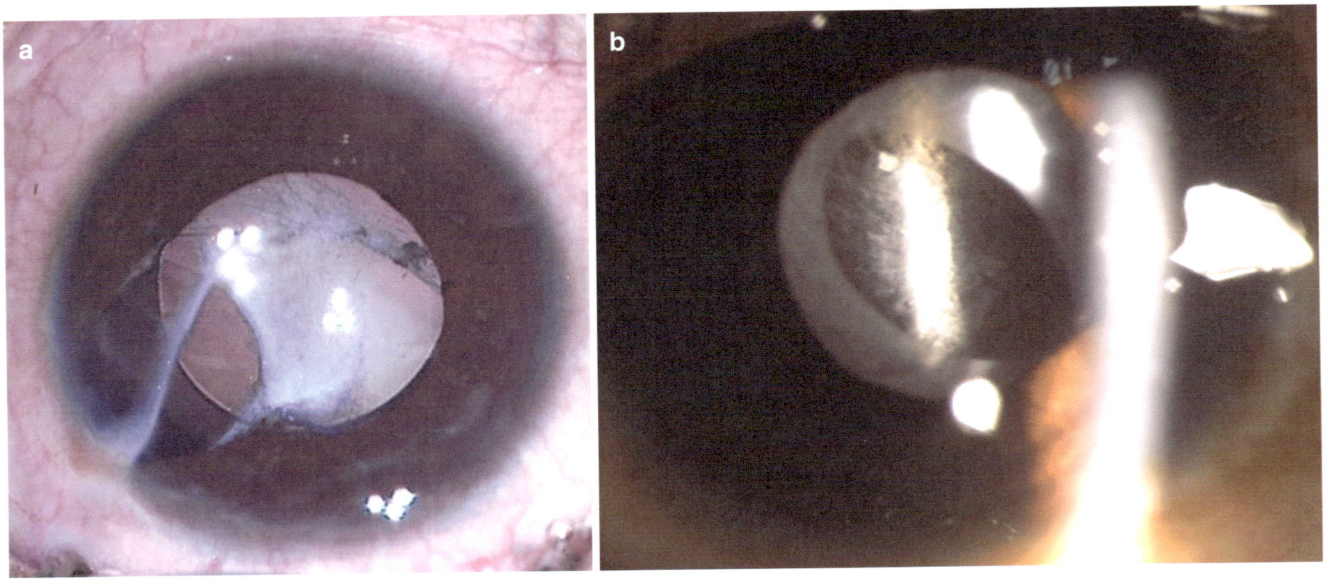

Fig. 15.11 Fibrotic type of VAO. (**a**) Anterior fibrotic VAO seen 4 months after surgery for post-traumatic cataract. (**b**) Posterior fibrotic VAO seen 1 year after surgery for intermediate uveitis

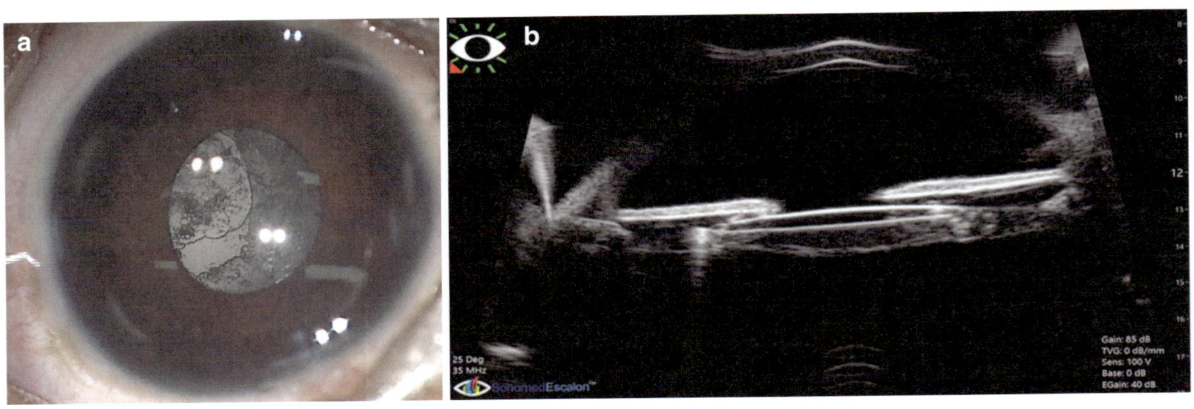

Fig. 15.12 Proliferative VAO with Elschnig pearl formation. (**a**) Clinical picture, (**b**) UBM of the same showing VAO posterior to IOL and intact posterior capsule

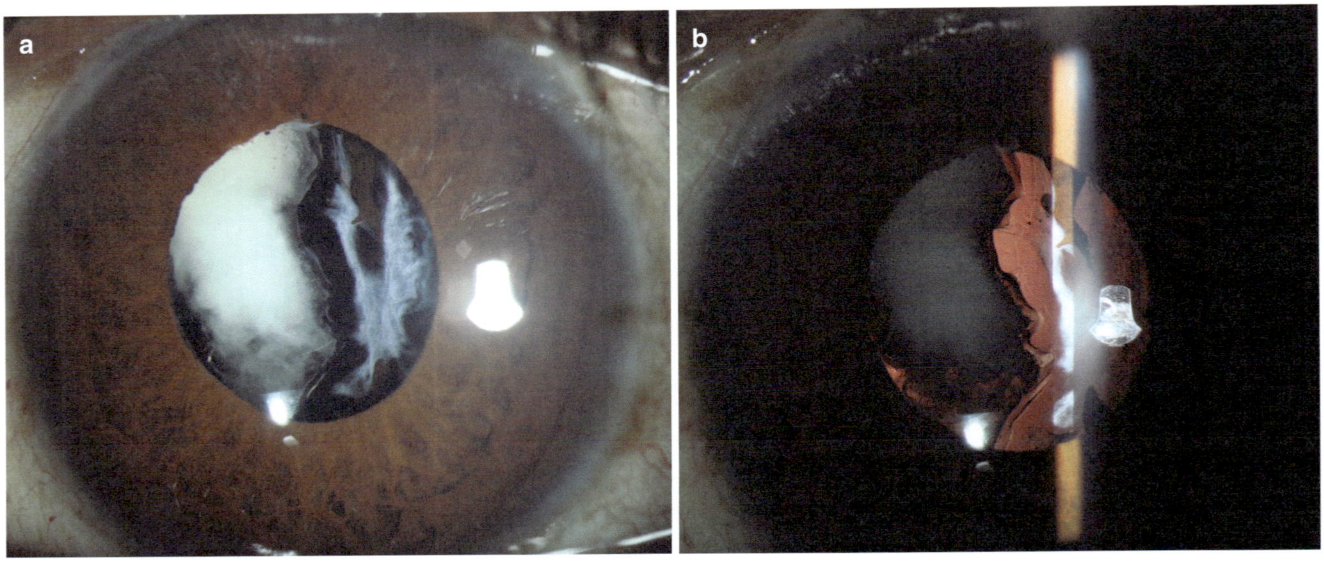

Fig. 15.13 Proliferative VAO with Soemmering ring seen in aphakic patient 20 months after surgery

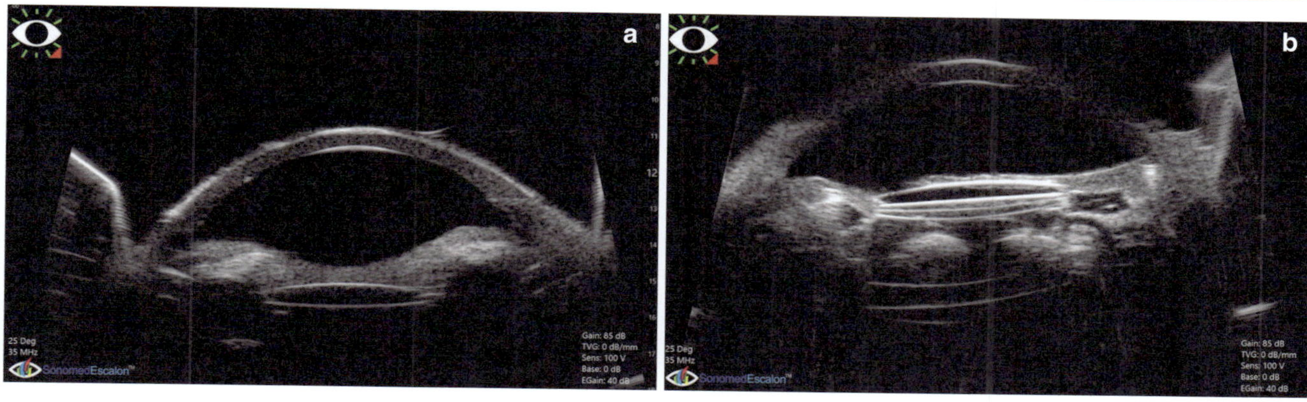

Fig. 15.14 UBM of dense VAO patients. (**a**) Anterior VAO seen, no VAO behind the lens, (**b**) combined anterior and posterior VAO

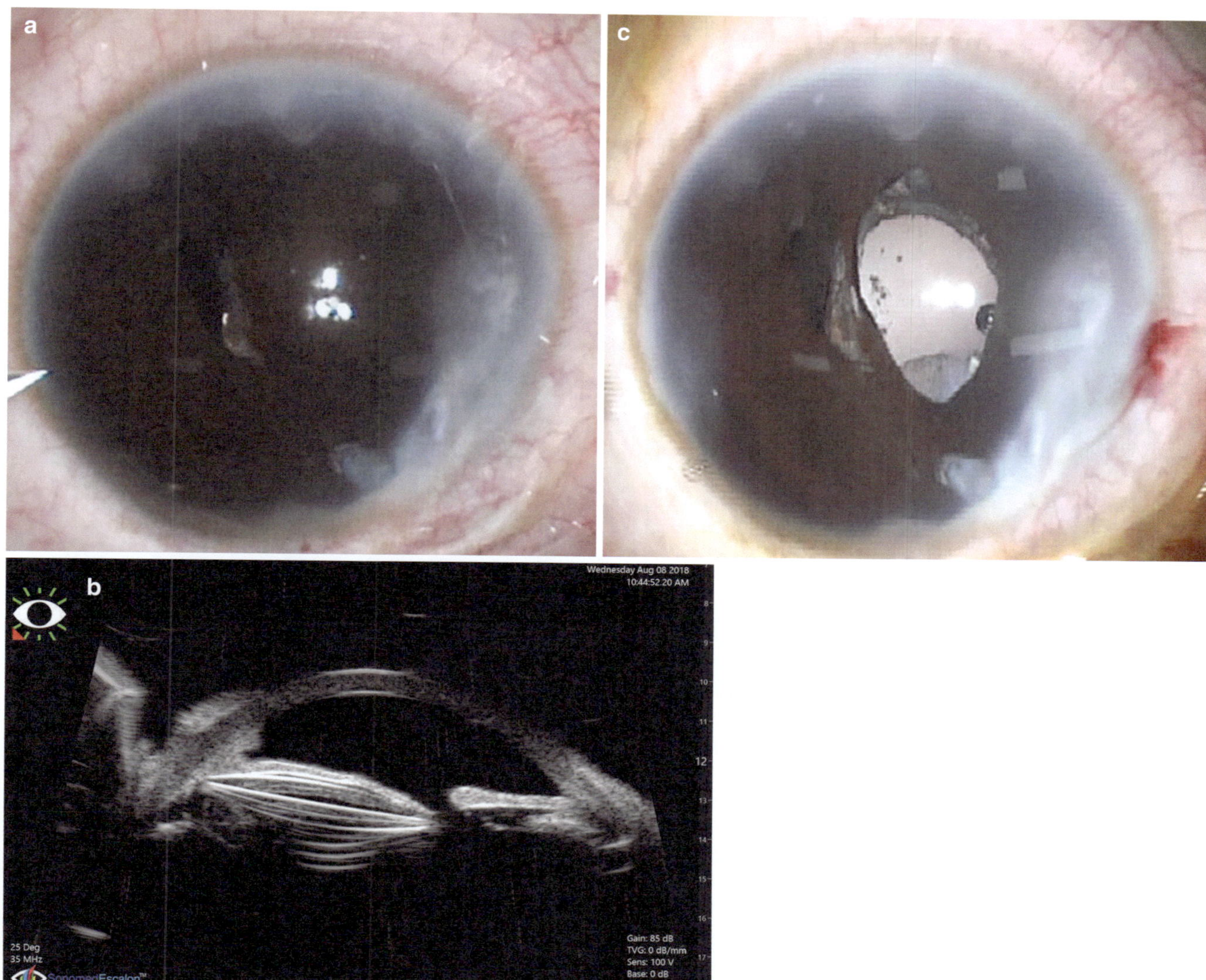

Fig. 15.15 UBM used in surgical planning in patient with dense VAO and eccentric pupil. (**a**) Preoperative clinical picture showing eccentric pupil, 270°, peripheral anterior synechiae and IOL not seen. (**b**) UBM of the same showing decentered IOL and anterior and posterior VAO. (**c**) Post-surgery picture—pupilloplasty with membranectomy from limbal and pars plana route has been done with minimum manipulation to attain clear visual axis

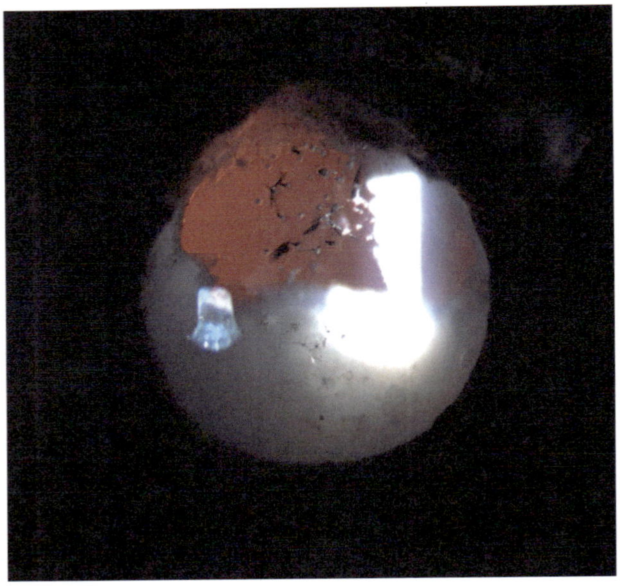

Fig. 15.16 Post Nd:YAG capsulotomy IOL pitting seen

15.5 Prevention of VAO: Lessons Learnt

Studies have well established the role of primary PCCC with anterior vitrectomy to effectively delay the secondary cataract formation in infants and children [17].

Anterior vitrectomy breaks the scaffold for the LECs that are actively proliferating and prevents deposition of metaplastic cells, thus preventing PCO formation [18]. Posterior capsulotomy is a must for all patients <6 years of age [18]. Vitrectomy can be deferred after 5 years of age [18].

The authors routinely perform PCCC with/without AV for all children operated for cataract at the age of less than 6 years and in special cases of older children with mental retardation, nystagmus or who are unable to follow up frequently.

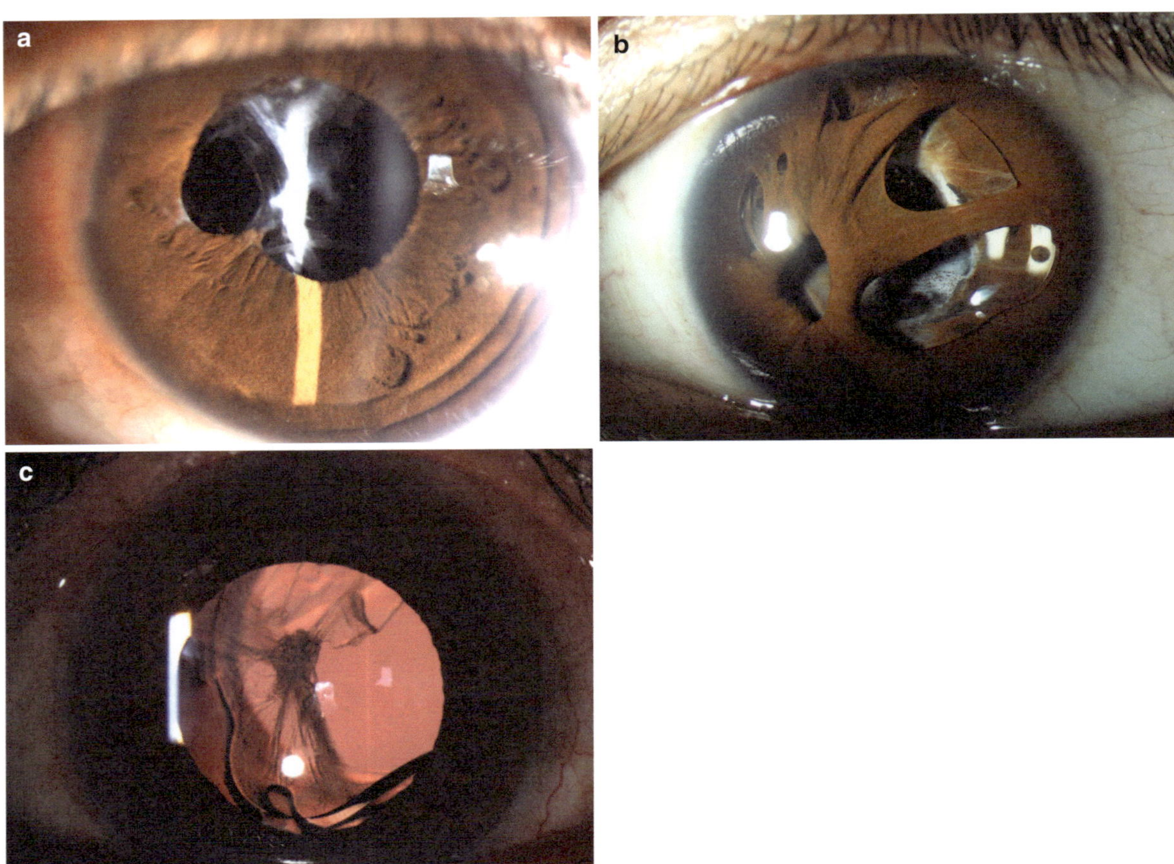

Fig. 15.17 Complicated cataract surgery with IOL malposition. (**a**) Inferiorly dislocated IOL with posterior capsular defect with posterior capsular opacification. (**b**) Universal IOL with anterior VAO due to iris overriding the IOL with posterior capsular opacification. (**c**) Hydrophilic foldable IOL in bag with anterior capsular fibrosis with inferior haptic protruding in the anterior chamber

References

1. McDonnell PJ, Zarbin MA, Green WR. Posterior capsule opacification in pseudophakic eyes. Ophthalmology. 1983;90(12):1548–53.
2. Wormstone IM. Posterior capsule opacification: a cell biological perspective. Exp Eye Res. 2002;74(3):337–47.
3. Saika S. Relationship between posterior capsule opacification and intraocular lens biocompatibility. Prog Retin Eye Res. 2004;23(3):283–305.
4. Knight-Nanan D, O'Keefe M, Bowell R. Outcome and complications of intraocular lenses in children with cataract. J Cataract Refract Surg. 1996;22:730–6.
5. Kuhli-Hattenbach C, Lüchtenberg M, Kohnen T, Hattenbach L-O. Risk factors for complications after congenital cataract surgery without intraocular lens implantation in the first 18 months of life. Am J Ophthalmol. 2008;146(1):1–7.e1.
6. Hosal BM, Biglan AW. Risk factors for secondary membrane formation after removal of pediatric cataract. J Cataract Refract Surg. 2002;28(2):302–9.
7. Peterseim MW, Wilson ME. Bilateral intraocular lens implantation in the pediatric population. Ophthalmology. 2000;107(7):1261–6.
8. Nishi O, Nishi K. Intraocular lens encapsulation by shrinkage of the capsulorhexis opening. J Cataract Refract Surg. 1993;19(4):544–5.
9. Heatley CJ, Spalton DJ, Kumar A, Jose R, Boyce J, Bender LE. Comparison of posterior capsule opacification rates between hydrophilic and hydrophobic single-piece acrylic intraocular lenses. J Cataract Refract Surg. 2005;31(4):718–24.
10. Lundvall A, Zetterstrom C. Cataract extraction and intraocular lens implantation in children with uveitis. Br J Ophthalmol. 2000;84(7):791–3.
11. Nishi O, Nishi K, Sakanishi K. Inhibition of migrating lens epithelial cells at the capsular bend created by the rectangular optic edge of a posterior chamber intraocular lens. Ophthalmic Surg Lasers. 1998;29(7):587–94.
12. Intraocular lens optic capture in pediatric cataract surgery. [cited 2018 Oct 28]. https://www.ncbi.nlm.nih.gov/pmc/articles/PMC6090124/
13. Bag-in-the-Lens Cataract Surgery. American Academy of Ophthalmology. 2015 [cited 2018 Oct 28]. https://www.aao.org/clinical-video/bag-in-lens-cataract-surgery
14. Atkinson CS, Hiles DA. Treatment of secondary posterior capsular membranes with the Nd:YAG laser in a pediatric population. Am J Ophthalmol. 1994;118(4):496–501.
15. Gilbard SM, Peyman GA, Goldberg MF. Evaluation for cystoid macu-lopathy after pars plicata lensectomy-vitrectomy for congenital cataracts. Ophthalmology. 1983;90:1201–6.
16. Hoyt CS, Nickel B. Aphakic cystoid macular edema; occurrence in infants and children after transpupillary lensectomy and anterior vitrectomy. Arch Ophthalmol. 1982;100:746–9.
17. Brady KM, Atkinson CS, Kilty LA, Hiles DA. Cataract surgery and intraocular lens implantation in children. Am J Ophthalmol. 1995;120(1):1):1–9.
18. Khokhar SK, Pillay G, Dhull C, Agarwal E, Mahabir M, Aggarwal P. Pediatric cataract. Indian J Ophthalmol. 2017;65(12):1340–9.

MIX
Papier aus verantwortungsvollen Quellen
Paper from responsible sources
FSC® C105338

If you have any concerns about our products,
you can contact us on
ProductSafety@springernature.com

In case Publisher is established outside the EU,
the EU authorized representative is:
Springer Nature Customer Service Center GmbH
Europaplatz 3, 69115 Heidelberg, Germany

Printed by Libri Plureos GmbH
in Hamburg, Germany